Chronic Pain FOR DUMMIES®

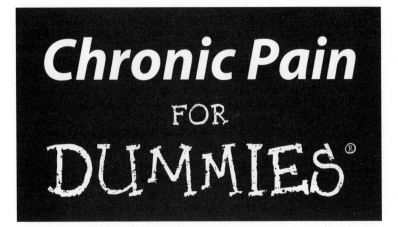

by Stuart S. Kassan, MD, FACP, Charles J. Vierck, Jr., PhD, and Elizabeth Vierck, MS

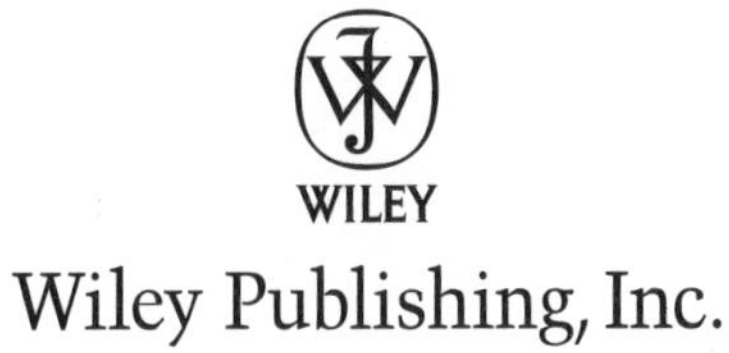

Wiley Publishing, Inc.

Chronic Pain For Dummies®

Published by
Wiley Publishing, Inc.
111 River St.
Hoboken, NJ 07030-5774
www.wiley.com

For general information on our other products and services, please contact our Customer Care Department within the U.S. at 800-762-2974, outside the U.S. at 317-572-3993, or fax 317-572-4002.

For technical support, please visit www.wiley.com/techsupport.

Wiley also publishes its books in a variety of electronic formats. Some content that appears in print may not be available in electronic books.

Library of Congress Control Number: 2008924959

ISBN: 978-0-471-75140-3

Manufactured in the United States of America

10 9 8 7 6 5 4 3 2 1

About the Authors

Stuart S. Kassan, MD, FACP: Dr. Kassan is a clinical professor of medicine at the University of Colorado Health Sciences Center. He is an internationally known expert in arthritis and painful conditions, such as lupus and Sjogren's syndrome. Dr. Kassan is a registered acupuncturist. In his current Denver-based rheumatology practice, he is active in both research and treatment of patients with conditions that are associated with significant pain.

Dr. Kassan has received numerous awards and honors for his work, most recently from the *Denver Business Journal* for excellence in patient care. He is on the national board of the Arthritis Foundation and is president of the Rocky Mountain chapter of the Arthritis Foundation.

Charles J. Vierck, Jr., PhD: Dr. Vierck has spent 40-plus years conducting leading edge research to better understand how our bodies feel pain. He is currently working with colleagues to develop new tools for diagnosing and treating fibromyalgia, a painful and debilitating disease that affects primarily women.

Now Professor Emeritus at the University of Florida School of Medicine, Dr. Vierck is the former director of the Center for Neurobiological Sciences in the University of Florida's McKnight Brain Institute. He has won numerous awards for his research and teaching, including the Javitz Neuroscience Investigator Award, a national prize for scientists. His articles appear regularly in *Pain* and *The Journal of Pain.* Dr. Vierck is coauthor of *Medical Neuroscience* (Saunders).

Elizabeth Vierck, MS: Dr. Vierck's sister is a well-known information specialist and writer on health and aging. She writes extensively and frequently about arthritis (all forms), inflammation, aging, and other diseases that involve chronic pain. Ms. Vierck is a Denver-based consultant and writes for many national aging and health organizations.

Ms. Vierck is a widely published author with 17 books and numerous other publications to her credit, including the *Complete Idiot's Guide to the Anti-Inflammation Diet* (with Dr. Christopher Cannon, Penguin), *Health Smart* (Simon & Schuster), *Aging* (two volumes, Greenwood), and *Keys to Understanding Arthritis* (Barrons). Ms. Vierck worked for the U.S. Senate for more than a decade, including the Special Committee on Aging and Labor and Human Resources Committee.

Ms. Vierck lives with chronic pain resulting from an aggressive form of osteoarthritis. She is long-time treasurer of the board of the Rocky Mountain chapter of the Arthritis Foundation.

Dedication

To our magnificent and patient spouses: Gail, Cheryl, and Craig. To the one in three Americans who live with chronic pain.

Authors' Acknowledgments

The authors would like to acknowledge the invaluable assistance of the following people and organizations: our talented agent, Marilyn Allen; our skilled and diplomatic acquisitions editor, Stacy Kennedy; our Dummies guru, Christine Adamec; our skilled and patient project editor, Kelly Ewing (we are in awe that you had took care of your two-month old baby and three other children and moved to a new home while skillfully managing this book); Penney Cowan of the American Chronic Pain Association; physical therapist par excellence, Andrea Vencl; general reviewer Michael L. Whitworth, MD, MS; illustrator Kathryn Born; and Alicia South, art coordinator.

We also want to thank the highly skilled production staff at Wiley: Reuben W. Davis, Alissa D. Ellet, Shane Johnson, Stephanie D. Jumper, Caitie Kelly, Kristie Rees, Toni Settle, Ronald Terry, and Christine Williams.

Publisher's Acknowledgments

We're proud of this book; please send us your comments through our Dummies online registration form located at www.dummies.com/register/.

Some of the people who helped bring this book to market include the following:

Acquisitions, Editorial, and Media Development

Project Editor: Kelly Ewing

Acquisitions Editor: Stacy Kennedy

General Reviewer: Michael L. Whitworth, MD, MS

Editorial Supervisor and Reprint Editor: Carmen Krikorian

Senior Editorial Manager: Jennifer Ehrlich

Editorial Assistants: Erin Calligan Mooney, Joe Niesen, Leeann Harney

Art Coordinator: Alicia South

Cover Photos: (c) Jessica Abad de Gail

Cartoons: Rich Tennant (www.the5thwave.com)

Composition Services

Project Coordinator: Kristie Rees

Layout and Graphics: Reuben W. Davis, Alissa D. Ellet, Shane Johnson, Stephanie D. Jumper, Ronald Terry, Christine Williams

Special Art: Kathryn Born

Proofreaders: Caitie Kelly, Toni Settle

Indexer: Potomac Indexing, LLC

Publishing and Editorial for Consumer Dummies

Diane Graves Steele, Vice President and Publisher, Consumer Dummies

Joyce Pepple, Acquisitions Director, Consumer Dummies

Kristin A. Cocks, Product Development Director, Consumer Dummies

Michael Spring, Vice President and Publisher, Travel

Kelly Regan, Editorial Director, Travel

Publishing for Technology Dummies

Andy Cummings, Vice President and Publisher, Dummies Technology/General User

Composition Services

Gerry Fahey, Vice President of Production Services

Debbie Stailey, Director of Composition Services

Contents at a Glance

Table of Contents

Part IV: Managing Your Pain with Lifestyle 209

Introduction

Chronic pain is pain that lasts for more than three months. It's stunningly common: One in three people have this type of pain.

If you have chronic pain, you're all too familiar with the constant intrusions it can make into your everyday life. However, you don't need to suffer. We wrote this book to give you tools to tame this unwelcome trespasser.

You can — and will — feel a lot better when you educate yourself about your condition, track your pain triggers, and use sound medical, complementary, and lifestyle approaches to control your chronic pain. These approaches work for many people, returning them to vitality and health. They can work for you, too.

About This Book

Our goals in writing this book are to help you understand and conquer your chronic pain. We give you the perspectives of a compassionate doctor, an avid researcher, and an informed chronic pain patient.

Conventions Used in This Book

The following conventions are used in this book:

- When this book was printed, some Web addresses may have needed to break across two lines of text. If that happened, rest assured that we haven't put in any extra characters (such as hyphens) to indicate the break. So, when using one of these Web addresses, just type in exactly what you see in this book, pretending as though the line break doesn't exist.
- New terms we're defining appear in *italics.*
- Sidebars — the text in grey boxes — include interesting asides, but you don't need to read them to understand the section in which they appear.

Foolish Assumptions

In writing this book, we assumed that you or a loved one has chronic pain. We also assume that you believe that knowledge is power and that you want to be armed with this power in order to conquer your pain.

How This Book Is Organized

Chronic Pain For Dummies is organized into six convenient parts.

Part I: Getting the Lowdown on Chronic Pain

In Part I, we paint the big picture of pain. We give you an overview of chronic pain and explain how it can be a disease all its own.

Because understanding the basics about the physical processes of pain can help you understand and adapt to your situation, in Chapters 2 and 3 we look at how pain develops inside your body. We also cover two important lifestyle consequences of chronic pain — chronic pain behavior cycles and caregiver stress. The first affects the person with chronic pain, and the second affects the loved one taking care of her.

Part II: Detailing Some Causes of Chronic Pain

Part II is where we describe the major diseases and injuries that can lead to chronic pain, as well as how these causes are diagnosed and treated. We provide details on the most common conditions that cause pain. But, remember: Just because you hurt all the time doesn't mean that you have one of these conditions!

Part III: Managing Your Pain Medically

In Part III, we cover the medical management of pain — from building your health-care team to considering surgery. Along the way, we give you the details about the benefits and side effects of a wide range of drugs used against chronic pain. We also give you guidelines for evaluating the effectiveness and legitimacy of complementary and alternative approaches to treating pain.

Part IV: Managing Your Pain with Lifestyle

Part IV gives you important suggestions for managing your chronic pain with your lifestyle. You should use these techniques in conjunction with the medical management of your condition. We also discuss how weight control and good nutrition directly affect your level of chronic pain and how to avoid a physical state known as *deconditioning.* We also cover the major sleep problems that can occur when you're in constant pain and what you can do about them. We present tools you can use to turn negative thoughts around and reduce your pain. Finally, we know that living with chronic pain means having to deal with the daily stress it creates. So, we provide information about techniques you can use to ease your stress levels.

Part V: Understanding Pain Throughout the Life Cycle

Part V presents helpful information about chronic pain at three important points in the life cycle: in children, the elderly, and at the end of life. Pain during each of these stages of life manifests itself in its own way and requires different solutions than during adulthood. So, we give you practical advice on detecting and managing pain during these critical times.

Part VI: The Part of Tens

This part covers helpful tips in lists of ten. We provide information on phony products and services that claim to cure chronic pain, sexuality and chronic pain, important sources of pain help, and ten things to avoid when you have chronic pain.

Icons Used in This Book

The icons we use in each chapter provide helpful information about the sentences or paragraphs that they appear next to.

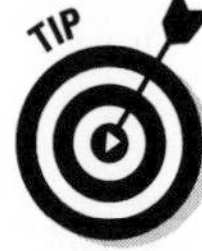

The tip icon gives practical suggestions that you can use to manage your chronic pain.

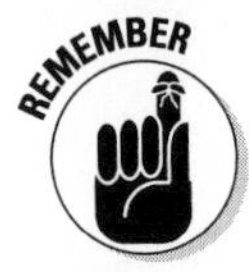

This icon marks information that it is important for you to pay attention to and remember.

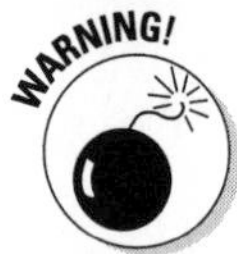

This warning icon warns you against something that could be harmful.

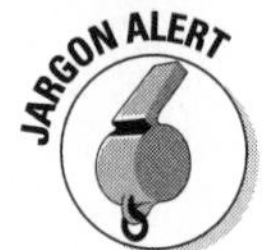

This icon marks a section that you can skip if you want to! It includes medical jargon that you don't really have to know to understand a topic.

Where to Go from Here

Chronic Pain For Dummies is a reference book. You don't have to read every page in order from the front to the back. And you don't have to remember anything from an earlier section to understand a later section.

However, you may want to read the first couple of chapters to get a basic understanding of chronic pain and then read the chapters or sections that apply to your specific chronic pain condition. (For example, if your problem is endometriosis, be sure to read Chapter 10. If your pain is caused by cancer, be sure to read Chapter 12.) Then use the Table of Contents or Index to find the chapters or topics most relevant to you.

For example, if you find that your current medications just aren't cutting the pain, go to Chapter 14 and look up the other options now available. Or would you like to know where to find a chronic pain support group? If so, go to Chapter 28, which gives you a handy list of resources. Or maybe you have a child with chronic pain and you want to know how to monitor her pain levels. Be sure to check out Chapter 23. One final note: Because the field of pain management is advancing very quickly, we also suggest that you use the extensive resources that we have listed in this book to find out about and stay on top of any new discoveries, techniques, and services that can help you tame your chronic pain.

Part I

Getting the Lowdown on Chronic Pain

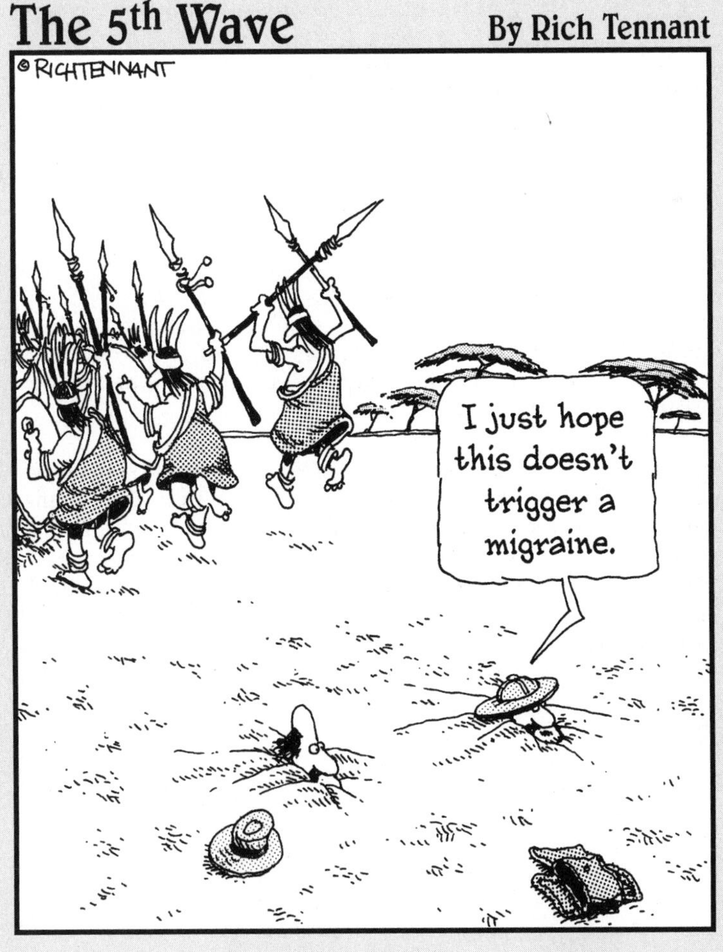
The 5th Wave
By Rich Tennant
© RICHTENNANT
I just hope this doesn't trigger a migraine.

In this part . . .

When you have chronic pain, your sensations can range from a small constant ache to excruciating and unrelenting pain. And these symptoms can be persistent, resistant, and insistent! The pain is always with you on some level, and it's often isolating.

In this part, we paint the big picture of chronic pain and how such annoying and nasty symptoms occur. We also celebrate the advances that have been made in the last couple of decades in managing chronic pain.

Because understanding the basics about the physical processes of pain can help you adapt to your situation, we describe pain pathways and other aspects of how pain works inside your body. We also describe the different types of chronic pain and cover two important lifestyle consequences of the problem: chronic pain behavior cycles and caregiver stress.

Chapter 1

Hurting That Doesn't Go Away

In This Chapter

- Understanding the solitude of chronic pain
- Recognizing common features
- Coping with chronic pain

Chronic pain is hurting that doesn't go away. But, as crazy as it sounds, suffering from chronic pain today is much better than developing the problem even ten years ago, when many doctors were afraid to give you pain meds. And dealing with chronic pain is certainly much better than a couple of centuries ago, when you may have had your veins opened to bleed the "bad humors" out of your body.

This chapter gives you an overview of what we know today about chronic pain — how it works, what it feels like, and how to manage it. We also cover the common characteristics of chronic pain and discuss how constant pain causes its own physical problems.

Just What Is Chronic Pain?

Medical professionals categorize pain as either *acute* or *chronic.* Acute pain is your nervous system's way of alerting you to an injury or other damage to your body's tissues (see Chapter 2). Acute pain gets your attention so that you'll take care of yourself fast. In fact, the word *acute* comes from the Latin word for needle, and if you've ever stepped on a needle, you'll agree that it's a good representation of acute pain. Acute pain usually goes away as the injury heals, although it may return for short periods.

Chronic pain is persistent pain. The word *chronic* comes from the Greek word for time. In medical terms, pain is chronic when it lasts three months or more.

Pain: The fifth signal

In the past, pain was often overlooked or ignored by doctors and other health-care professionals because it couldn't be measured, and they couldn't do much about it. Doctors treated the condition causing the pain and not the pain itself. However, that approach is changing so that now *both* the condition and the pain that it causes receive equal attention.

In fact, the concept that pain is a fifth vital sign is now a mainstream idea. Four vital signs — temperature, pulse, respiration, and blood pressure — are routinely taken by medical professionals to determine how a patient is doing. Pain becomes the fifth measure of a patient's status.

When pain becomes chronic, your body's pain signals keep firing for weeks, months, or years, even though the damage that set them off may have long since healed (see Chapter 2). The pain may have been caused by an injury, and, for unknown reasons, your body never turned off its pain switch. Or the pain may have an ongoing cause, such as arthritis, cancer, or nerve damage (see Part II). You also may have multiple causes of chronic pain, which is particularly common for older adults.

One big difference between acute and chronic pain is when you have acute pain, you usually know *why* it hurts. (Some examples of acute pain are broken bones, kidney stones, and childbirth.) When you have chronic pain, you may have no idea what's causing the hurting. The bone has healed, the stone has passed, and the baby is now walking and talking, but you still have lingering problems in the areas where the acute pain occurred.

In addition, many people with chronic pain aren't even aware that an injury ever occurred in the first place. (And, indeed, maybe there was no injury to begin with!) For them, the pain appears to slam in from out of the blue, like a sudden tornado that levels a house.

Whether you know the source, chronic pain is a sensation without purpose. It has no biological function, and its usefulness as a warning system has long since passed or never existed. Ironically, while chronic pain has no purpose, it's still often difficult to treat. The medical term for this type of pain is *treatment resistant pain.* Experts at the Cleveland Clinic describe chronic pain this way: It persists, resists, and insists: It persists beyond the expected healing time, resists interventions (treatments), and it also insists upon being recognized.

Chronic Pain Is a Solitary Experience

Life with chronic pain is a solitary, and often lonely, experience. Compare this hypothetical experience to that of chronic pain:

You and your husband are hiking in the mountains and get stuck in a cold, hard rain. You have five miles to go to reach your car. Lunch was four hours ago, and in your pack is only 8 ounces of water, chewing gum, and an apple. And, oh yeah, you forgot your raincoats. (This stuff actually happens to otherwise smart people.) So you just keep going. And going. And going. And the cold hard rain never stops.

Two and a half hours later, you finally reach your car. When you arrive, you each know how the other feels. You're both exhausted, cold, wet, and hungry. And you're both very relieved that you lived through the experience and your heated cabin — the one with the hot tub — is only a mile away. Later that night, you share a good, long laugh about the experience. For years, you two enjoy telling the story of "the day we almost died on the mountain."

Chronic pain is very different from this shared experience. You're up on that mountain all alone. And when you return to your cabin, there may be no heat and no hot tub. And there's no shared laughter.

Yes, chronic pain is a solitary experience. Each person feels chronic pain differently, even people who have identical injuries or illnesses. Consider good friends Lou and Matt. They both have a nerve condition called peripheral neuropathy (see Chapter 11). Lou's symptoms are nerve pain, tingling, and numbness. Matt's symptoms are muscle cramps and frequent falls due to loss of muscle control. They both know that the other person has chronic pain from the same disease he has, but their symptoms are very different.

Because pain is so subjective, it can be difficult to diagnose and treat. There's no blood test for pain, no pain urinalysis, no pain pulse. It's up to you — in your role as a chronic pain patient — to describe your pain to doctors and other medical professionals who work to help you. The good news is that there are many effective ways to deal with chronic pain, which we cover throughout this book, but particularly in Parts III and IV where we cover managing and living with chronic pain.

Checking Out Common Characteristics of Chronic Pain

Chronic pain is a solitary experience, yet it's also a universal one. About one in three Americans suffer from chronic pain. (Read more about the numbers of people with chronic pain in Chapter 3.)

Chronic pain: Making headway every day

Scientists and the medical community are continually learning about what causes chronic pain, and we can celebrate these advances in understanding the following points:

- Scientists and the medical community have amassed tremendous knowledge about the causes of chronic pain, including new research that shows that extended periods of pain *change* the physiology of the central nervous system. This knowledge impels doctors to address pain problems swiftly and effectively when they occur so that they don't lead to chronic pain.
- Research and advances in medical treatment of pain-causing conditions have dramatically improved treatment for many painful conditions, such as rheumatoid arthritis and fibromyalgia.
- Organizations such as the American Chronic Pain Association help sufferers with the latest information on treatments, support groups, advocacy efforts, and more. (Chapter 28 includes a contact list of these resources.)
- Pain management receives much more attention in medical schools, which means newbie docs are better armed to tackle chronic pain. Some states require completion of an educational program in pain management to receive a medical license.
- Acceptance of using opiates to control severe chronic pain, when appropriate, has greatly reduced unnecessary suffering for many people.
- Many new pain treatments are on the horizon. For example, researchers are studying new classes of drugs to treat pain more effectively. They're also looking at the possibility of implanting cells that release powerful painkillers in the spinal cord. If you have severe back pain, you may be ready to sign up for this treatment now! But, unfortunately, it's not available yet. In another five to ten years, expect major breakthroughs.

How do you tell when your pain is chronic? The Cleveland Clinic and other prestigious medical institutions have identified specific characteristics of chronic pain, including the following:

- Your pain doesn't go away.
- You've had lots of medical "work-ups," and yet no cause for the pain has been identified.
- You've tried lots of different medicines to control your pain, and yet the pain doesn't go away.
- You may have undergone numerous surgeries, and yet your pain still doesn't go away.
- You've visited doctors or other health providers over and over again in an attempt to find relief, but your search for relief has been futile.

Don't worry if these symptoms don't apply to you. They don't make your chronic pain more or less real. (In fact, you should be glad. Who wants them?)

People with chronic pain also may have the following symptoms: tense, tight muscles; an inability to get around; a lack of energy/fatigue; changes in appetite; sleep problems; depression, anger and/or anxiety; and fear of further injury.

What Chronic Pain Feels Like

If you have chronic pain, at some point, you realized part of your body has been hurting way too long. Maybe you have ongoing pain in your hip, and you're beginning to limp. When you first noticed the pain, you thought it was related to that day you fell on the ice in the driveway. But that was a year ago. Your bruised hip has long since healed, and yet the pain is still with you. You go to the doctor, who takes an X-ray and discovers that you have significant arthritis in your hip, which was probably irritated by the fall, but is a problem on its own.

In another example, your daughter, age 4, comes home from a Halloween party with a crushing headache. You attribute it to a sugar overdose. You take care of her, and she recovers. But a couple of weeks later, she has another severe headache. And three weeks after that, she has yet another one. Her pediatrician eventually diagnoses your child with chronic migraine headaches.

Chronic pain is not only persistent, resistant, and insistent, but it also seems ruthless. It's always with you on some level. It either doesn't give you a break, or it gives you very brief respites, fooling you into thinking you're all better and then returning with a wallop — regardless of whether you have an important sales presentation that afternoon, it's your son's birthday, or your plane to the Caribbean is about to take off.

Sensations of chronic pain range from a small, constant ache to excruciating pain. Your chronic pain may feel like one or more of the following feelings: aching, burning, crushing pain, dull pain, electrical-like pain, flu-like symptoms, jabbing pain, mental fogginess, numbness, piercing, prickling, sharp pain, shooting pain, soreness, stiffness, stinging sensations, throbbing, tightness, tingling, or vise-like pain.

Most people with chronic pain experience more than one of these feelings. For example, many people with fibromyalgia (see Chapter 4) have flu-like pain, aching, and stiffness. And people with rheumatoid arthritis (also covered in Chapter 4) may struggle with aching, stiffness, weight loss, and *mental fogginess* (a term used to describe confusion and forgetfulness).

Educating Yourself on How Pain Works

Why are you having pain? What's happening physically? Pain is caused by an exchange of information between three major systems in your body: your peripheral nerves, spinal cord, and brain. (Chapter 2 covers these systems in more detail.)

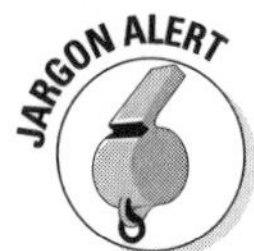

Peripheral nerves contain fibers that bring pain impulses to the spinal cord. Many of them have ends that sense danger, such as a cut or burning. These fibers are called *nociceptors,* and you have millions of them throughout your body.

Different types of nociceptors have different jobs. For example, some, nociceptors detect heat, while others watch out for pricks of pain, and still others respond to pressure. Once they detect these qualitative sensations, nociceptors then send pain signals to your spinal cord.

Your spinal cord is home to special cells that either wave the signals on through to the brain or turn them away like a door slamming shut on a gate. Your spinal cord cells also release chemicals during this alert phase. (You can read a discussion of this whole process in Chapter 2.)

The pain signals that *are* waved through to your brain arrive at the thinking and emotion centers where your brain then decides what on earth is causing the problem, whether it's worth getting anxious about, and what, if anything, to do about it.

Sometimes this complicated pain system crashes, kind of like a malfunctioning computer, yet the electricity keeps humming because the power's still on. The result is that your nerve/spinal cord system continues to send danger signals to your brain even though the real threat has long since passed (or maybe never existed in the first place).

Of course, this section describes chronic pain in a very rudimentary way. You can read more about the inside workings of pain in Chapter 2. (You need to know some basics about the pain enemy before you can vanquish her!) Chapter 3 also covers chronic pain in general.

Constant Pain Causes Its Own Damage

Constant pain causes its own damage, and medical science is just beginning to understand just how toxic the effects are. In fact, many pain experts say that the pain has become its own disease.

What happens is that the presence of pain changes the peripheral nerve/spinal cord/brain system that we mention in the previous section, causing the pain itself to get worse. As a result, treating the pain, as well as the underlying disease or injury, is key to preventing even more pain. (You can read more about this idea in Chapter 2.)

Living with Chronic Pain

The fact that pain is subjective and complicated means that it's up to you to take charge of your own care and treatment. You should understand enough about what causes your pain so that you can be on top of the best treatments (see Part II).

You also should discover how to do as much for yourself as you can, including the following:

- Developing a great pain management team (see Chapter 13)
- Tracking and avoiding your own individual pain triggers (see Chapter 17)
- Relieving your pain with lifestyle changes, such as maintaining a nutritional diet, exercising, and minimizing stress (see Part IV)

Managing your pain medically

When you have a chronic pain condition, you need to take control and gather a team of experts to help you find relief. (See Chapter 13 to find out how to assemble this team.) You need to find medical professionals and paraprofessionals who will work with you on different aspects of your pain condition. (Think of them as your own anti-pain team.)

For example, your group may include a primary-care physician (PCP), a specialist such as a neurologist or rheumatologist, and perhaps a physical therapist and a dietician. Your team also may contain some alternative practitioners, such as an acupuncturist or massage therapist. (Read more about alternative means to alleviating your chronic pain in Chapter 15.)

Your pain management team should work with you to find the right medicines and treatments that give you pain relief. (You can read more about medications for chronic pain in Chapter 14.)

Some people with chronic pain may need surgery, which is a tough decision for anyone to make. Read Chapter 16 for advice on how to make the choice for or against surgery.

Helping yourself with lifestyle changes

Your chronic pain can be made better or worse by your lifestyle. Not eating a healthy diet, being under- or overweight, not getting adequate exercise on a regular basis, and being stressed out can all make your pain worse. Chapter 3 and other s in Part IV cover many aspects of lifestyle and its relationship to pain. Here are the key concepts:

- **Track your pain triggers and avoid them.** Pain triggers are things in your life — such as overdoing exercise or missing too many hours sleep — that can set off a pain cycle. Keeping a pain log can help you identify your particular pain triggers. When you know what your own personal pain triggers are, you can avoid them, and you'll feel better! See Chapter 17 to learn a variety of techniques for keeping track of your pain triggers.
- **Purge "empty calories" from your diet and follow sound nutritional principles.** The key principle of a healthy diet is to eat a well-balanced variety of wholesome foods so that you'll take in all the nutrients required for good health and disease prevention. A healthy diet also means only occasionally eating white rice, white bread, potatoes, white pasta (pasta made from refined flour), soda, and sweets for special occasions. Check out Chapter 18 for more information on how to follow a nutritional diet.
- **Get physical!** If you don't get adequate exercise for an extended period of time (weeks, months, or longer!), you develop a physical state called *deconditioning.* The No. 1 rule for exercise and chronic pain is to do as much as you can as often as you can. (For more on exercise and chronic pain, read Chapter 19.)
- **Develop sound sleeping habits and beat fatigue.** Sleep loss can make you much more sensitive to pain. One study found that sleep deprivation caused by continuous sleep disturbances throughout the night increased spontaneous pain and impaired the body's ability to cope with it. Chapter 20 gives you information about major sleep problems that can cause or aggravate pain and what you can do about them.
- **De-stress your life.** When you have chronic pain, every day you must deal with the stress it creates. The best approach is to curb your stress as much as you can, whenever you can. From meditation to praying, numerous techniques can help reduce both your stress and pain. Read Chapter 22 to discover other stress-reduction techniques.

- **Cope with aging demands.** Are you older than 65? Sadly, the older you get, the more likely you are to suffer from some form of chronic pain. This news doesn't mean you should just give up and park your chair permanently in front of the TV! Absolutely not! Read Chapter 24 for great ideas about how to cope with the pain that often comes with aging.
- **Help your child in pain.** Few sights are more heartbreaking than watching a child in pain. If you're a parent, you wish you could take on your child's pain yourself, but you know you can't do that. Read some helpful advice on how you can help your child in Chapter 23.

Researching what's causing your pain

If you've been diagnosed with a condition causing your pain — such as migraine headaches (see Chapter 6), fibromyalgia, or post herpetic neuralgia — it's important to find out more about the disease and the best ways that your doctor can help you treat it. This knowledge ensures that you're doing everything possible to reduce your pain. If you don't have a diagnosis of what's causing your pain, it's important to seek one.

Part II covers the most common causes of chronic pain, ranging from arthritis (4) to back pain (5) to cancer (12.). These s describe symptoms of the diseases and give you the latest information on finding the best medical specialists to assist you.

If you've suffered a serious injury or a stroke, be sure to read Chapter 7 for advice on this chronic pain problem. Is severe burn pain your problem? Check out Chapter 8.

Some people never discover the cause of their pain, which is frustrating for everyone involved, from the patient to the doctor. For example, back pain, even when it's severe, is notorious for not displaying any known cause during a physical examination by a doctor, on imaging tests such as magnetic resonance imaging (MRI) scans and X-rays, or even during surgery. The pain is real, but it's not easily detectable.

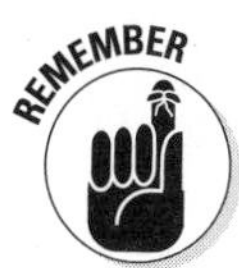

Even if you don't know the source of your pain, it's important to work with a medical team to make sure that you're maximizing your options for treatment. (See Chapter 13 to find out how to assemble your anti-pain team.)

Chapter 2

Discovering How Pain Works

In This Chapter

- Discovering the nervous system
- Tracing chronic pain in the peripheral nervous system
- Seeing chronic pain in the central nervous system
- Understanding the vocabulary used to describe the physiology of pain

If you suffer from chronic pain, you probably perceive pain as your constant enemy and may wonder what on earth has gone wrong with your body. How did pain transform itself from a friendly, early warning system into a chronic troublemaker? This chapter helps answer these questions by exploring the physical aspects of chronic pain.

Understanding the basics of how your nervous system processes pain can also help you understand and adapt to your own situation. Your pain isn't merely a bad sensation. It also motivates (or demotivates) you. It produces strong emotions and its own set of reflexes. For example, pain can wake you up from the deepest sleep if it's severe enough. These effects occur because your pain pathways commingle with all parts of your nervous system. This chapter also explores this phenomenon.

Touring the Nervous System

The first step toward understanding the physiology of pain is to consider how pain signals travel from the location of an injury to your brain, where feelings of pain are formed. This knowledge provides you with a framework to comprehend how malfunctions can occur along the route (the pain pathway) from the injury to "ouch" locations in the brain.

First, you need basic information about the route that pain pathways follow in the nervous system. The nervous system is divided into two parts:

- The brain and spinal cord, also known as the central nervous system (CNS), shown in Figure 2-1.
- All the nerves that go to and from the CNS, called the peripheral nervous system (PNS), also shown in Figure 2-1. Figure 2-2 shows a typical pain pathway.

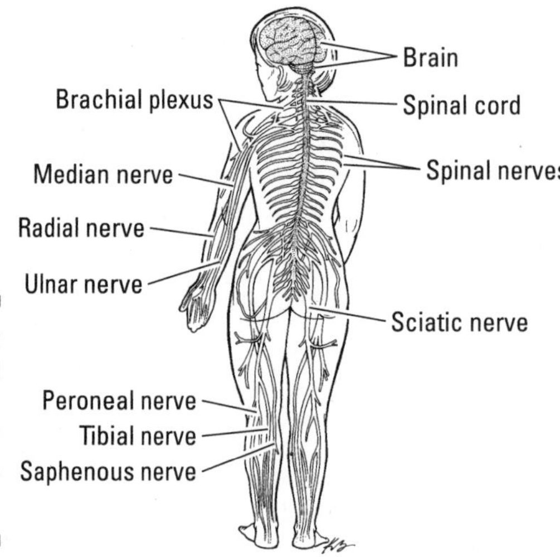

Figure 2-1: The central and peripheral nervous systems.

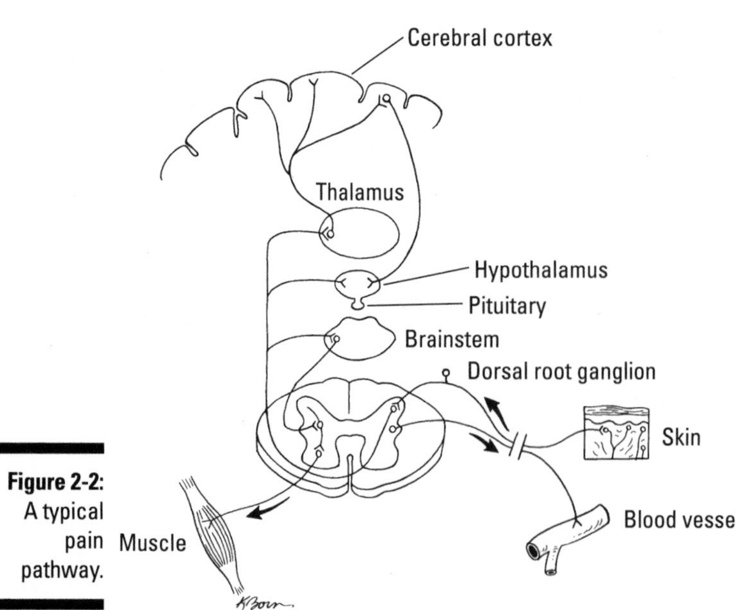

Figure 2-2: A typical pain pathway.

The PNS includes two types of neurons:

- *Efferents* send impulses *away* from the CNS. Some of the efferents go to *(innervate)* muscles and are called motor neurons, and others innervate visceral structures (autonomic neurons).
- *Afferents* send impulses to the CNS. They're also called *sensory nerves.* They affect and inform the CNS, telling your body what's going on, both inside and outside.

All neurons, including sensory neurons, are comprised of three parts:

- **Cell body,** which contains the nucleus of the cell and makes substances that keep the cell alive and running.
- **Dendritic tree,** which includes extensions of the cell body in the CNS that bring information in. Peripheral sensory neurons are unusual. Instead of having dendrites, they have a long axon that brings information from places, such as the skin, back to the cell body.
- **Axons,** which usually are located at the opposite end of the neuron from the dendrites. They carry information *away* from the cell body (see Figure 2-3.)

Cell bodies of sensory afferents are located near the spinal cord, forming a cluster of cells called the *dorsal root ganglion.* A long axon brings information from the skin or other tissues to the cell body, and a short axon enters the spinal cord (refer to Figure 2-3).

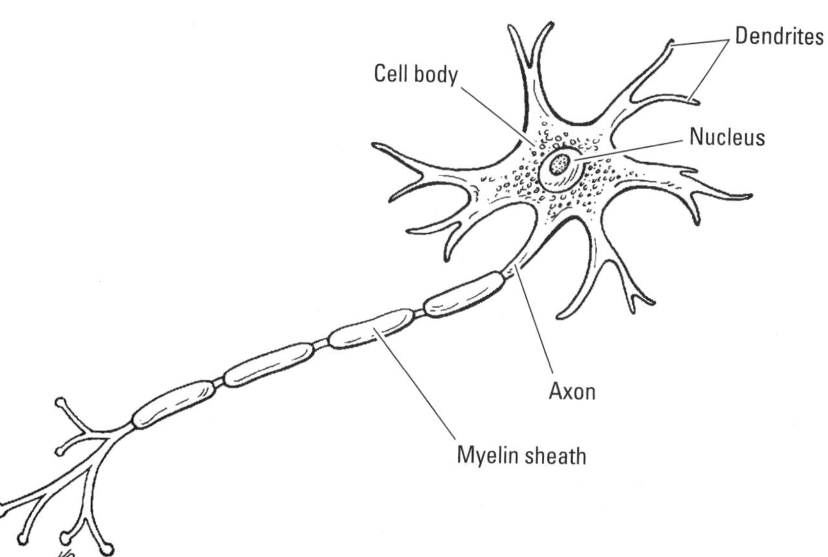

Figure 2-3: Neurons.

Some of your sensory axons receive and carry the news that you're hurt, whether the injury occurred from a car crash, a stroke, or a bee sting. Sensory nerve fibers send a pain alert to your spinal cord. Peripheral nerves (part of the PNS) that contain the long axons of afferents also contains motor axons (efferents) running from the spinal cord to your muscles. These motor axons manage your responses, such as when you swat an annoying fly or run away from a swarm of bees.

Peripheral nerves not only carry sensory and motor axons. They also are home to efferent axons from the spinal cord to body structures, such as your blood vessels or your stomach. These efferents are part of the autonomic nervous system. We talk about the sympathetic division of the autonomic nervous system because it produces stress reactions to pain.

Targeting the axons responsible for chronic pain

The peripheral endings of sensory nerves contain a variety of nerve endings called *receptors.* They transform different kinds of energy, such as touch, cold, or heat, into neural impulses (also called *action potentials*). These impulses from receptors responsive to painful stimuli (called *nociceptors*) carry messages to your pain pathways in the CNS.

The axons of sensory neurons differ by size and the degree of myelin on them. (*Myelin* is a substance that covers and protects nerves.) The largest axons are encased in a myelin sheath, which makes them big and fast. In fact, their impulses can rush forward at speeds of up to 40 miles an hour, faster than you can drive your car in a school zone. These fast and large axons are called *A-Beta fibers.*

Small axons with some myelin respond to painful stimulation. They're your warning system for acute pain. For example, they're fast enough to set off a withdrawal reflex to make you snatch your hand back from a hot burner. These axons are called *A-Delta fibers.*

The smallest axons, called C fibers, have *no* myelin, and they conduct information very slowly (about 3 miles an hour). These axons are the most plentiful, and they can reach any tissue. C fibers are responsible for the pain you feel if something touches the cornea of your eye or you have a toothache. Knowing this information, you probably aren't surprised to discover that a lot of chronic pain comes from activation of C fibers.

Electrically charged impulses

When a peripheral receptor responds to a stimulus, such as a pin prick, an electrically charged impulse rushes right through the nerve, heading toward the spinal cord. The impulse blasts through the nerve's cell body and into the spinal cord.

Your central nervous system contains

- **Your spinal cord:** When a sensory impulse has passed through axons of your peripheral nervous system and reaches your spinal cord, it communicates with cells in the dorsal horn of the spinal gray matter. (Gray matter of the CNS contains cell bodies of neurons.) The points of interaction between axons and cell bodies (or dendrites) are called *synapses.* Many synapses live on each spinal cell. The electrical signal from each sensory axon causes chemicals, called *neurotransmitters,* to be released at the synapse. These neurotransmitters attach to receptors on cells in the spinal cord, causing them to send messages along their axons. This relay race goes from cell to cell to numerous destinations in the CNS, depending upon which CNS pathway the axons travel in.
- **Your brain:** Some spinal cells receive information from the small partially myelinated neurons, the A-Delta neurons, and also from very small un-myelinated C sensory neurons sensitive to painful stimulation. These pain sensitive afferents are called nociceptors. The spinal cells with synapses from nociceptors send axons to the other side of the spinal cord, where they turn toward the brain.

The next synapse for this pain pathway is in a part of the brain called the *thalamus,* which has regions assigned to different sensory systems.

Sending pain messages to the brain

The main pain pathway from the spinal cord to the thalamus is called the *spinothalamic tract.* (That's a mouthful, and it takes plenty of neurons to help you say it!) Cells in the thalamus that receive spinothalamic input then send axons to the cerebral cortex.

The cerebral cortex tells you a lot about different aspects of pain you're experiencing. For example:

- It gives you qualitative information. (Is it cold or hot on your skin, or are you experiencing a muscle cramp or stomachache?)
- It gives you quantitative information. (How painful *is* it?)

- It tells you *where* the pain is and how big an area it involves. (For example, your entire forehead hurts intensely.)
- It assesses how much the pain bothers you. (Your pain is tolerable, or it makes you miserable.)

Responding to pain

A few more aspects of pain pathways can lead to chronic pain or effects of chronic pain. Axons of the spinal cells that receive pain signals branch out through the CNS where they perform different actions. Some actions are important to understanding pain:

- Some branches go to the brain stem located between the spinal cord and the brain (also called the cerebrum). Nuclei in the brain stem regulate sleep and wakefulness. Input to these regions arouses you and can prevent you from sleeping. Loss of sleep can be a major problem for people with chronic pain.
- The brain stem is a major player in controlling your muscular tone and coordinating reflexes that contribute to all your movements. For example, the brain stem coordinates your withdrawal from a painful stimulus in a way that prevents you from falling over. It also governs your reflexes and can inhibit them; for example, it keeps withdrawal reflexes from going off time and time again if the pain doesn't stop. Unlike the alarm on a timer, which doesn't stop until someone turns it off, your brain is smart and turns the withdrawal reflex off after awhile.
- The brain stem inhibits reflexes with axons in pathways that descend to your spinal cord. There is some spillover of inhibition to spinothalamic cells in the spinal cord. Therefore, some scientists think the brain stem may play a role in regulating pain.
- Systems within the brain regulate stress reactions. One form of stress, called *psychological stress,* activates both the hypothalamus and the pituitary gland, which in turn leads to activation of the sympathetic nervous system. The result can be increased pain.

Producing Chronic Pain in the Peripheral Nervous System

When you stub a toe, maybe you curse and grab your hurt foot, while hopping up and down on the other foot. If you reflect on what you felt, you'll find that you experienced two distinct pain sensations.

First, A-Delta fibers gave you immediate feedback that you hurt yourself once again by stubbing your toe on that same table leg that hasn't moved since the last time you bumped into it. (Maybe now is a good time to move it!) The input from these sensory nerves may even have been fast enough to help you reduce the force that you applied to the poor toe.

Second, you likely felt a later pain sensation from C fibers that didn't seem all that useful. The late C fiber pain is the one that causes you to curse the table that hurt your toe. This delayed pain from an injury tells you about the severity of the injury and motivates you to do something about it. For example, it keeps you from injuring the toe further by continuing to walk or run around while the pain is active.

Scientists have rigorously studied how injuries generate pain that persists until healing is complete. This form of pain, known as *acute pain,* is understood by most people as "par for the course" for minor injuries. How long the pain lasts depends on how much force was involved, whether or not you broke your toe, and so on.

Chronic pain is a very different story. Even if an injury appears to have healed, a variety of adaptations of the body to the injury can set in motion changes that result in chronic pain. Some of these attempts of the body to deal with injury can go wrong and are important for understanding why chronic pain can develop.

Injury to your body sets in motion your immune system, which is your body's defense system against disease and injury. In turn, your immune system mobilizes inflammation. A staggering array of inflammatory cells are released at and near the injury, and nociceptors (especially C fibers) are uniquely able to respond to these chemicals. A slight stub of a toe protected by a shoe yields a low level of inflammation that clears up quickly. A forceful stub of a bare toe in the dark turns the toe lovely shades of purple and causes swelling and sensitivity for a few days.

Here's where things get interesting. It turns out that when C fibers respond to pain, they also turn on inflammation, which itself is another source of pain. In other words, pain begets more pain. As long as you have inflammation, you have activity in nociceptors and vice versa. This process is the culprit behind some types of chronic pain, which is like a stubbed toe with endless inflammation.

The following sections describe some reasons why chronic pain can develop.

Chronic phantom pain from nerve injury

If an injury to a nerve completely interrupts the flow of information to the nervous system, common sense says you should feel nothing in the area where the damaged axons have peripheral terminals.

This thinking is true, but only to a point. If you stimulate skin in the damaged area, you may have no sensation of touch, cold, heat, or pressure. However, people who have lost their arms or legs report that *phantom* sensations occur where the limb *used* to be. For example, after amputation of a limb, most people feel or imagine that the limb is still present, sometimes in a distorted form. Then after some time, the phantom sensation actually can become painful.

Paradoxically, the healing process itself may create pain. When peripheral axons are damaged, the portion closest to the spinal cord is still connected to its cell body, and it survives, but the part close to the skin that's separated from the cell body deteriorates (degenerates). Like a plant seeking the sun, the axons attempt to grow toward their old target from the injury, and they can ordinarily reach it, make new receptors, and reestablish nearly normal sensations.

This process, called *regeneration,* works best when a nerve is crushed rather than cut across, because the nerve's coverings are preserved, providing channels for growth. However, in the worst case, when the nerve is cut and its normal target is gone, as in limb amputation, a tangle of regenerating axons, called a *neuroma,* forms. Neuromas can create the sensation of pain.

Normally, axons in sensory nerves don't conduct impulses unless their receptors are stimulated. Axons in nerves are insulated from one another, and no synapses communicate between axons or cell bodies in the dorsal root ganglion. In other words, they don't usually talk. However, this system in a neuroma goes crazy, and two things happen:

- The ends of axons in the neuroma start acting wildly, which is called *spontaneous activity.*
- The axons start talking to each other (even though, normally, they give each other the silent treatment).

Sensations generated by spontaneously active nerves are felt at (referred to) the sites where the terminals and receptors used to be (such as an amputated leg). This situation is because the brain is fooled into thinking that the damaged axons are responding to the same stimuli that *normally* activated them *before* the nerve was injured. The activity within a neuroma can even be interpreted by the brain as *feeling* like the pain of the original injury that set off this unfortunate series of events in the body.

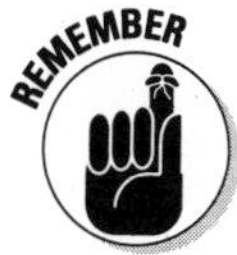

Neuromas can form at the site of a nerve injury even if the nerve is not severed and the limb is not amputated. If this occurs, pain is felt in that nerve's *innervation territory* (where it's peripheral receptors are). And — here is the really, really important thing to understand — activity within the pain pathways produced by some abnormal source is what you're usually dealing with when you have chronic pain.

Adrenaline

Adrenaline is always present to some degree in your body. Adrenaline is usually a good thing because it mobilizes our resources to deal with dangerous and injurious situations. However, following a nerve injury, even if the nerve is not severed, it becomes very sensitive to any release of adrenaline (also known as *epinephrine*) in the surrounding area, which is the case for axons that have been cut as well as those that are damaged but still in one piece. This situation is called *sympathetically maintained pain* because release of adrenaline normally occurs with activation of the sympathetic nervous system.

Nerve entrapment

If nerves are stretched or pinched continually, axons can be damaged and can become spontaneously active. This condition is called *nerve entrapment.* For example, *sciatica* is usually caused by pressure on the sciatic nerve from osteoarthritis or disc protrusion in the lumbar spine.

Nerve entrapment is an example of how any condition that irritates a nerve can cause chronic pain. Also, diabetes can lead to pain due to constant nerve trauma caused by the disease and made worse by inflammation.

Tracking Chronic Pain in the Central Nervous System

While the PNS is the communicator of sensory news, the CNS receives the news and responds to it. Activity in the CNS in response to pain signals can amplify and extend pain, causing two issues:

- **Central reorganization:** Unlike peripheral neurons, the axon of CNS neurons typically goes in one direction. For numerous reasons, central axons don't regenerate when severed, and the cell body can eventually die. If an injury damages CNS axons that communicate between the spinal cord and the thalamus, cells in the thalamus will no longer receive normal messages. When central cells lose their normal inputs, they become spontaneously active. As a result some people develop severe chronic pain following injuries that cause damage to the spinothalamic tract. Examples are spinal cord injury and post-stroke pain.

  Here is the reason why cells become spontaneously active: Losing input is traumatic for CNS neurons. For one thing, they suffer structural damage caused by the loss of synapses that normally come from the axons that are now damaged. Also, substances that normally nurture the health of cells are lost. As a result, the cell that has lost its input *(is deafferented)* becomes sick. One good way to think of the spontaneous activity of deafferented neurons is as cries for help!

  Long tracks of axons in the CNS don't renew themselves following an injury. However, some reorganization of synaptic connections occurs for cells that lose their input. Therefore, when cells in the CNS have lost their peripheral nerve supply, it's likely that new inputs come to them over time. If the output of the cell was interpreted as pain, any new input also can trigger pain. Alternatively, the "right" inputs can get rid of the spontaneous activity and alleviate pain. Therefore, reorganization should probably be directed by training rather than left to chance.

- **Central sensitization:** Two types of inflammatory reactions in the central nervous system can contribute to chronic pain:

  - When nociceptors are doing their thing, and particularly when their activity is caused by a peripheral injury, support cells called *microglia* are attracted to the region. Microglia are the immune cells of the CNS, and they release inflammatory chemicals that sensitize spinal cells to overreact when pain messages come in from sensory nerves.

  - Another form of pain coming from inflammation is similar to nerve entrapment or diabetic trauma to a peripheral nerve. (See the section "Nerve entrapment," earlier in this chapter.) Axons in the CNS are usually myelinated for fast conduction, even though the cell body for these axons may receive input from unmyelinated nociceptors. When the myelin of these axons deteriorates for any reason, microglia come in to clean up the damage, and the axons become spontaneously active. Multiple sclerosis involving demyelination of CNS axons can be associated with such pain.

- *Glutamate* is the primary neurotransmitter for nociceptors and therefore for pain. The higher the alarm setting from the nociceptor, the more glutamate released in the spinal cord.

  Copious amounts of glutamate may seem sufficient to feel pain, but the spinal cord also has a built-in amplifier for input from the bad guys — C fibers. Unmyelinated nociceptors release a variety of transmitters. One of these transmitters, substance P, initiates a cascade of events that increases pain if the discharge from C nociceptors persists over time. (Remember Substance P by thinking "P" is for pain.) The amplification of pain by C nociceptors is called *temporal summation.*

Most chronic pain involves input from C fibers, plus temporal summation, causing double trouble. So, when someone with chronic pain stubs a toe, the pain is likely to be exaggerated. This exaggerated pain, called *hyperalgesia,* usually lasts longer than normal pain because the sensitized cells in the CNS continue to discharge after receiving input from the stubbed toe.

In addition to its role in initiating of temporal summation, substance P spreads out readily from its site of release in the spinal cord to nearby neurons not receiving input from nociceptors at the moment. ("Hey guys, we're hurting!") As a result, the areas surrounding a source of painful input become hypersensitive to stimulation. This process is called *secondary hyperalgesia.*

With some pain conditions, a light touch or mild heat can produce severe pain. A possible explanation is that some cells in the pain pathways are so sensitized that even input from the usually blah A-beta afferents set them off. Painful responses to nonpainful input are called *allodynia.*

Chapter 3

When Pain Becomes Chronic

In This Chapter

- Identifying different types of chronic pain
- Seeing the cycle of chronic pain
- Overcoming major effects of chronic pain
- Acknowledging caregiver stress

Until recently, all pain was viewed solely as a symptom of disease. The philosophy toward pain was, "Treat the health problem, and you automatically treat the pain." Today, experts report that chronic pain itself is often the villain that must be pursued and tackled. In fact, the medical term for chronic pain is *maldynia,* which means your pain has become its own disease as a result of changes in the nervous system. Even though the original cause of the pain is gone, the pain itself remains.

Unlike normal pain that can point to an untreated medical problem, in most cases, chronic pain has no useful biological function. Not only is it without purpose, but the condition often takes on its own puzzling life; for example, it may be constant or may come and go. It may be hellish on Monday and more tolerable on Tuesday. It may move around, ending up far from its source, which is sometimes known as *referred pain.*

Chronic pain may respond to medications one day, and then, the next day, little relief comes from the same treatment that worked yesterday. Your frequent pain can lead to problems with relationships, lack of sleep, depression, and more. In this chapter, we cover common problems that may occur with chronic pain and what you can do about them.

Assessing Different Types of Chronic Pain

Chronic pain is pain that recurs or persists for three months or longer *or* pain related to an injury expected to either continue or worsen. Your body's response to injury, which may generate severe but temporary pain, may initially cause chronic pain. If these injuries don't heal properly and the pain generator *(nociceptors)* continues to be stimulated, changes can occur in your nervous system.

These changes at the molecular level can be quite dramatic and may even include genetic alterations. One of the most frustrating aspects of chronic pain is that no known cause may exist. In fact, in the case of low back pain, doctors can't identify the cause in up to 85 percent of individuals — talk about frustrating!

Chronic pain falls into different types of relentless hurting, which are described in the following list. Unfortunately, you or a loved one may have more than one type of chronic pain.

- **Somatogenic pain** is caused by physical diseases and disorders. Somatogenic pain is divided into two different types of pain:
  - *Nociceptive pain* occurs when pain-sensitive nerve endings called *nociceptors* are activated or stimulated. (See Chapter 2 for more information on nociception and nerve endings.) Most nociceptors are located in the skin, joints, muscles, and the walls of internal organs. Nociceptors are smart; they're specialized to detect different types of painful stimuli, such as heat, cold, pressure, toxic substances, sharp blows, or inflammation.
  - *Neuropathic pain* is the result of damage to or malfunction of the nervous system. It may involve the central nervous system or the peripheral nervous system or both. (See Chapter 2 for descriptions of the two types of nervous systems.) Neuropathic pain can occur after a stroke or spinal cord injury or may be caused by diabetes.
- **Psychogenic pain** occurs when psychological and emotional factors influence the intensity of the pain. You're not imagining it, and the pain is real, but the explanation for the pain is a mystery. Examples of chronic pain problems that are thought to be psychogenic are frequent headaches, low back pain, atypical facial pain, and pelvic pain of unknown origin.
- **Somatoform disorders** have some of the marks of real conditions, but the condition doesn't fully explain the individual's symptoms. In other words, these disorders completely baffle the doctors and the patient. Examples of somataform disorders are *body dysmorphic disorder* (a preoccupation with a real or imagined flaw in appearance), *conversion disorder* (neurological symptoms, such as paralysis, that aren't caused by a neurological disease), and *hypochondriasis* (obsessive worry about having a serious illness).

Looking at Behavioral Cycles

You may describe your pain with phrases such as, "Today is a bad pain day," "Today is an okay day," or "Today is a better day." Chronic pain waxes and wanes, and you may notice that as your pain intensifies, your mood goes downhill. Alternatively, if you're in an okay or a good mood, your pain may not seem so bad.

For many people, chronic pain means that their day-to-day activities become difficult (or impossible) to perform. This limitation can result in a negative cycle in which the more pain you're in, the more you limit yourself, which also creates more pain.

Whatever type of chronic pain you have, it can lead to self-defeating behavioral cycles that perpetuate *more* chronic pain. Just what you don't want!

Figure 3-1 shows how the chronic pain behavioral cycle works. The cycle is made up of the following five phases:

- **Phase 1: Inactivity.** In this phase, you're in pain, so you limit what you'd normally do. You cancel a trip to visit your mother because it means two hours in a car, which will make you even more stiff and sore. You put off carrying the laundry downstairs to the laundry room, because just thinking about it makes you tired. You don't make dates to play tennis.
- **Phase 2: Catching up.** In phase 2, you feel okay. You may hop (well okay, you move into) the car and drive to visit your mother. You do the laundry, making many trips up and down the stairs. You make a date to play tennis. Life is good.
- **Phase 3: Inactivity.** In phase 3, the day after you've visited your mother, done the laundry, and all your other catch-up activities, you wake up stiff and sore. "Ouch! I did too much," you say. You slow down. You cancel that tennis date.
- **Phase 4: Repeating the cycles.** You may repeat this scenario many times as you try to adjust to life with chronic pain. It becomes a vicious cycle: You feel better. You do more. You feel worse. You slow down.
- **Phase 5: Deconditioning.** Phase 5 refers to the deconditioning that your body suffers as you get out of shape in response to your pain. The time you spend slowing down makes you tired and weak, which is an irony of chronic pain. You try to protect yourself through slowing down, but this inactivity actually damages and weakens your body. Among other things, it causes your muscles to weaken, which gives you less stamina and makes you tired. See the sidebar "Avoiding deconditioning" for some specifics.

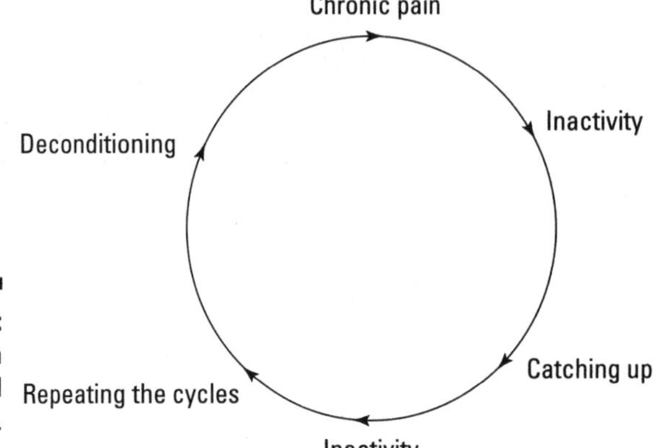

Figure 3-1: Chronic pain behavioral cycles.

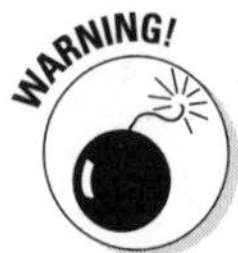

A danger of the pain cycle is that you may spend more time alone. Your tennis buddies don't call anymore because you've cancelled one too many games, and they've given up on you. Your family has gotten used to doing things for you and without you. They think they're helping out by filling in for you and not forcing you to go. They don't realize that the more helpless you become, the more pain you'll experience.

Managing Flare-Ups

Chronic pain worsens, and then it improves. This waxing and waning pattern repeats, again and again. *Flare-ups* are those times when your chronic pain is most intense. For example, on a 0-to-10 pain intensity scale, a flare-up may be a time when your pain is a 7 or higher.

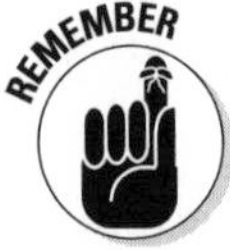

You're most likely to use pain medications during chronic pain flare-ups. While use of pain relievers can be the right thing, it's important to have other strategies in your anti-pain war chest. Don't rely on drugs alone.

Flare-ups are often the result of pain triggers. Two major categories of pain triggers reflect your physical and emotional states.

The first category includes activity or inactivity triggers, such as

- Staying in one position too long (such as sitting or standing for an extended period of time)
- Repetitive movements performed frequently and for long periods of time
- Movements that strain your body (lifting or pulling a heavy object)
- Bad posture, such as slumping over, and stressing painful areas

Avoiding deconditioning

If you have chronic pain, you know how easy it is to become a couch potato. Here are a few consequences of deconditioning:

- Muscle deterioration (atrophy)
- Stiff joints
- Loss of calcium from bones (leading to osteoporosis)
- Increased risk of heart disease and diabetes
- Loss of red blood cells
- Decrease in sex hormones and the production of sperm
- Decreased resistance to infection (reduced immune functions)
- Obesity
- Depression

Too negative for you? Turn this list around to consider a few *advantages* of becoming active:

- Increased joint flexibility
- Improved muscle tone
- Strong muscles
- Increased aerobic and cardiovascular fitness
- A desirable weight and fat ratio
- Release of *endorphins* (the feel good hormones that counteract depression and pain).

Sounds great doesn't it? Who wouldn't want these things? If you agree, then flip to Chapter 19 to read about exercises for people with chronic pain.

The way to avoid these triggers is obvious: Do the opposite. For example, make sure that you don't stay in one position for too long. If your job involves sitting for long periods of time, get up and move around frequently to loosen up. If you're slouched over, sit up straight.

Emotional triggers represent a second type of pain activator. It's important to minimize or prevent unnecessary emotional stress and find better ways to cope with it. (For more information, see Chapter 17.)

Another form of prevention involves heeding your own personal early warning signs. You may become aware of body sensations, such as migraine auras or a sudden inability to move your neck, that give you advance notice of flare-ups. Don't ignore these signs! Instead, try the techniques we recommend in Part III of this book.

Fighting Side Effects of Chronic Pain

You may be one of the lucky ones: You're able to manage your pain and keep it from taking over your life and the lives of your loved ones. But many people who live with chronic pain run into some major trouble. They can become physically and emotionally overwhelmed. They may drink too many cocktails at night to "take the edge off" or run through all their painkilling drugs before the prescription can be renewed. Their lives spiral out of balance.

Chronic pain often has serious side effects, such as weight changes, depression, and problems with stress and sleep. The following sections talk about these major side effects and what you can do to fight them successfully.

Dealing with weight gain or loss

Obesity is a major problem in America, and 66 percent of adults in the United States are either overweight or obese. Deconditioning is all too frequently a consequence of chronic pain. (For more on deconditioning, see the section "Looking at Behavioral Cycles," earlier in this chapter.)

Not everyone overeats when they're in pain. Some people eat much less and lose weight. Although weight loss sounds great to most people, losing weight because you've stopped eating a healthy diet is not a good idea. Some conditions that cause chronic pain, such as gastrointestinal problems, can cause weight loss. Weight loss can be as dangerous as weight gain, but for different reasons. Underweight individuals may have poor physical stamina and a weak immune system, leaving them open to infection. If you or a loved one has unexplained weight loss, you need to see a physician for a medical diagnosis.

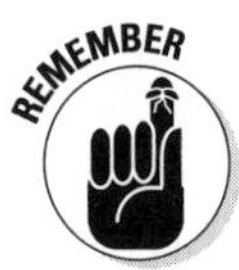

Maintaining a healthy weight can help you prevent weight-related diseases, such as heart disease, diabetes, arthritis, and some cancers, all of which can cause chronic pain.

Tackling depression and a negative self-image

Chronic pain can generate negative emotions, such as anger, frustration, and fear. Probably the most common emotional result is depression, and at least half of all people with chronic pain experience depression. People with weight changes (see the preceding section) may also be depressed, because eating more or less is a symptom of depression. Chronic pain may also cause physical qualities that overlap with those of depression, such as moving slowly, having trouble getting adequate rest, and feeling fatigue. A negative self-image usually accompanies depression. But the good news is that these problems are readily treatable.

If you or a loved one has symptoms of depression that linger for several months and that stay the same or worsen, you may be in the throes of a serious depression.

The first step toward beating depression is to accept that you or your loved one needs help. The good news is that depression can be treated.

Knowing when you need help

Are you unsure if you're depressed? Here's a list from the National Institute on Mental Health of common signs of depression. If you have several signs lasting more than two weeks, see your doctor.

- Persistent sad, anxious, or "empty" mood
- Feelings of hopelessness and pessimism
- Feelings of guilt, worthlessness, and helplessness
- Loss of interest or pleasure in hobbies and activities that were once enjoyed, including sex
- Decreased energy, fatigue, and feeling slowed down
- Difficulty concentrating, remembering, and making decisions
- Insomnia, early-morning awakening, or oversleeping
- Appetite and/or weight loss or overeating and weight gain
- Thoughts of death or suicide; suicide attempts
- Restlessness and irritability
- Persistent physical symptoms that do not respond to treatment, such as headaches, digestive disorders, and chronic pain

Fashioning a positive self-image

Your *self-image* is the sum of your opinions of yourself. Do you think you are smart, funny, and beautiful (or handsome)? If so, you're unusual. Most people are very critical of themselves. And, on top of that, the limitations that accompany chronic pain can damage your self-image. So work on accentuating the positive aspects of yourself rather than fixating on what's wrong with you.

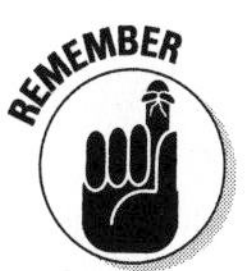

Your self-image directly affects how you feel about yourself and interact with others. It also influences the way you react or respond to the stresses of life. Learning to have a positive relationship with an imperfect body is key to improving your self-image. And the better your self-image, the better you'll manage your pain.

Reinventing your view of you

Develop a healthier and more accurate view of yourself. A healthy self-image starts with learning to accept and love yourself.

The following steps are recommended by the Cleveland Clinic to foster a positive self-image, with some of our own thoughts added:

- Take a realistic self-image inventory. Focus on the positives instead of your weaknesses.
- Set realistic and measurable goals, such as losing a pound a week, rather than fixating on the 20 pounds that you need to lose.
- Confront thinking distortions, such as "I can't ever lose weight." (See Chapter 21 for more information.)
- Identify childhood labels. Did Johnny down the street laugh at your limp when you were a kid? Get over it.
- Stop comparing yourself to others. They have their weaknesses and strengths, too. Try to improve from where *you* are now.
- Develop your strengths. And play down your weaknesses.
- Learn to love yourself. Trite but true: If you love yourself with all your limitations, others will also.
- Give positive affirmations. Stop moaning and groaning or acting sick!
- Remember that you are unique.
- Learn to laugh and smile.
- Remember how far you have come. (And celebrate it.)

Reducing stress and getting some sleep

Stress and lack of sleep make chronic pain worse, although pain itself is a powerful stressor. Yes, this merry-go-round is another vicious cycle associated with chronic pain. You need to break out of the cycle if you have one or both problems. Imagine that you're locked in a small, cold and gray cell, a cell of stress. Let yourself feel bad and sad. Then imagine yourself deciding to break out. You punch out of that cell, which now has the consistency of cardboard. You're free! This imagery may help you feel empowered.

De-stressing your life

Chronic pain is nerve-wracking. Your body automatically tries to fight pain. Then, pain itself creates physical, emotional, and psychological tension. As if that wasn't bad enough, physical tension increases your muscle tension where it hurts.

Not fair, you say! We agree. And it's a big reason why reducing stress is so important for the person with chronic pain.

On top of that sorry state of affairs, your body systems, such as your central nervous system, heart, and immune system, also react to tension. Your mind and emotions respond to the whole mess with increased worry, anger, sadness, frustration, and so on. All these factors escalate your pain.

Another source of stress is the yucky consequences that chronic pain can have on your life and the lives of your loved ones. For example, chronic pain can

- Impact your ability to work and, therefore, your financial security.
- Limit family activities and social life.
- Limit the fun things you do on your own and that give you satisfaction, such as hobbies and recreational activities.
- Harm your self-esteem and feelings of self-worth.

For tips on overcoming stress, see Chapters 21 and 22. Among the things we recommend are taking advantage of proven stress-reduction techniques, such as meditation and self-hypnosis.

Solving sleep problems

Sleep problems are yet another vicious cycle: Pain causes sleep problems. These sleep difficulties lead to increased sensitivity to pain, increased stress, and so on. And this challenge can be worsened by other factors, such as medications you take for pain, some of which can reduce sleep quality; how much exercise you get; and your daily diet.

Lack of sleep makes pain worse and increases stress, yet it's very difficult to sleep when you have pain. If this cycle sounds like your situation, you're not alone. A Gallup poll found that 62 percent of people with chronic pain say that they wake too early because of pain and are unable to fall back to sleep.

A variety of sleep disturbances, including difficulty falling asleep and waking frequently during the night, are common for people who are hurting. If you or a loved one has chronic pain, your sleep may also be less restful than it would be otherwise.

Insomnia is the most common sleep problem. If you have insomnia, you have trouble falling and staying asleep. Insomnia can last for days, months, or even years. According to the National Institutes of Health, signs that you're having trouble sleeping include

- Taking a long time to fall asleep
- Waking up many times during the night
- Waking up early and being unable to fall back to sleep
- Waking up tired

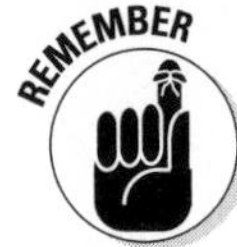

Your chronic pain may be only one cause of your insomnia. Other problems, such as worrying about your health or medical bills, can contribute to sleeplessness. And sometimes insomnia is a side effect of a medication or an illness.

Insomnia may become a bad habit. Develop new behaviors that will help you get the good night's sleep your body needs. See Chapter 20 for information on how to develop these habits.

Maintaining balance

One of the costs of chronic pain is that it can throw your life out of balance. Taking care of your pain condition may take up a lot of your time and energy, which you have to factor in with all your other commitments, such as working, taking care of your family, or enjoying retirement.

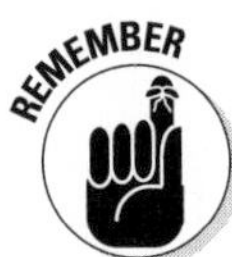

After you face up to having a serious chronic pain condition, you may need to reassess your lifestyle. Take an honest look at what you do on most days. How much time do you spend working, with your family or relaxing? Are you able to devote time every day to exercise? Do you set aside time to take care of yourself and your pain-causing condition? If not, you may need to rethink your schedule.

Keeping Relationships on Track

Chronic pain impacts you physically and emotionally and also affects your relationships with others. Your pain affects everyone you love, everyone who loves you, everyone whom you work with, and everyone whom you play with in some way, whether it's because you have less time for them or they're upset by how the pain is obviously taking over your life. In most cases, they want to help! Most families and other social structures, such as work colleagues and friendship networks, experience significant stress when chronic pain hits one of their members. The following sections address issues you may encounter in your relationships, as well as ideas on how to maintain good connections.

Dealing with relationship problems

Following are just some of the common relationship problems that can occur for people who have a chronic pain condition:

- **Withdrawal:** Particularly during flare-ups, many people with chronic pain would rather be by themselves and end up isolating themselves from family and friends.
- **A short fuse, taking out frustration and anger on those around you:** Anger and frustration about your pain are natural responses. But if you take these emotions out on people you care about, it can cause serious relationship conflicts.
- **Trouble asking for and receiving help:** One of the most difficult things about being dependent is that it can be hard to ask for and receive help. This situation is also problematic for the person who's the helper. In short, the dynamic between the giver and receiver of help sometimes can be awkward and cause considerable stress in the relationship.
- **Difficulty in sexual relationships:** Some people with chronic pain develop sexual problems. Medications, pain, and fatigue can all decrease sex drive. Read Chapter 27 for ideas on how to enhance your sex life when you have chronic pain.

Maintaining communication

One of the keys to resolving relationship conflicts is to give both time and attention to problems when they crop up. Often visiting a trained therapist can help. Here are some resources:

- The **American Association for Marriage and Family Therapy** offers guidance materials and links to locate qualified therapists in local areas. Web site: `http://www.aamft.org`
- The **American Psychological Association (APA)** in Washington, D.C., is the largest scientific and professional organization representing psychology in the United States. Its membership includes more than 150,000 clinicians and other professionals. Obtain a referral to a psychologist in your area by calling 1-800-964-2000. The operator will use your zip code to locate and connect you with the referral service of the state psychological association. Web site: `www.apa.org`
- Members of the **National Association of Social Workers (NASW)** help people in their own environments by looking at different aspects of their life and culture. Search for a clinical social worker near you by entering your city, state, and/or zip code into NASW's drop-down menu on its Web site: `www.helpstartshere.org/common/Search/search.asp`

Acknowledging caregiver stress

What if you're not the one in severe pain but instead you're someone who cares about that person? For lack of a better word, you're the *caregiver,* even if the main care giving is holding the ill person's hand when she's feeling really bad. Sometimes the caregiver feels stressed, and it's important to acknowledge this fact.

Research suggests that the physical and emotional demands on caregivers put them at greater risk for health problems. These facts are from the National Institutes of Health:

- Caregivers are more at risk for infectious diseases, such as colds and flu, and chronic diseases, such as heart problems, diabetes, and cancer.
- Depression is twice as common among caregivers compared to noncaregivers.
- Caregivers supply nearly 257 billion dollars a year in services for their loved ones, such as transportation, supervision, financial management, and so on.

Caregivers juggle many roles. Besides assisting a loved one, most are married or living with a partner, have a paid job, and also care for a child or an elderly person. If you're a caregiver, you may go through the same cycles as your loved one with chronic pain. Like them, you're losing control over your daily life: Maybe your wife is no longer the confidante she used to be because she's absorbed with her pain, and consequently, you feel lonely and sad. Maybe your loved one is grumpy and takes it out on you, which can be very hard to take. You're trying to help, and your head gets bitten off! Even when you know it's the "pain" that is talking, it still hurts.

If you're a caregiver, watch for signs that this role is stressing you out too much. These common signs of caregiver stress are from the American Academy of Family Physicians (AAFP):

- Feeling sad or moody
- Crying more often than you used to
- Having a low energy level
- Feeling like you have no time for yourself
- Having trouble sleeping, or not wanting to get out of bed in the morning
- Having trouble eating, or eating too much
- Seeing friends or relatives less often than you used to

- Losing interest in your hobbies or the things you used to do with friends or family
- Feeling angry at the person you are caring for or at other people or situations

In addition, you may get little or no thanks from the person you're caring for, which can add to your feelings of stress and frustration. Realize that these feelings are perfectly natural. AAFP points out that some doctors regard caregivers as *hidden patients* because of the stress and strain on them. Talk with your doctor about your feelings. Stay in touch with your friends and family members. Ask them for help in giving care.

If you're a caregiver but you don't take care of yourself and stay well, you won't be able to help the people you love.

Many communities offer caregiver support groups that provide you an opportunity to share information and feel connected to others providing care, just like you. Support groups are often organized through churches, synagogues, recreation centers, and Area Agencies on Aging. Your local social services or aging office can direct you to a support group.

Part II

Detailing Some Causes of Chronic Pain

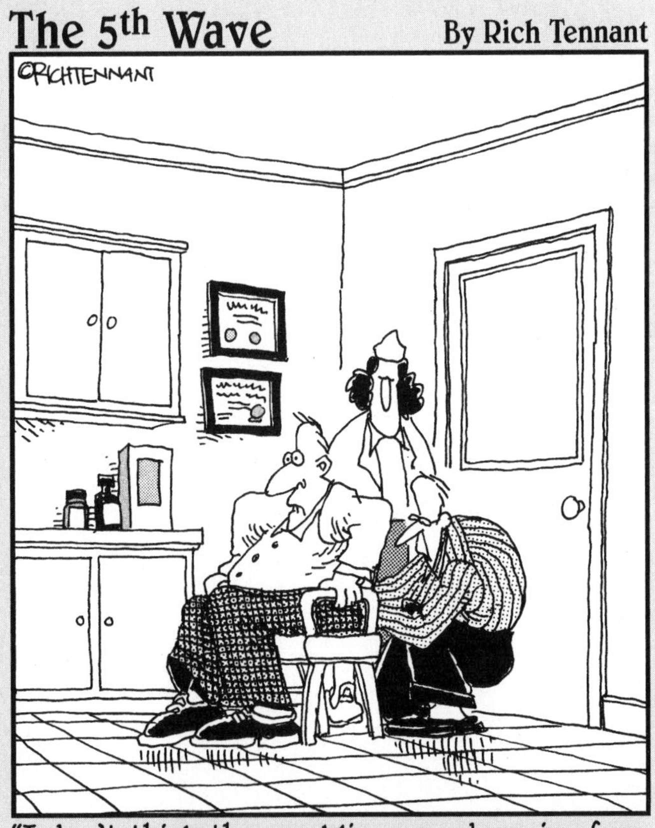

"I don't think the crackling sound coming from your lower back is as serious as you thought. Just relax, and I'll have this Rice Krispie Square out of your back pocket in no time."

In this part . . .

Part II describes the major diseases and injuries that can lead to chronic pain, as well as how these causes are diagnosed and treated. We cover the most common forms of arthritis, headaches, and cancer pain, to name just a few.

Remember that just because you hurt all the time doesn't mean that you have one of these conditions! In fact, you may have chronic pain and never know the cause. (How frustrating is that?) Or your pain may be caused by a less common condition that we didn't cover.

Chapter 4

Arthritis and Its Cohorts

In This Chapter

- Understanding arthritis
- Reviewing the major types of arthritis
- Finding out how arthritis is diagnosed
- Identifying techniques for using your body wisely

It can sneak up and strike you suddenly and without warning. You *were* okay yesterday, but today you're hurting. Or it can overtake you in small, increasingly painful steps — you noticed a sore knee a year ago, a painful shoulder about six months ago, and soreness in your wrist a month ago. None of them has gone away.

It's arthritis, the leading cause of disability in the United States. Tragically, arthritis can strike as early as infancy, although most people with arthritis are middle-aged or older adults.

This chapter includes general information about arthritis and what you can do about it. We cover the most frequently occurring form of arthritis, osteoarthritis, along with nine other common types of the disease.

Sneaking Up on You: Arthritis

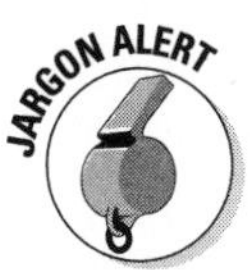

Most people think of arthritis as a disease that affects the *joints* (the intersection where two bones meet). But the term *arthritis* actually is a catchall term for more than 100 medical conditions that affect not only your joints, but your muscles and bones as well. In fact, some conditions, such as rheumatoid arthritis and psoriatic arthritis, can attack the entire body.

According to the National Institutes of Health, common symptoms of arthritis are pain and stiffness in your body, trouble moving around, and swelling in your joints.

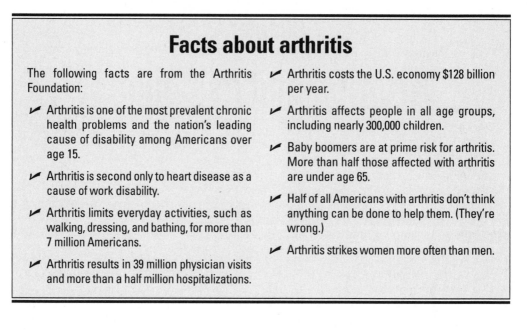

Facts about arthritis

The following facts are from the Arthritis Foundation:

- Arthritis is one of the most prevalent chronic health problems and the nation's leading cause of disability among Americans over age 15.
- Arthritis is second only to heart disease as a cause of work disability.
- Arthritis limits everyday activities, such as walking, dressing, and bathing, for more than 7 million Americans.
- Arthritis results in 39 million physician visits and more than a half million hospitalizations.
- Arthritis costs the U.S. economy $128 billion per year.
- Arthritis affects people in all age groups, including nearly 300,000 children.
- Baby boomers are at prime risk for arthritis. More than half those affected with arthritis are under age 65.
- Half of all Americans with arthritis don't think anything can be done to help them. (They're wrong.)
- Arthritis strikes women more often than men.

Treatments for arthritis vary according to the type. In other words, what works for rheumatoid arthritis doesn't work for gout. You can read about specific treatments in the upcoming sections on different types of arthritis. General treatments are used by people with all arthritis types, such as popular painkillers to treat pain and inflammation. In addition, most doctors recommend that overweight people lose weight. And everyone should exercise. (Read more about exercise in Chapter 19.)

The Most Frequent Form: Osteoarthritis

Linda, 35, says most of her osteoarthritis pain is in her knees, and it's often hard to walk. Diana, 55, says her arthritis is primarily in her back. As with Linda, Diana has trouble walking, but her problem is severe back pain caused by osteoarthritis. (Read more about back pain in Chapter 5.)

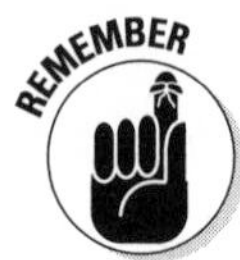

The hallmark of *osteoarthritis* (OA) is damage to one or more joints. Osteoarthritis is the most commonly occurring form of arthritis. The troublemaker in the joint is the *cartilage,* which is a rubbery, fibrous, dense connective tissue that cushions the joint. The cartilage — which usually protects joints from the wear and tear of daily walking and other activities, as well as general aging — breaks down (see Figure 4-1). The result is that the bones of the joint rub against each other, causing inflammation. As the disease progresses, joints become painful, stiff, and limited in motion.

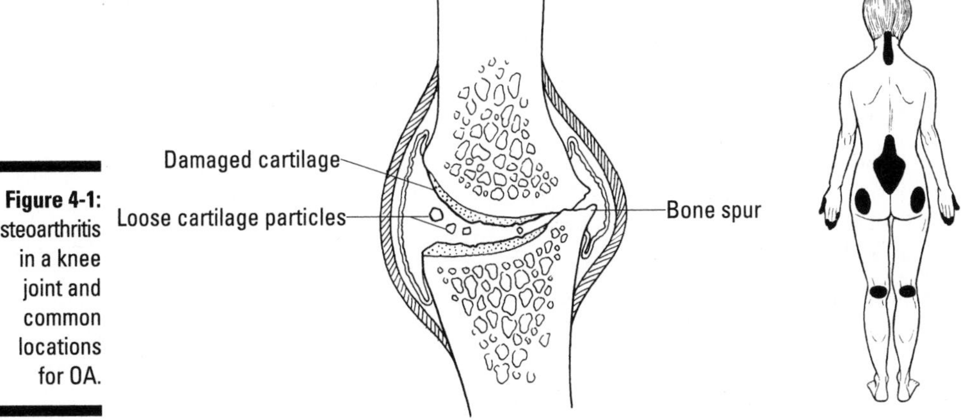

Figure 4-1: Osteoarthritis in a knee joint and common locations for OA.

Osteoarthritis is often thought of as an older person's disease. And, indeed, the line, "Live long enough, and you'll get osteoarthritis" is mostly true. However, younger people sometimes develop this form of arthritis, usually due to sports injuries or accidents. For example, football players can develop osteoarthritis in their knees, and tennis players can develop it in their shoulders. (Many people mistakenly believe *tennis elbow* is caused by osteoarthritis, but it's actually due to an injury of the muscle and tendon area around the outside of the elbow.)

What causes or triggers osteoarthritis is a mystery, but some risk factors are known. According to the National Institutes of Health, key risk factors are

- A genetic defect in joint cartilage
- Being overweight
- Getting older
- Joint injury
- Joints that are not properly formed (such as hip dysplasia)
- Stresses on the joints from certain jobs and playing sports

If you have any of these symptoms, you may have osteoarthritis:

- A crunching feeling or the sound of bone rubbing on bone
- Stiffness in a joint after getting out of bed or sitting for a long time
- Swelling or tenderness in one or more joints

If these symptoms are interfering with your daily life, talk with your doctor about them right away.

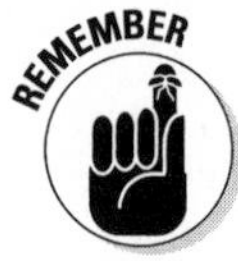

While medications for pain relief are usually necessary, the most important treatment for osteoarthritis is a joint-friendly lifestyle. Eating a healthy diet, maintaining a healthy weight, avoiding joint damage, and lessening the stress in your life are all keys to managing osteoarthritis. (For information on these topics, see Chapters 18, 19, and 21.)

Painful Joints and More: Rheumatoid Arthritis

Rheumatoid arthritis (RA) is called a systemic disease because it not only affects joints, but also muscles such as the lung and heart. It causes pain, swelling, and stiffness, and these symptoms are usually worse in the morning.

RA is known as a symmetrical disease. If one knee has rheumatoid arthritis, usually the other knee has it, too (although one knee may be worse than the other). RA can affect any joint in the body and often attacks more than one joint. People with this disease often feel sick, and they're tired. (They're also sick and tired of having rheumatoid arthritis!) Sometimes they have chronic fevers.

If you develop RA, you may have it for only a few months, or for a year or two. Or you may have times when the symptoms get worse *(flares),* and times when they get better *(remissions).* Some people develop a severe form of the disease that lasts for many years or a lifetime. This type of RA can cause serious joint damage.

The damage that occurs with RA is different from damage caused by OA, which is described in the preceding section. With RA, the synovial membrane that surrounds the joint is inflamed and swollen, and infected cells move in and attack both the vulnerable bone and cartilage (see Figure 4-2). The cartilage becomes thin, the joint space narrows, and the joint capsule is inflamed.

Anyone can develop rheumatoid arthritis, although women are more likely to suffer from it than men. RA often starts in middle age and is most common in older people. But children and young adults can also have rheumatoid arthritis (For more information on the various types of arthritis that children may develop, see Chapter 23.)

Doctors don't know exactly what causes RA, but they do know that with this form of arthritis, the person's immune system attacks its own body tissues. Possible causes include

- Genes (passed from parent to child, but don't blame Mom or Dad; if they could've stopped this gene from getting to you, they would've!)
- Lifestyle factors, such as smoking and obesity

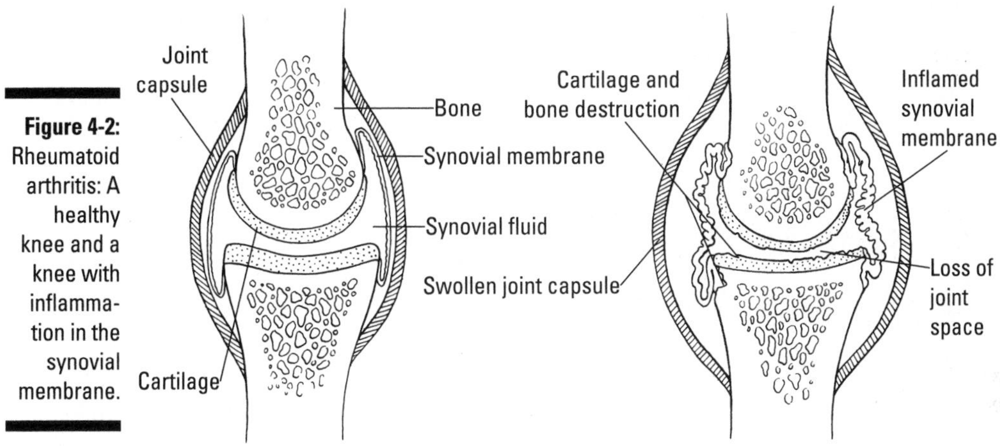

Figure 4-2: Rheumatoid arthritis: A healthy knee and a knee with inflammation in the synovial membrane.

Most people with rheumatoid arthritis take medicine on an ongoing basis to relieve pain, reduce swelling, and stop the disease from getting worse. In addition to pain relievers generally used by people with other types of arthritis, other specific types of medications, such as disease modifying antirheumatic drugs (DMARDs), provide tremendous relief for people with RA. These medications are often used alongside NSAIDs and/or prednisone to slow down joint destruction. Examples of DMARDs are methotrexate, azathioprine, chloroquine, and hydroxychloroquine.

The biological response modifier is another type of drug used to treat RA. Medications in this category inhibit proteins called cytokines, which contribute to inflammation. Examples of biological response modifiers include etanercept (Enbrel), inflixamab (Remicade), and adalimunab (Humira). Another drug used to treat rheumatoid arthritis is anakinra (Kineret). This medication blocks *interleukin 1,* a protein seen in excessive levels among patients with rheumatoid arthritis.

Sick and Tired of Fibromyalgia

Fibromyalgia is a disease that causes muscle pain and tenderness. This condition has been not-so affectionately nicknamed *fibro.* The muscle pain can be anywhere and is often characterized as whole-body. Specific places on the neck, shoulders, back, hips, arms, and legs — called *tender* points — hurt when pressure is placed on them, and the presence of these tender points is used as a diagnostic test. Figure 4-3 shows these tender points.

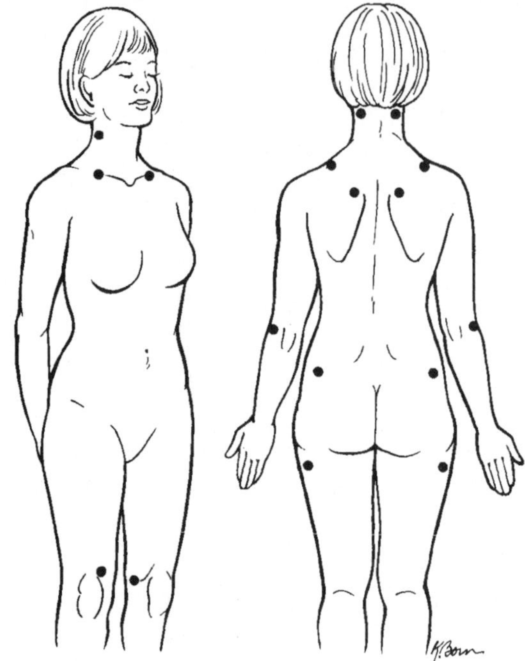

Figure 4-3: Fibromyalgia tender points.

Often, sufferers of fibromyalgia have a previous history of some other chronic pain condition, such as whiplash pain, temporomandibular pain, rheumatoid arthritis, irritable bowel syndrome, repetitive strain injury, headache, back pain, and interstitial cystitis.

Fibro affects as many as 1 in 50 Americans, but women are much more likely to have the disease than men. Also, women with a family member with fibromyalgia are more likely to have this condition.

Because people with fibromyalgia frequently score high on psychological tests of anxiety or depression, it may appear that anxiety or depression caused the muscle pain. However, pain itself generates psychological distress. The bottom line is that stress is important for understanding and dealing with fibro.

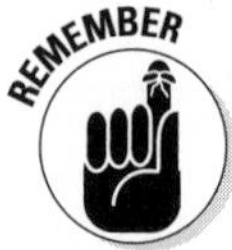

If you or a loved one has fibro, relaxation training is beneficial (see Chapter 22). Any technique that improves blood supply to muscles helps, such as exercise (see Chapter 19). Exercise is difficult to sell to people with fibro, because it hurts in the short term although it helps over the long haul. Learning to pace the exercise and adjust the amount of exercise day to day based on symptoms of fibro can be helpful. The relatively new drug Lyrica has helped some people with fibromyalgia. Opiate narcotics aren't very useful for most patients with fibromyalgia.

Chronic stress and fibromyalgia

Chronic stress, whether it's psychological stress or stress stemming from a focal pain condition, works through complex circuits in the brain to activate the hypothalamus and the sympathetic nervous system. The long name for the central organizing centers of stress is the hypothalamic-pituitary-adrenal (HPA) axis. This fight-or-flight system mobilizes you in a short-term crisis. When long-term stress and activation of the HPA axis occurs, it has widespread effects that can explain not only fibromyalgia, but also other associated conditions. Chronic stress can increase pain sensitivity anywhere in the body. Even pain from stimulation of the skin is exaggerated for some fibro patients.

Both stress and pain interrupt sleep (see Chapter 2), and sleep deprivation is a significant problem for people with fibro. Also, sleep loss is a major stressor (see Chapter 20). Sleep deprivation and stress together can cause impaired memory (called *fibro fog).*

Sympathetic activation from chronic stress reduces the blood supply to muscles *(peripheral vasoconstriction).* Females are more susceptible to this effect, contributing to the high incidence of fibro among women. Many fibro patients have *Raynaud's syndrome,* with symptoms of reduced peripheral blood supply (such as cold hands).

Long-term reduction of blood supply to the muscles (ischemia) makes the pain receptors (nociceptors) more sensitive to pressure, an important characteristic of fibro. In addition, it sensitizes a peripheral receptor responsible for muscular fatigue. A condition called *chronic fatigue syndrome* (CFS) is commonly associated with fibro. (CFS is a syndrome that involves debilitating fatigue, which makes physical exercise or mental activity very difficult.)

Input to the CNS from muscle nociceptors is a very potent source of central sensitization (see Chapter 2). This process is a vicious cycle: Any focal pain condition can eventually produce widespread muscular pain, which increases central sensitivity to both the focal pain and the widespread pain.

Overlapping Conditions: Polymyalgia Rheumatica and Temporal Arteritis

Polymyalgia rheumatica (PMR) and temporal arteritis often strike together. *Polymyalgia rheumatica* is a form of arthritis that causes low-grade pain in the large joints. When asked to describe their pain, people with PMR often point to their entire hip or shoulder rather than to specific tender points. Stiffness and muscle pain are common with the disease. Other symptoms include fatigue, night sweating, lack of appetite, a slight fever, and depression. PMR affects both sides of the body, and more than one area may be stricken.

PMR has symptoms that can be confused with fibromyalgia (see preceding section). However, fibro usually strikes women in their 30s and 40s, and PMR is more common in older adults.

Temporal arteritis is an inflammation of the lining of your arteries. (Temporal arteritis is also called giant cell arteritis.) The *temporal arteries,* which supply blood to part of the head, are most often affected. The disease is potentially very damaging and can lead to violent headaches and even blindness. PMR and giant cell arteritis overlap in many cases.

White women over age 50 have the highest risk of developing the two conditions. While people with PMR may also develop giant cell arteritis, if you're over age 50, arteritis can strike even if you don't have PMR.

Anti-inflammatory drugs and rest are used to treat PMR. Corticosteroids are used to treat both diagnosed PMR and temporal arteritis. Without treatment, these conditions can progress with devastating consequences, such as blindness and/or stroke.

TMJ Dysfunction: It's All about Your Jaw

TMJ is an abbreviation for the temporomandibular joint, the technical term for the joint between the lower jaw and the temporal bone of the skull (see Figure 4-4).

TMJ results from your jaw not functioning properly, leading to tenderness, pain, a clicking sound when you move your mouth, and/or locking of the jaw. TMJ may cause headaches, earaches, and dizziness.

People who get TMJ usually have arthritis in the joint and/or clench (or grind) their teeth, but the pain can come from the muscles used to chew and close the mouth and doesn't always involve the actual joint.

To treat TMJ, rest your jaw by eating soft foods, such as yogurt and applesauce (which are very nutritious foods). Be sure you avoid clenching or grinding your teeth and use ice packs when the condition really bothers you. If you have symptoms of TMJ, talk them over with your dentist. He may suggest using a mouth guard or refer you to an otolaryngologist (head and neck surgeon) or oral (dental) surgeon.

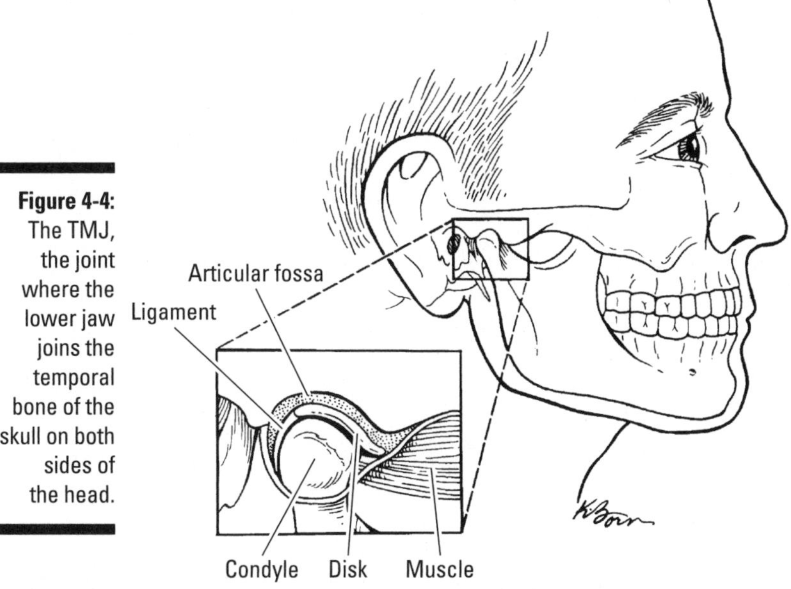

Figure 4-4: The TMJ, the joint where the lower jaw joins the temporal bone of the skull on both sides of the head.

Sniffling Over Soft Tissue Diseases

Soft tissue syndromes affect the tissues surrounding joints, causing pain, swelling, and inflammation. These syndromes can affect any area of your body, such as your shoulder, elbow, or lower back.

Soft tissue syndromes have many names, depending on where they occur in the body. One of the best-known syndromes of this type is *myofascial pain syndrome* (MPS), a chronic pain problem that may involve a single muscle or an entire muscle group. The pain may burn, stab, ache, or nag. The pain from MPS may also be *referred,* which means that it does not occur at the source, but travels to another place in your body.

Scientists aren't sure what causes MPS. The most well-known theory is that a muscle injury causes a painful tender point.

If any of these traits apply to you, you may be at risk for MPS:

- Abnormal bone or muscle structures
- Bad body posture
- Overuse or injury of a joint or muscle

MPS can also strike in association with other diseases or conditions, such as fibromyalgia, described earlier in the chapter in the section "Sick and Tired of Fibromyalgia."

The primary treatment for MPS is to stop overusing the muscle or muscle group that has been injured. Other treatment options are

- Massage therapy
- Physical therapy
- *Stretch-and-spray therapy,* which involves spraying the painful muscle with a coolant and then stretching it
- Trigger point injections of pain-relieving drugs

Lupus: When Your Immune System Attacks You

With *lupus,* something goes wrong with your immune system and attacks your healthy cells and tissues. The antibodies present in this process cause inflammation and pain. They also damage many parts of the body, such as the joints, skin, kidneys, heart, lungs, blood vessels, and brain. Inflammation is considered the primary feature of lupus.

For many people, lupus is a mild, but painful disease affecting only a few organs. For others, it may cause serious problems and can even cause death.

Lupus comes in many different types. The most common type, *systemic lupus erythematosus,* affects many parts of the body. Other types of lupus are

- **Discoid lupus erythematosus,** which causes a skin rash that doesn't go away
- **Drug-induced lupus**, which is caused by some medications such as procainamide (Pronestyl), and quinidine (Quinaglute), used to control abnormal heart rates
- **Neonatal lupus,** a rare type of lupus that affects newborns
- **Subacute cutaneous lupus erythematosus,** which causes skin sores on parts of the body exposed to sun

The Lupus Foundation of America (LFA) estimates that 1.5 to 2 million Americans have a form of lupus. More than 90 percent of people with lupus are women. Lupus usually strikes women in their childbearing years, between ages 15 to 45 years. In the United States, lupus is more common in African-Americans, Latinos, Asians, and Native Americans than Caucasians.

Many people can do well when treated for lupus. If you have lupus, getting plenty of rest and wearing sun block to protect against sun exposure are key measures to avoid flare-ups. For information on treatment and other concerns about lupus the following Web sites are great resources:

- **Lupus Foundation:** www.lupus.com
- **Lupus Research Institute:** www.lupusresearchinstitute.org

Too Dry for Too Long: Sjogren's Syndrome

Sjogren's syndrome is an autoimmune arthritic disorder that causes severe dryness in the mouth and eyes. It may also affect other organs in the body. Sjogren's comes in two types: primary and secondary. Primary Sjogren's syndrome strikes by itself. People who develop secondary Sjogren's have another disease, such as rheumatoid arthritis, and they develop dry eyes and mouth as a result of that disease. Secondary Sjogren's is usually less severe than primary Sjogren's.

Most people who get Sjogren's syndrome have passed age 40, and 9 out of 10 sufferers are women. Sjogren's syndrome is sometimes linked to rheumatoid arthritis, described in the section "Painful Joints and More: Rheumatoid Arthritis," earlier in this chapter.

According to the National Institute of Arthritis and Musculoskeletal Disease (NIAMS), treatment for the dry eyes of Sjogren's may include

- Hydroxypropyl methylcellulose (Lacriserts), a prescription drug that wets the eye surface and keeps natural tears from drying out fast. It comes in a small pellet placed in your lower eyelid. When you add eye drops, the pellet melts and forms a film over your own tears, trapping moisture.
- Artificial tears that come in different thicknesses and are available over-the-counter.
- Chewing gum or sucking on hard candy to help your glands make more saliva. Sugar-free gum and candy are best. (But be careful about chewing gum because it can cause TMJ!)
- Eye ointments, which are available over-the-counter, are thicker than artificial tears. They protect the eyes and keep them wet for several hours. They can blur vision, so you may want to use them while you sleep.
- Sipping water or a sugar-free drink often to wet your mouth.
- Surgery to shut the tear ducts that drain tears from the eye.

In addition, your doctor may prescribe pilocarpine (Salagan) tablets to treat dryness of the mouth and throat, Evoxac to treat a dry mouth, or cyclosporine ophthalmic solution (Restasis) to treat dry eyes.

An important resource for people with Sjogrens is the Sjogren's Syndrome Web site at `www.sjogrens.org`.

Giving Up Gout

Gout, also known as metabolic arthritis, is a painful condition caused by crystals of uric acid that settle into tissues of the body. *Uric acid* is a breakdown product of *purines* (organic compounds), which are present in many foods. Gout may be caused by an inherited abnormality in the body's ability to process uric acid.

Gout is known for its recurring, extremely painful attacks of joint inflammation (arthritis). Chronic gout can lead to deposits of hard lumps of uric acid in and around the joints, as well as decreased kidney function and kidney stones. Almost 20 percent of people who have gout develop kidney stones.

Gout is a menace for about 1 million people per year in the United States. Nine out of ten gout victims are men. In women with gout, the onset usually occurs after menopause. Certain characteristics are common in people who develop gout, including

- Abnormal kidney function
- Abnormal metabolism of uric acid
- Excessive weight gain
- High blood pressure
- Moderate to heavy alcohol intake
- Obesity

If NSAIDs or corticosteroids don't control gout symptoms, your doctor may consider prescribing colchicine. This drug is most effective when taken within the first 12 hours of an acute attack. For chronic gout attacks, your doctor may prescribe allopurinol (Zyloprim) to treat high levels of uric acid and reduce the frequency of sudden attacks. (See Chapter 14 for information on NSAIDs and corticosteroids.)

If you have gout, avoid high-purine foods, such as sweetbreads, liver, meat extracts such as Oxo or Bovril, herring, and scallops, which can increase uric acid levels.

Bones Silently Turning to Powder: Osteoporosis

Osteoporosis is a common and painful condition that can disfigure and disable its victims. It weakens bones and can cause spontaneous fractures. In fact, in the advanced stage, doctors sometimes say that their patient's bones have "turned to powder." The signature worst symptom of osteoporosis is fractures, primarily of the spine, hips, and wrists. Many physical characteristics commonly associated with aging — such as a stooped posture, shrinking height, and thick waist — are actually caused by osteoporosis. So it's not surprising that many people think of osteoporosis as a condition of older age. Actually, however, osteoporosis begins in the early adult years, and steps to thwart it should start then.

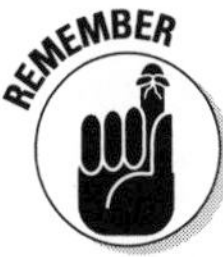

Osteoporosis is often called silent because bone loss occurs without symptoms. People may not know that they have osteoporosis until a sudden strain, bump, or fall causes a bone to break.

Ten million people in the United States have osteoporosis. Millions more have low bone mass, or *osteopenia* (not as bad as osteoporosis, but bad enough), placing them at increased risk for more serious bone loss and subsequent fractures

These characteristics put people at high risk for osteoporosis:

- A family history of osteoporosis
- Decreased consumption of dairy products
- Endurance athlete, including running and dancing
- A medical condition such as inflammatory small bowel disease or celiac disease
- Taking a medication that blocks calcium absorption, such as a steroid
- Heavy cigarette smoker
- Heavy consumption of alcohol
- Older age
- Partially or totally immobilized
- Physically inactive
- Poor eating habits and/or an eating disorder
- Strenuous dieter and/or faster

Osteoporosis isn't curable, but it is treatable. Two important preventive and treatment measures are a diet adequate in calories, calcium, vitamin D, and protein, and secondly, weight-bearing exercise. (See Chapters 18 and 19 for information on diet and exercise.)

Medications and other substances can prevent and treat the bone-robbing condition. They include

- Biophosphonates (Aredia and Zometa), which can increase bone density and can help in preventing osteoporsosis caused by use of corticosteroids
- Calcitonin, which reduces the risk of bone fractures
- Estrogen supplement therapy
- Selective estrogen receptor modulators (Ralozifene), which also can increase bone density
- Strontium ranelate (Protelos), popular in Europe, to treat osteoporosis
- Parathyroid hormone (Teriparatide), which can increase bone density
- Vitamin D and calcium, to help reach and keep maximum bone density

The National Osteoporosis Foundation's Web site at www.nof.org is a valuable resource for people with osteoporosis.

Diagnosing Arthritis

Whichever form of arthritis you have, the diagnosis and treatment requires a hands-on approach. Your doctor will examine your tender joints and muscles, move them around, and ask you to describe your symptoms.

Your doctor may also order lab tests to help diagnose the cause of your pain and other symptoms. Most lab tests are performed on your blood, which is like a script that holds many clues to what's going on throughout the body. Other tests may require urine, joint fluid, or pieces of skin or muscle. Your doctor will study your tests to confirm a diagnosis, monitor the progress of your disease, determine whether a medication is working, or look at whether any drugs you're taking are causing any problems.

Doctors also use tests to see whether your disease is getting better, flaring, or progressing. For example, tests called sed rates and C-reactive protein tests can show whether inflammation is under control.

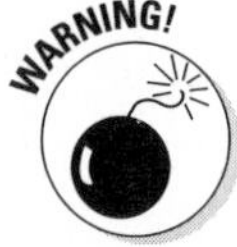

Many people with arthritis take pain-killing and disease-modifying drugs on an ongoing basis. If this is the case for you, it's important to have regular lab tests to see whether the drugs are causing any problems. Some medication side effects aren't noticeable until they do significant damage to the liver or kidneys, so it's better to be safe than sorry.

Specific tests for arthritis

You may hear people with arthritis talk about their sed rates or CRP levels. The following tests help your doctor diagnose arthritis and show how you're doing.

- **Antibodies to CCP:** This test looks for an antibody called anticyclic citrullinated peptide, which can diagnose rheumatoid arthritis. The antibody is almost never present in people who do not have RA.
- **Antinuclear antibody (ANA):** This sensitive blood test can detect autoimmune diseases, including SLE, STU polymyositis, scleroderma, Sjogren's syndrome, and rheumatoid arthritis.
- **C-Reactive protein (CRP):** CRP is a blood test that identifies inflammation.
- **Erythrocyte sedimentation rate (ESR or sed rate):** This blood test looks for a marker of inflammation. It measures how fast red blood cells fall to the bottom of a tube of blood.
- **HLA tissue typing:** This blood test can diagnose two less common types of arthritis, ankylosing spondylitis and Reiter's syndrome.
- **Joint fluid tests:** This test is for abnormalities, such as uric acid crystals or infectious agents, in joint (synovial) fluid.
- **Rheumatoid factor (RF):** This test for RA looks at gamma globulin, a component of blood.
- **Skin biopsy:** Some forms of arthritis involve the skin. Biopsies of skin can tell the presence of lupus, psoriatic arthritis, and other conditions.
- **Uric acid:** This test looks at the levels of uric acid in the blood in order to diagnose gout.

Keep in mind that lab tests don't catch everything. You may have a disease, such as RA, but the lab tests show nothing. For example, 15 to 20 percent of people with RA never have a positive rheumatoid factor. And on the flip side, lab tests may be positive for a disease that you show no signs of (and thank goodness for that!). (See the sidebar "Specific tests for arthritis" for a description of the test for rheumatoid factor.)

In addition, no lab tests are available for some forms of arthritis, such as OA. (See the sidebar for tests for other types of arthritis.) Other tests, including X-rays and magnetic resonance imaging, are used to diagnose such diseases as well as to check on further deterioration.

Considering Surgery

Most people with arthritis never need joint surgery. But when other treatment methods don't lessen pain, or you have major difficulty moving and using your joints, surgery may be necessary. (You can read more about surgery in general in Chapter 16.)

Resources for people with arthritis

Some important resources for people with arthritis include

Arthritis Foundation (AF), P.O. Box 7669, Atlanta, GA 30357-0669; phone 1-800-568-4045; Web site `www.arthritis.org`. The AF is a national, voluntary health agency seeking the causes, cures, preventions, and treatments for the more than 100 forms of arthritis. AF has 150 chapters and service points nationwide.

National Institutes of Health of Arthritis and Musculoskeletal and Skin Diseases (NIAMS), Bldg. 31, Room 4C02, 31 Center Dr. - MSC 2350, Bethesda, MD 20892-2350; phone 301-496-8190; Web site `www.niams.nih.gov`. Part of the National Institutes of Health, NIAMS supports research into the causes, treatment, and prevention of arthritis and provides information on research progress. Its Health Information Web pages provide valuable information for people with arthritis.

***Arthritis For Dummies*, 2nd Edition,** Barry Fox, Nadine Taylor, Jinoos Yazdany, Wiley. This book is for the millions who suffer from arthritis, as well as their family members and friends.

Types of surgery for arthritis include

- **Arthrodesis:** Surgery to fuse a vertebrae or other joint.
- **Arthroscopic surgery:** A minimally invasive procedure in which a small viewing instrument, an arthroscope, is used to look at the joint. It is usually an outpatient procedure used both for diagnosis and treatment.
- **Injections:** Rheumatologists and orthopedic surgeons inject substances such as glucocorticoids and hylauronic acid into painful joints in order to provide pain relief.
- **Joint replacement:** A major surgery in which damaged joints are removed and artificial joints are inserted in their place. Common examples are knee and hip replacements.
- **Synovectomy:** A surgical procedure to remove the lining of the joint (synovium).

Focusing on Healthy Joints

You can act to protect your joints and even prevent some forms of arthritis, such as OA, and lessen the damage from others, such as RA.

- **Maintain your ideal body weight.** The more you weigh, the more stress you put on your joints, especially your hips, knees, back, and feet. (See Chapter 18 for tips on eating a healthy diet.)

Use your body wisely

The way you carry your body largely affects how much strain you place on your joints. Proper body mechanics allow you to use your body more efficiently and conserve your energy.

- Stand up straight. Mom was right! Good posture protects joints in the neck, back, hips, and knees.
- When sitting, the proper height for a work surface is 2 inches below your bent elbow. Make sure that you have good back and foot support. Your forearms and upper legs should be level with the floor.
- If you type at a keyboard for long periods and your chair doesn't have arms, consider using wrist or forearm supports. An angled work surface for reading and writing is easier on your neck.
- When standing, the height of your work surface should enable you to work comfortably without stooping.
- Increase the height of your chair to decrease stress on your hips and knees as you get up and down.
- To pick up items from the floor, stoop by bending your knees and hips. Or sit in a chair and bend over.
- Carry heavy objects close to your chest, supporting the weight on your forearms.
- Use your big joints. When lifting or carrying, use your largest and strongest joints and muscles to avoid injury and strain on your smaller joints.
- Don't try to do a job too big for you to handle. Get another pair of hands to help.
- Don't give your joints the chance to stiffen up — keep moving. When writing or using your hands, release your grip every 10 to 15 minutes. On long car trips, get out of the car, stretch, and move around at least every hour. While watching television, get up and move around every half hour.
- Balance periods of rest and activity during the day. Work at a steady, moderate pace and avoid rushing. Rest before you become fatigued or sore. Alternate light and moderate activities throughout the day and take periodic stretch breaks.

- **Avoid pain triggers.** Find out how to tell the difference between the pain of arthritis and pain from overusing or misusing a joint. If you can identify an activity that stresses a joint, stop that movement as much as possible. See Chapter 17 for tips on avoiding pain triggers.
- **Move each joint through its full range of motion at least once a day to help you maintain freedom of motion in your joints.** For tips on how to take your joints through their range of motions, see Chapter 19.
- **Exercise!** Exercise protects joints by strengthening the muscles around them. Strong muscles keep your joints from rubbing against one another, which wears down cartilage (and hurts!).

Chapter 5

My Aching Back

In This Chapter

- Understanding back pain
- Accepting the mysteries of back pain
- Exploring treatment options
- Adapting to back pain

At least once in your life, you've probably winced with pain and moaned, "Ouch, my sore back!" Back pain is so common that it's the No. 2 reason why people visit doctors. (Headaches beat out back pain for the No. 1 spot.)

Sore backs that are long-lasting are frustrating for many reasons. First is the pain itself. It's an intruder — and an unwelcome and constant companion. Two other maddening characteristics of chronic back pain are that the cause (or sometimes the causes, if more than one factor is involved) is often unknown, *and* back pain can often severely limit activities at work, at home, and at play.

Although an ongoing sore back is just no fun at all, it's not all gloom and doom either. Whether you know what caused your back pain or not, you can use many effective treatments and techniques to lessen and manage your pain, even if you can't completely cure it. We cover many of these treatments and techniques in this chapter and Parts III and IV in this book.

If you follow the guidelines in this book, you may need to be cautious about lifting, twisting, and performing some other actions. But you likely can resume many tasks that you love, such as playing ball with your children and joining your buddies on the golf course. And you may even take up some new and fun activities like yoga or Pilates, which are great for your back.

Identifying Who Gets Chronic Back Pain

Maybe you're like Sandy, whose back really hurts nearly every day from her chronic arthritis problem. Or you may be more like Jim, who somehow twisted his back getting out of the car, and found the pain excruciating. The doctor treated him for a pulled muscle, which helped for awhile, but every so often, the pain comes back again. In Lori's case, she woke up one day with severe back pain and has no idea why she has it — and the reason for her pain has her doctor stumped as well. Fortunately for Lori, proven treatments can improve chronic back pain, even when the cause is unknown.

The back and spine are two of the strongest parts of the human body. Even so, because of day-in-and-day-out wear and tear on the back, at some point in life, nearly everyone has a sore back. But, what about back pain that *never* altogether leaves? Studies show that one in five adults have chronic, low back pain, which is the most common form.

Some people are more inclined to have back pain than others. Randy Shelerud, M.D., director of the Spine Center at the Mayo Clinic in Rochester, Minnesota, says that people with the following traits are especially likely to develop chronic back pain:

- **Taller height:** Studies demonstrate that people prone to back pain have a greater standing height than people who are not.
- **Overweight or obese:** Additional weight puts stress and strain on the spine and muscles.
- **Smoking cigarettes:** Smoking leads to degeneration of the discs of the spine.
- **Poor muscle strength and conditioning in the lower back:** Weak muscles are less able to support the spine.
- **Age 45 to 64:** The older you are, the more likely you are to have arthritis in the spine or degenerative joint disease.

Looking at the Back's Delicate Anatomy

To understand back pain and why it's laid claim to your life, you need to know a little bit about your spine and the other parts of your body that are associated with it.

If you're reading this chapter, you or someone close to you probably knows the woes of back pain, and you probably want to skip right away to the part about how to make it go away. However, we encourage you to at least scan this section on anatomy. It'll help you better understand how to manage your sore back or will help you to help your loved one to understand what you're going through.

Your back is supported by your quite remarkable spine, which provides your body with strength and flexibility and also surrounds and protects your spinal cord and nerves. Your spine is a canal that runs down the length of your back from your brain to your bottom. It's made up of bones, ligaments, tendons, large muscles, weight-bearing joints, and highly sensitive nerves. (See Chapter 2 for more details on human anatomy.) The following sections look at each part of the spine, shown in Figure 5-1.

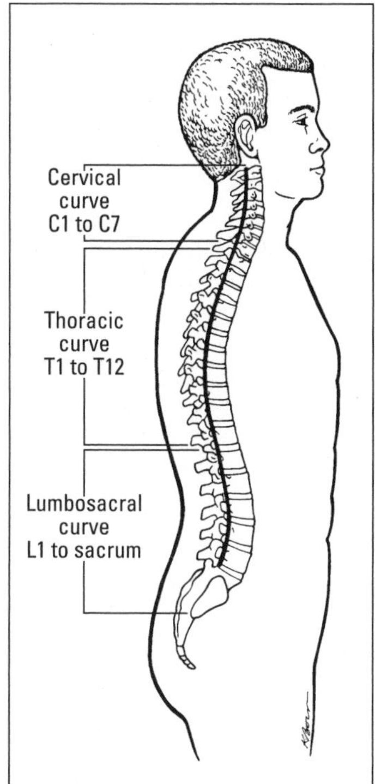

Figure 5-1: Anatomy of the spine.

Vertebrae

The bones in your spine are called *vertebrae,* and they are held together by ligaments. The normal adult spine has 32 vertebrae, each stacked on top of each other:

- **Cervical vertebrae:** These seven vertebrae in the neck area hold up your neck.
- **Thoracic vertebrae:** These 12 vertebrae are located in the middle back and extend forward as the ribs.
- **Lumbar vertebrae:** These five vertebrae, located in the lower back, are the largest ones, and they carry most of your body's weight. That's why so many people with back pain report pain in this area.

- **Sacrum:** These five vertebrae, located below the lumbar vertebrae, are fused together as one section. They attach the spine to the pelvis.
- **Tailbone:** These three vertebrae, located at the very bottom of the spine, are also fused.

Facet joints

The joints between adjacent vertebrae are called *facet joints.* The facets are bony knobs that meet between each vertebra. They link the vertebrae together and make it possible for them to move against each other. The facet joints give the spine its flexibility.

Spinal cord

Your spinal cord is comprised of cells and nerve-like pathways or tracts that run from the bottom of your brain stem all the way down to your lower back. Part of the central nervous system, the spinal cord is protected by the vertebral column, which is formed by the vertebrae.

Discs

Between each vertebra are discs that cushion them and serve as spacers. They safeguard the openings where the nerves exit the spinal cord.

Muscles, tendons, and ligaments

The muscles running up and down your back play an important role in supporting your spine so that you don't collapse like a jellyfish. When these muscles are strong (in other words, when you're "physically fit"), they support and protect your spine and help you move around with ease. But if these muscles become weak (through lack of exercise, aging, or other reasons), then your spine is more vulnerable to injury, and your mobility is also more limited.

The muscles in your stomach area and trunk also help support your spine and give it good mobility. In addition, tendons connect your muscles to your bones, and ligaments join your vertebrae together.

Describing Chronic Back Pain

Chronic back pain ranges from a general vague soreness to a recurring sharp severe pain, with all variations of pain in between. Stiffness is a common complaint of back sufferers, especially in the morning. For many people, the pain is located in the lower back (lumbar region). Although the pain is undeniably a problem, often the biggest concern with backaches is the havoc they can play with your everyday life.

For example, is it difficult to perform your everyday activities, such as grocery shopping or walking your dog? Do you have trouble moving around at work? Is it uncomfortable to sit at a computer for long periods of time?

Chronic back pain commonly hits (and stays with you) in one of two ways:

- **Constant:** It's present for more than three months.
- **Recurring:** The pain stays for long periods of time. Then it leaves (hooray!), but later it comes back yet again. This maddening pattern continues, for months or longer.

Chronic back pain may get worse when you move your back, sit down, or lift something weighing more than 10 or 20 pounds. The pain often improves when you "take a load off," meaning that you reduce the amount of weight that your spine has to support. Often, doing something simple, such as getting off your feet or putting down a heavy bag, can help. (And if you're a woman carrying a purse, clean it out at least once a week! Those loose coins can add unneeded pounds to your burden.)

Is it hard to carry your bags through airports? Maybe you've even given up flying because you don't want to make your back problem worse by carrying around heavy bags. Get suitcases with wheels that you can move much more easily than the bags you must lug around.

Taking a Look at the Causes of Back Pain

The bad news is that, for the vast majority of people, the cause of back pain is and will remain a mystery. In fact, only 15 percent of people with back pain have a diagnosis that specifically explains the cause. Knowing this fact can be discouraging. Simply put, if you and your doctor don't know what's causing your back pain, how do you go about treating it?

Fortunately, doctors use proven treatments and activities that can help lessen back pain even when the cause of your pain is unknown. (That's the good news.) We discuss these issues in the "Diagnosing and Treating Your Chronic Back Pain" section, later in this chapter. The following sections look at some common causes of back pain.

Behaviors

You can't control your gender or your age. (As mentioned in the section "Identifying Who Gets Chronic Back Pain," earlier in this chapter, middle-aged and older people have a greater risk for back pain than men or younger people.) But you *can* control some factors, such as smoking, being overweight, and not being fit. These causes are so important that we include them in the following list of behaviors that can cause chronic back pain. According to the Mayo Clinic:

- Positioning yourself awkwardly, such as twisting around too far
- Not stretching or not stretching correctly, both before and after exercising
- Attempting to lift heavy items or lifting them improperly (such as using your back, instead of your legs, to lift the weight)
- Carrying around heavy objects, such as computer cases
- Performing numerous repetitive motions, such as lifting and bending, which strain your back muscles
- Standing or sitting with poor posture
- Being overweight
- Having poor "core" muscle strength (The core consists of the abdominal, lower back, and pelvic muscles around your trunk.)
- Being overweight and not exercising regularly
- Smoking

Lifestyle factors

Some common causes of back pain may not be within your control — especially if they're tied to your livelihood:

- Demanding physical work, such as construction
- Repetitive heavy lifting
- Repetitive work of other kinds that includes a lot of bending or twisting
- Staying in one position for a very long time, such as sitting at a computer screen for hours and hours

Sometimes your job induces back pain. Maybe you don't want to quit your job, so what can you do instead? If you have to sit for long periods at the computer, be sure to take regular breaks, at least a few minutes every hour. Stand up, stretch, and shake out your body. Okay, you may look funny. But you may also find that you've started a new trend at work!

Common health conditions

When a doctor can diagnose the source of back pain, the cause is usually one of the following conditions:

- **Muscle spasms:** A strain or sprain can cause your back muscles to shrink and the blood flow to decrease, both of which cause pain. Fibrous connective tissue (fibrosis) may grow in the muscle.

  Injured muscles may also spasm or knot up to keep you from using that part of your body while it heals. Often the pain doesn't strike right away, but instead it lurks in the background and then sneaks up on you later and pounces, long after you've forgotten what may have caused it.

- **Osteoarthritis:** Sometimes back pain is caused by osteoarthritis (OA) of the spine (see Chapter 4). This condition is often called *spondylosis.* OA causes the discs between the vertebrae to collapse. Without the discs to cushion the space between the vertebrae, the joints (facets) abrade against each other, which can cause pain and stiffness.

  Ironically, your body may try to make up for the collapse of the discs by creating new bone (called *bone spurs*), which can pinch your nerves and cause significant pain.

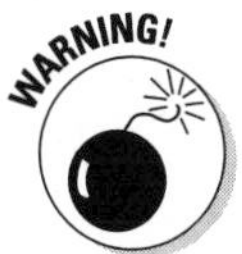

  Being significantly overweight increases the chance of getting OA in the spine, so try to keep your pounds down to a reasonable level.

- **Osteoporosis:** As you age (especially if you're a woman), your bones are more likely to lose calcium, causing them to fracture easily. This condition is known as *osteoporosis.* If you have osteoporosis, even routine activities like grocery shopping and cleaning can cause low back pain. And a fall can lead to a very painful broken back or hip. Medications for osteoporosis can help, as well as a routine level of caution. (For more information on osteoporososis, see Chapter 4.)

- **Herniated discs:** Sometimes the discs in your spine come apart and stick out of the spine. This condition is called a *herniated, ruptured,* or *slipped disc.* If the disc pinches one of the nerves coming out of the spinal cord, it can cause a great deal of pain. The sciatic nerve, which runs from your spinal cord to your leg, is most commonly affected by herniation. This condition is called *sciatica.*

- **Spinal stenosis:** Over time, the spine may narrow, a condition called *spinal stenosis.* The narrowing can put pressure on the spinal cord and/or nerves. In general, spinal stenosis can cause cramping, pain, or numbness in your legs, back, neck, shoulders, or arms. It may also cause loss of sensation in your extremities and sometimes causes problems with bladder or bowel function.
- **Spondylolisthesis:** If one of the vertebrae moves out of place and touches the bone below it, the resulting condition is called *spondylolisthesis.* The slipped bone, usually in the lower back or neck, can pinch a nerve and cause pain.
- **Degenerative disc disease:** Sometimes the spinal discs lose their essential internal moisture that acts like fluid in a shock absorber. Once the fluid is gone from the middle of the disc, the external disc starts to buckle from the weight formerly carried by the middle of the disc. The disc begins to bulge, and then it cracks.

Diagnosing and Treating Your Chronic Back Pain

The first step toward diagnosing what's going on with your back is to find the right doctor to help you. (See Chapter 13 for more information on selecting a good doctor.)

To find out what's going on with your spine, your doctor may order tests, such as X-rays, a magnetic resonance imaging (MRI) scan, a computerized tomography (CT) scan, or a discogram, which is a special X-ray examination that involves injecting dye into the affected disc. These tests can help you and your doctor establish a diagnosis, and decide on a treatment plan.

When developing a treatment plan for chronic back pain, having realistic expectations is extremely important. The hard truth is that chronic back pain usually doesn't go away forever. However, you can do many things to lessen and manage your back pain. Your goal should be to get to a point where you can function and have a normal or close-to-normal quality of life, despite your sore back. We cover some major actions that you can take to achieve that goal in the following sections.

Hurry up and wait

A common approach to both acute and chronic back pain is "watchful waiting." We know, we know. You want to feel better *now* — even if that means having less pain instead of being completely pain-free. Who could blame you?

But the truth is that often it takes awhile, sometimes a long while, for sore backs to heal to a more tolerable level of pain.

Waiting doesn't mean that you try to pretend your pain isn't there and that you basically do nothing. Instead, it means that you wait and watch to see whether taking over-the-counter painkillers, stretching, and protecting your back from further injury lessens the hurting and stiffness enough so that you can enjoy life without resorting to taking heavy-duty prescribed drugs and/or having surgery.

Most people don't realize it, but when back pain is severe, a short period of bed rest is okay. However, more than a couple of days of down time actually does more harm than good.

Judicious exercise and stretching

Exercise therapy is really the best choice that you can make to strengthen and heal the muscles and other tissues surrounding your spine so that they can better support your back, give it the flexibility you need, and prevent future pain.

We emphasize the word *therapy* in the term *exercise therapy.* In this sense, therapy means performing exercises specifically designed to strengthen and improve sore backs. The exercises should be supervised by physical therapists or other professionals who'll ensure that you're doing them correctly and that you're not injuring yourself by doing too much or performing the exercises the wrong/painful-inducing way.

Hot and cold therapy

Heat and cold can soothe sore backs and help reduce inflammation. If you injure or irritate an already sore back, as soon as possible, apply a cold pack for up to 20 minutes at a time. (You don't need anything fancy. Put the ice in a plastic bag and then wrap the bag in a cloth or towel to keep a thin barrier between the ice and your skin.) Continue applying ice as long as you have pain spasms.

When things settle down, switch to using heat from a heating pad, hot towels, or a heat lamp. The heat from the pad, towels, or lamp helps loosen up your tight muscles.

Don't use a heat application longer than 20 minutes.

Support braces or belts

You may want to consider using a brace or back belt to support your spine, particularly when you're lifting anything especially heavy. And some people with fragile spines — particularly those with advanced osteoporosis (see Chapter 4) — must wear them to prevent injury. If you're not in the latter category, but are considering wearing a brace or belt to reduce pain, be sure to discuss this option with your doctor first and be cautious about using these supports too often or too long. Research studies are inconclusive about whether braces or belts reduce pain and stiffness, and they can cause your muscles to weaken.

If you do decide to use a brace or back belt, they are available without a prescription at pharmacies and medical-supply stores. In some cases, your doctor may write a prescription to have a device specially made to fit your particular circumstances.

Medications

Medications for chronic back pain range from taking over-the-counter painkilling drugs (a common strategy) to taking narcotics, which should be used only when absolutely necessary and for limited periods of time. Always try nonprescription pain killers first. (See Chapter 14 for an overview of these drugs.)

Surgical procedures

Most people don't need surgery for back pain. However, when your back pain has a known cause and all other approaches have been exhausted, surgery can provide welcome relief. (Read more about surgery in general in Chapter 16.)

Here are the major types of surgeries for back pain:

- **Laminectomy and laminotomy:** With these procedures, part of the vertebrae are removed.
- **Fusion:** Two vertebrae are welded together. This surgery has a long recovery time, but it's used for many patients with back pain.
- **Disc replacement:** The Food and Drug Administration (FDA) approved this therapy of removing the old disc and replacing it with an artificial disc in late 2004. It's still unknown how effective it is.

If you need back surgery, find out whether your surgery can be performed in a minimally invasive manner. Using a laparoscopic surgical technique, the surgeon reaches your spine from the front rather than through the back. This technique avoids the need for long incisions, and the spinal nerves and cord do not have to be set aside to remove a disc. Therefore, there is less risk of pain caused by the surgery, and the recovery should be faster.

Complementary and alternative therapies

We cover complementary and alternative therapies for chronic pain in Chapters 14 and 15. Many therapies we describe in these chapters are great for managing chronic back pain. They include the techniques that physical therapists, occupational therapists, recreational therapists, fitness instructors, and massage therapists — all people interested in improving back pain — use effectively. Other important approaches to look over in Chapter 15 are acupuncture, biofeedback, and chiropractic care.

Chapter 6

Head Cases: Migraines and Other Types of Craniofacial Pain

In This Chapter

- Telling the difference between primary and secondary headaches
- Managing migraines
- Discovering other major types of chronic headaches
- Finding help for chronic headaches

Just before one of Mona's horrible migraines strikes her, she gets fuzzy in the head and can't think straight. Sometimes she sees weird jagged patterns, which means that a really bad headache is on its way. Tim, on the other hand, has severe cluster headaches that cause his eyes to water like crazy and give him excruciating pain for about 45 minutes each time — then it's over. Sandy has frequent tension headaches, and when they hit, she feels like some evil genie has placed an invisible rubber band around her head and is steadily and maddeningly tightening it, probably laughing like crazy the whole time.

Maybe you can relate to the headache problems of Mona, Tim, or Sandy. Headaches are one of the most common chronic pain conditions, and 45 million Americans suffer from chronic headaches, according to statistics from the American Chronic Pain Association. Seven in 10 people have at least one headache a year.

All headaches are caused by the activity of pain fibers that innervate blood vessels within the brain, its fibrous covering (called the *dura*), or muscles that support the head. The good news is that often people can learn to identify their own headache triggers and work to avoid the things that set them off, whether it's a type of food, severe stress, or another trigger. And if you can't avoid a trigger, at least you can have your medication or treatment at the ready.

Distinguishing Between Primary and Secondary Headaches

Experts define headaches as either primary or secondary headaches. *Primary headaches,* such as migraine and tension headaches, aren't caused by other diseases, but happen on their own. Genetics is thought to play a role in primary headaches, particularly in the case of migraines and tension headaches. In contrast, *secondary headaches* are caused by diseases or injuries. Examples are headaches that are caused by tumors or an infection.

Both types can hurt a lot, and sometimes a secondary headache hurts more than a primary one.

If you suffer from frequent headaches, here's a little self-test to help you determine whether you're suffering from a primary or secondary headache. When a headache attacks, ask yourself this question: "Are the symptoms of this headache different from the headaches I usually get? Or, is this headache just like those I usually get?" Ongoing (old) headaches tend to be primary. New headaches or those with different symptoms tend to be secondary headaches. (This little test is only a generalization and not a hard and fast rule. For example, you may have never had migraines, and sometimes they suddenly appear in your life.)

Resources for people with chronic headaches

The Internet offers helpful resources for people with chronic headaches. Check out the following Web sites:

American Headache Society (AHS) Committee for Headache Education (ACHE): ACHE is sponsored and directed by the American Headache Society, a professional society of health-care providers dedicated to the study and treatment of headache and face pain. Educational information on headache topics such as migraine, headache treatments, diary cards, nonpharmacological management, and trigger avoidance are available on this site (www.achenet.org).

National Headache Foundation: NHF is an information resource for headaches sufferers, their families, and the health-care providers who treat them. You can contact NHR at 1-888-NHF-5552 or visit its Web site at www.headaches.org.

National Institute of Neurological Disorders and Stroke (NINDS): NINDS conducts and supports research on brain and nervous system disorders, including headaches. Its Web site (www.ninds.nih.gov/about_ninds/ninds_overview.htm) provides information on numerous clinical trials in headache research.

If you're having symptoms that point to a secondary headache, don't write them off as "just another headache." Secondary doesn't mean "not important." The thing is, primary headaches are almost never life-threatening — they can be stunningly painful and make your life miserable — but they're rarely medical emergencies. In contrast, serious illnesses, such as brain tumors or meningitis, can cause secondary headaches, so you need to attend to them.

Avoiding Tension Headaches

Most headaches are *tension headaches,* which are headaches caused by tensed muscles in the shoulders and/or the neck. If you suffer from tension headaches, you probably experience two or three of them a month. But you may be among the unfortunate few who have headaches two weeks out of every four, or even more often. Ouch! Tension headaches usually appear gradually, and they can last from hours to days.

Many people can't concentrate when they have a tension headache because of the very distracting pain. Tension headaches (see Figure 6-1) are often accompanied by strain in the muscles of the head, neck, and shoulders. Many people compare the pain of a tension headache to a vise squeezing their heads. The pain usually occurs on both sides of the head, and it's a constant, dull pain. Most tension headaches strike during the daytime and worsen over the day's events. You rarely wake up with a tension headache.

Tension headaches can be triggered or worsened by stress, tiredness, loud noise, and/or bright light or glare. Other triggers are eyestrain, temporomandibular joint dysfunction (TMJ) (see Chapter 4), and neck pain, covered in the section called "Paying Attention to Neck Pain," later in this chapter.

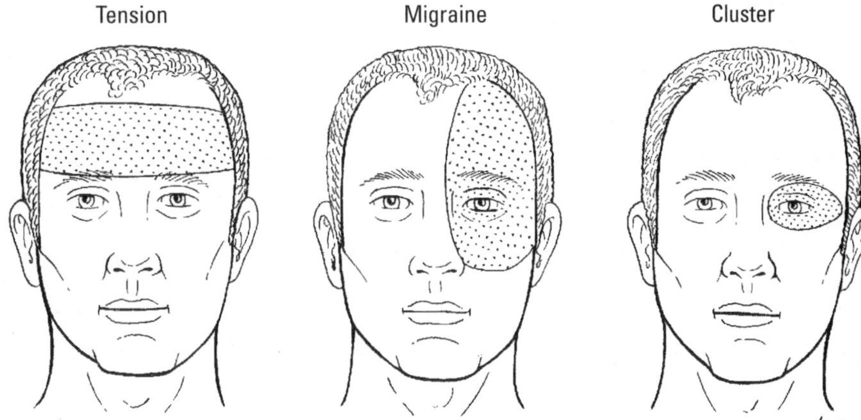

Figure 6-1: Three common types of headaches.

Diagnosing tension headaches

The International Headache Society (IHS) has developed standards, which are widely accepted around the world, for diagnosing tension headaches. According to the IHS, tension headaches last from 30 minutes to seven days and are accompanied by at least two of the following criteria:

- A pressing/tightening, as opposed to a throbbing or pulsating quality
- Mild or moderate intensity (which may interfere with, but doesn't prevent, activity)
- A headache that occurs on both sides of the head
- The head pain isn't aggravated by walking, climbing stairs, or similar routine physical activity

You usually don't have nausea and vomiting with a tension headache (although you may lose your appetite).

Treating tension headaches

Tension headaches are usually treated with pain relievers such as aspirin and acetaminophen. Research by the Diamond Headache Clinic in Chicago has found that 200 mg of caffeine helps some people once a headache is triggered. (Although caffeine is usually bad for you, it occasionally can help you.) If these measures don't work, your doctor may recommend trying specific medicines used for migraines. (We cover these medicines in the next section, "Managing Migraine Headaches.") In addition, some doctors recommend tricyclic antidepressants, a type of medication that — although referred to as an antidepressant — has a variety of medical uses such as treatment of neuropathic pain, irritable bowel syndrome, and headaches.

Watch out for caffeinated drinks

If you drink a lot of soda with caffeine or you're a heavy consumer of coffee or tea, you need to know that heavy doses of caffeine may be the cause of your chronic headaches. A study in *Cephalgia* (a headache journal for professionals) in 2003 reported that after children who drank a lot of soda every day were tapered off caffeine, all but 3 of the 36 participants experienced a complete remission of their severe chronic headaches. You're not a child, but maybe caffeine is the unknown villain in your chronic headache problem.

Don't stop drinking all sodas immediately, but instead taper off slowly and substitute water. Hopefully, your headaches will be much fewer — or even gone altogether!

Many people with tension headaches find that when they get adequate rest and sleep their headaches occur less often and are less intense. You can read about techniques to help you sleep well and tackle fatigue in Chapter 20.

Injections of *Botulinum toxin type A (Botox),* a neurotoxin that blocks the ability of nerves to make muscles contract, helps some people. (Yes, it's the same Botox that's used by people who want to eradicate their facial wrinkles. Maybe you can have a smooth forehead and fewer migraines!) Botox actually eases tension headache pain for some people. But eventually, without further treatments, the headaches (and the wrinkles) come back.

Treating tension headaches with medicines, such as nonsteroidal anti-inflammatory medications (NSAIDs) and caffeine on an ongoing basis can actually cause more headaches or make the headaches that you have get even worse. This condition is called *rebound headache* or *daily headache syndrome.* The treatment for rebound headaches is to steadily taper off all headache medications. Limiting how much medicine you take is key to preventing rebound headaches.

Managing Migraine Headaches

Migraines are so much more than just a headache. Yes, they involve head pain, usually on one side. But the pain can be brutal, and it's often accompanied by nausea, vomiting, and very high sensitivity to light and noise. Often these symptoms are extremely severe.

The typical migraine appears on one side of the head and generates a throbbing pain (refer to Figure 6-1). Migraines usually build up gradually and may last from several hours to (gasp!) a couple of days. However, sometimes they strike suddenly, and they're agonizing from the starting point.

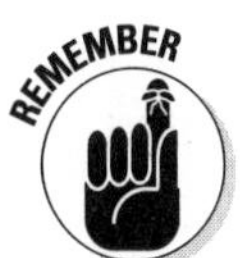

A headache may not follow the classic migraine pattern, but it may still be a migraine headache. For some people, migraines encompass both sides of the head and cause a dull pain rather than a throbbing pain. Fortunately, such nontypical migraines usually respond to treatments for migraines.

Triggers for migraines include foods or drinks such as chocolate and certain wines, stress, the environment, odors/perfumes, emotions, medications, and hormonal fluctuations. Ironically, relaxation after stress can trigger this type of headache.

Some sufferers know when a migraine is about to strike because it is preceded by a sensory distortion called an *aura,* which includes visual disturbances such as flashing lights, zig-zag lines, or disturbed vision.

Migraine headaches are three times more common in women than in men, and some women experience migraines just before or during their periods. They may finally receive some relief from migraines during pregnancy, only to be slammed again with migraines soon after Junior is born, when their menstrual cycle resumes. Migraines often begin during the teenage years.

Diagnosing migraine headaches

IHS developed the standard for diagnosing migraines and migraines with and without auras. If the symptoms of either type are painfully familiar to you, be sure to discuss them with your primary care physician.

In general, chronic migraines without aura last 4 to 72 hours and have at least two of the four following characteristics:

- It's located on one side of the head
- It has a throbbing quality
- The pain is moderate or severe, to the point that it inhibits or prohibits daily activities
- The pain is aggravated by using the stairs or doing routine physical activity
- During the headache, at least one of the two following symptoms occur: an acute sensitivity to light, sound, nausea, and/or vomiting

Rare migraines

Some people suffer from rare forms of migraines:

- *Basilar artery migraine,* which may cause combinations of temporary blindness or visual disturbances, dizziness, an inability to talk, a loss of balance, ringing in the ears, tingling and/or numbing in the arms and legs, disequilibrium, a temporary loss of consciousness, or confusion. These symptoms, in turn, are followed by a throbbing headache, usually in the back of the head, which may be accompanied by nausea and vomiting.
- *Ophthalmoplegic migraine,* pain around the eye, accompanied by nausea, vomiting, and double vision.
- *Abdominal migraine,* which affects children of families with a history of migraine. The child has stomach pain, nausea, and vomiting. They frequently have migraine headaches as adults.

A migraine with aura is experienced by people who've had at least two headaches with a minimum of three of the following signs:

- Visual disturbances.
- An inability to speak.
- At least one aura symptom that develops gradually over more than four minutes or two or more symptoms that occur in succession.
- No aura symptom that lasts more than 60 minutes.
- The migraine follows the aura. (It may also simultaneously begin with the aura.) The advantage of the aura and the delayed headache is that it gives you warning time to take your medication and stave off the worst pain.

Treating migraine headaches

If your migraine headaches are interfering with your daily life, treatment should include organizing your lifestyle so that you're away from your triggers as much as possible. Even daylight and everyday noises, such as children playing and dogs barking, can trigger excruciating pain. Your doctor may also suggest that you take preventive medications.

When migraines strike, many people find it helpful (and others say it's absolutely necessary) to rest in a quiet, darkened room until their symptoms lessen. Some migraine sufferers lie in bed and pull the covers over their head or wear masks to block out as much light and sound as possible. Painkillers such as aspirin or naproxen can provide relief, particularly when taken as soon as the headache starts. The earlier you take them, the better.

If migraines make you nauseous and/or cause you to vomit, taking medicine by mouth may not work. In this case, other options are available, including taking medications rectally or intravenously. Your doctor can also prescribe a type of medication called an *antiemetic* to stop nausea and/or vomiting.

Your doctor may also prescribe other medications effective for migraines. They include triptans, which block the release of chemicals that trigger migraine pain (Imitrex, Zomig, and others); dihydroergotamine, a drug which narrows veins and arteries; and butalbital (Fiornal or Fioricet), a barbiturate.

Some people with migraines experience nasal congestion, runny eyes, or other symptoms that may suggest a sinus headache. These headaches should not be confused with sinus headaches because they won't respond to medical treatment for sinusitis. (For more on sinus headaches, see the upcoming section "Suffering from Sinus Headaches.")

Preventing migraines

If you get migraine headaches more than two or three times a month, then preventive treatment should be at the top of your to-do list. The first step is to identify and stay away from your headache triggers as much as possible. (You can read about identifying and side-stepping pain triggers in Chapter 17.) Your doctor may also prescribe medications such as beta-blockers to block the release of adrenaline, which can trigger migraines, or she may order an anti-seizure medication called Divalproex, which can help prevent migraines. Typically, migraine sufferers take these medications at a time when the headaches usually strike, such as before a menstrual period or on weekends.

Some people with migraine headaches experience weekend headaches or headaches brought on by sleeping more than usual. If weekend headaches are a problem for you, avoid sleeping in on weekends. Try to wake up at the same time on weekends as you do during the week.

Too little sleep is also a problem for migraine sufferers. People who get migraines need sufficient sleep. In fact, fatigue is one of the most common triggers of migraine headaches. In other words, playing poker until 3 a.m. and then getting up at 6 a.m. to go fishing is a no-no if you get migraine headaches.

In addition, some patients with migraine headaches believe that certain foods trigger the condition. However, not all people with migraines have dietary triggers, and sensitivity to certain foods differs for each migraine sufferer. In other words, chocolate may trigger a migraine for you, but not for your coworker who also gets migraines. His triggers may be peanuts and wine, which don't bother you at all. (Read the sidebar on common migraine triggers for more information.)

Are you a chocoholic? Sometimes chocolate is a migraine trigger, but don't go on the wagon right away. Just savor a smaller than usual amount of chocolate for a week or so and note whether your migraines decrease in frequency or severity. If not, your beloved chocolate probably isn't a trigger, so it's a keeper.

Keep a diary of the foods you eat and the drinks you consume and eliminate any suspicious foods from your diet so that you can see whether their absence eases the frequency and severity of your headaches.

Common migraine triggers

According to the National Headache Foundation, certain foods may trigger migraine headaches; if they trigger migraines in you, avoid them. All the foods in this list contain *tyramine,* a substance that's produced in the natural breakdown of the amino acid tyrosine. Tyramine levels increase in foods when they're aged or aren't fresh.

- Ripened cheeses, such as Cheddar, Emmentaler, Stilton, Brie, and Camembert (American, cottage, and cream cheese, as well as Velveeta, are okay.)
- Herring (pickled or dried)
- Chocolate
- Anything fermented, pickled, or marinated
- Sour cream (no more than 1/2 cup daily)
- Nuts, peanut butter, or foods such as crackers or cookies that contain nuts
- Sourdough bread, breads and crackers containing cheese or chocolate
- Broad beans, lima beans, fava beans, or snow peas
- Foods containing monosodium glutamate (MSG), such as soy sauce, meat tenderizers, and seasoned salt
- Figs, raisins, papayas, avocados, or red plums (no more than 1/2 cup daily)
- Citrus fruits (no more than 1/2 cup daily)
- Bananas (no more than 1/2 banana daily)
- Pizza (because of the cheese)
- Excessive amounts of tea, coffee, or cola beverages (no more than 2 cups daily)
- Sausage, bologna, pepperoni, salami, summer sausage, or hot dogs
- Chicken livers

Suffering from Sinus Headaches

Some people suffer from a chronic inflammation or infection of the sinuses *(sinusitis),* which causes a severe headache. They may be allergic to a variety of items, ranging from cats and dogs to dust and many other possible allergic triggers. If this is your situation, try to determine what you're allergic to (ask your doctor for help) and if you can, avoid that trigger. If that means you need to stay away from Fluffy or your partner's beloved cat, then do it! It's better than walking around with a very bad headache most of the time.

If you have sinusitis you may need antibiotics. Your doctor may also prescribe a nasal spray to help keep your nasal passages clear.

Understanding Cluster Headaches

Middle-aged men are the primary victims of *cluster headaches.* Often, these headache sufferers have one attack a day for one to three months. Then, happily, they go into remission for months to years. However, some unfortunate people have cluster headaches with no interruption.

Cluster headaches usually occur at the same time and often wake up their victims in the middle of the night. Pain always occurs on one side of the head and in and around the eye (see Figure 6-1). The pain of a cluster headache is severe, but usually (whew) only lasts about 30 minutes to one hour. People experiencing cluster headaches are usually anxious and restless. Other symptoms include nasal congestion, a watery discharge from the nose, watery eyes, and a condition called *Horner's syndrome,* which causes a droopy eyelid and contraction of the pupil of the eye.

Diagnosing cluster headaches is based on its distinctive group of symptoms and by ruling out other problems. Because cluster headaches are so frequent and severe, they can make it impossible to work, care for children, or carry out day-to-day tasks.

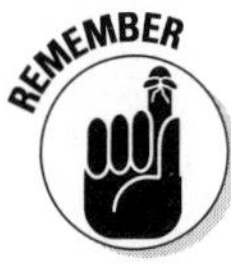

Prevention is extremely important. You and your doctor can head off cluster headaches (pun intended) with some of the same medicines used for migraine headaches, such as acetaminophen, aspirin, and a triptan. Oxygen inhalation also helps many people when they're having an acute attack. So, it is important to discuss treatment options with your doctor.

Tackling Thunderclap Headaches

Thunderclap headaches get their names for how they arrive: Boom, just like a thunderclap. One minute you're fine, and the next minute, you have a severe headache. The pain of thunderclap headaches peaks in a minute or so and then, blessedly, fades over the next few hours. A less severe headache may follow.

Thunderclap headaches occur most frequently in women older than age 45. These headaches are secondary headaches that can have serious causes, such as bleeding in the brain or a blood clot in the sinuses. If you ever experience a thunderclap headache or think you may be having one, seek immediate medical attention. If bleeding in the brain is causing the headache, you may need emergency surgery.

Emergency headaches

If you have any of the following symptoms, seek immediate medical care:

- A sudden, severe headache, unlike one you've ever had (which may be due to bleeding in the brain and is a medical emergency for many reasons, including the fact that it can cause severe damage to the brain)
- A headache that strikes after heavy exercise (which may also be caused by bleeding in the brain)
- Fever and neck stiffness associated with the headache (which may be due to bacterial meningitis or viral encephalitis)
- Seizures or lessening of mental function, which may be symptoms of brain tumors
- Weakness of the arms, legs, or face muscles, which may suggest a *transient ischemic attack* (a short interruption of blood flow to the brain)
- A recent head injury, which may be causing bleeding in the brain
- A new headache associated with nausea, vomiting, and visual changes
- Alcoholic beverages (The National Headache Foundation recommends that you limit yourself to two normal size drinks selected from Haute Sauterne, Riesling, Seagram's VO, or Cutty Sark)

Paying Attention to Neck Pain

Neck pain is just that: a pain in the neck, and far too often also in the shoulders, arms, and head. It affects about 10 percent of the population each year.

Neck pain may be caused by a *whiplash injury,* where the neck is jerked forward and back in a car crash. It may also be caused by changes in the spine due to arthritis, aging, or muscle strain. Often, the cause of neck pain is occupational and may be brought on by sitting at a computer desk for long periods of time.

If the problem is your computer, make sure that your monitor is set so that your eyes naturally hit about the middle of the screen. If not, adjust your chair and your screen until they do. Make sure that your knees are slightly lower than your hips.

Some simple suggestions can considerably ease neck pain:

- Keep your head back, over your spine, to reduce neck strain.
- Take frequent breaks if you drive long distances or work long hours at your computer.

- If you grind or clench your teeth during sleep, consider using a night brace, available from your dentist.
- Don't tuck your phone under your chin. Use a headset or speakerphone for long conversations.
- Pull your shoulder blades together and then relax. Pull your shoulders down while leaning your head to each side to stretch your neck muscles. Stretch your neck frequently if you work at a desk. Shrug your shoulders up and down.
- Sometimes acupuncture helps. Read about acupuncture in Chapter 15.
- Stretch and strengthen the muscles that support your neck, which helps make the job of holding up your head easier. Walking provides a workout for the neck muscles. These simple movements can translate into much less pain!

For many years the standard treatment for neck pain was wearing a brace to hold up the head and give the neck a rest. Now experts know that movement is critical to keeping the neck and surrounding muscles healthy. However, if you have severe neck pain, it's important to exercise your neck only under the supervision of a physical therapist or other medical professional. Deep massage is also helpful for people with chronic muscular neck pain.

Chapter 7

The Odd Couple: Injuries and Strokes

In This Chapter

- Understanding complex regional pain syndrome
- Exploring the different types of spinal cord injury pain
- Thinking about the pain associated with strokes
- Identifying the different types of brain injury

Jack was driving home after working late Friday night when his car was violently rear-ended by a drunk driver. Jack survived the accident, but he suffered an injury to his left leg. He recovered well after rehabilitation. But months later, Jack was stricken in his left leg with a very painful condition known as *complex regional pain syndrome.* About the same time, Marie, one of Jack's coworkers, suffered a major stroke. Months later, she, too, was stricken with pain in her left leg — different causes, but the same end condition.

This chapter covers major chronic pain conditions that result from injury to the peripheral nerves, the spinal cord, or the brain, regardless of whether the injury is from a car accident or other injury or from a stroke.

You need to know a few caveats about the pain-causing conditions discussed in this chapter. After an injury has healed, a lot is known about the previous harm to the body, but much remains still undiscovered. You may ask your doctor a question like "Why do I have post-stroke central pain, but my mother, who had a similar stroke years ago, didn't have it?" The answer is that no one really knows why. In this chapter, you discover what *is* known today about pain conditions that result from damage to the nervous system.

Getting the Lowdown on Complex Regional Pain Syndrome (CRPS)

Complex regional pain syndrome is long-term pain that may strike after an injury to an arm or a leg. The hallmark of complex regional pain syndrome (CRPS) is pain that's through the ceiling and agonizingly painful when compared to the feeling from the trigger that set it off, which may be something as ordinary as a cool breeze brushing against your shirt. (Some people never identify the trigger.) On a scale of 1 to 10, the pain from CRPS is about a 50. Unfortunately, the pain of CRPS gets *worse* over time. It may not even show up until long after the damage has healed. (For more information about CRPS, see Chapter 11.)

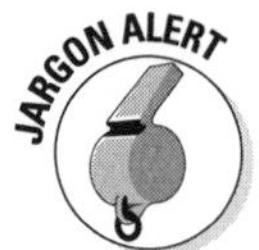

CRPS is also known as *reflex sympathetic dystrophy* or *causalgia,* a Civil War term that described intense pain felt by some soldiers long after their wounds healed.

CRPS probably doesn't have only one cause, but instead this medical syndrome may result from *many* causes with similar symptoms. Scientists know that injured nerves can become active spontaneously, sending impulses to the spinal cord even without painful stimulus. This abnormal activity depends on inflammation and scarring with constriction of the nerve and other factors that are difficult to detect (diagnose). In short, the sympathetic nervous system can be a culprit that's maintaining the chronic pain of CRPS. (See Chapter 2 for information about the sympathetic nervous system.)

Identifying CRPS requires considerable skill and guesswork on the part of the neurologist or other diagnostician. No specific test is available to diagnose the condition; the common thread is the excruciating pain felt by you or our loved one. As a result, CRPS is diagnosed by first ruling out other conditions. For example, doctors may use bone scans to identify changes in the bone and in blood circulation.

Symptoms of CRPS may include color changes in the arm, hand, leg, or foot. The changes may vary from red to white to blue at different times, and there is excessive hair loss over the painful extremity. The skin may become very thick, and a significant amount of swelling may occur in the affected extremity. Excessive sweating may occur over the affected area, and usually the sufferer feels severe burning pain.

If you discover you have CRPS, you may be one of the lucky ones who recovers spontaneously from the symptoms. However, some people have unremitting pain and crippling, irreversible physical changes despite treatment. Some doctors believe that early treatment is helpful in limiting the severity of the disorder.

Treatment is focused on lessening pain and includes techniques you read about in this book, such as physical therapy, surgery, and medication. (See Chapter 11 for more information about treatments for CRPS.)

Suffering a Spinal Cord Injury (SCI)

The spinal cord contains cells with axons that form pathways to the brain for conducting information from your body. Also, it contains pathways from the brain to cells in the spinal cord that control your movements. The spinal cord is surrounded by bones (vertebrae which make up the spinal column or back bones). (Read more about the spinal cord and its role in carrying information to and from your brain in Chapter 2.)

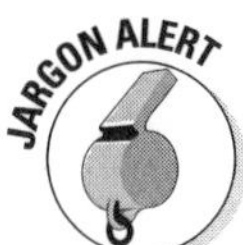

Spinal cord injury (SCI) includes injury to the cord itself, as well as to one or more vertebrae. Severe damage to the cord can eliminate intentional movements controlled by all the regions of the spinal cord below the injury. All sensations from below the injury can also be lost.

Because the treatments differ, you need to understand the distinction between a spinal cord injury and the type of back injury pain that is specifically caused by pinched nerves (for example, by ruptured discs). Even if you break a vertebra or vertebrae, you may still not have injured the spinal cord, but chances are you will have pinched nerves. And the pinched nerves can cause pain in regions supplied by nerves coming in between the injured vertebrae. This type of pain is called *at-level* (at the level of injury) or *segmental.* (Chapter 5 covers issues concerning chronic back pain.)

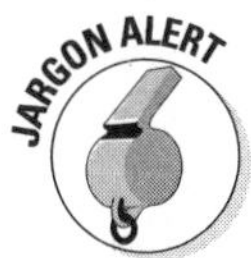

If you have segmental pain, you may develop *allodynia* and *hyperalgesia* in the painful region. *Allodynia* is pain caused by something that usually does not elicit pain, such as shaking hands with someone. *Hyperalgesia* is an extremely painful reaction to something minor, such as a soft breeze, that would normally only hurt a little.

If you're unlucky enough to have vertebrae that are so badly crushed or displaced that they constrict and damage your spinal cord, the damage can cause the cells in the pain pathways of your spinal cord to go haywire, resulting in pain. (Yes, we know that haywire is not an accepted medical term. But we thought we'd use something a little more descriptive than abnormal spontaneous activity, which is what scientists call it when, for no detectable reason, cells in the pain pathways send pain messages to the brain. See Chapter 2 for more information on abnormal spontaneous activity in pain pathways.)

These haywire pain messages can result in chronic pain that is felt below the injury called *below-level pain.* This type of pain is often described by victims as horrible.

If you have pain from a SCI, you may hurt severely at times and have little or no pain at other times. Pain may come and go with your daily circumstances. For example, fatigue, weather changes (particularly cold), and stress can all affect your pain levels.

Research has shown that your level of injury and how you were injured can determine whether you develop chronic pain after a SCI. Paradoxically, lower levels of injury tend to mean more pain, while higher levels mean less pain.

Treatments for SCI are similar to those for other pain conditions, including techniques you read about in this book, such as physical therapy and medication. Surgery may be necessary to repair vertebral displacement or other causes of traction on the spinal cord. SCI can cause ulcers, *spasticity* (a condition in which some of the body's muscles are continuously contracted) and other health problems, which in turn can cause chronic pain.

Dealing with Central Post-Stroke Pain

A *stroke* occurs when blood can't reach the brain, either because blood is blocked from getting through a vessel or a blood vessel bursts. The result is an injury to the brain, hence the popular term for stroke: *brain attack.*

Five percent of the people who have a brain attack develop *Central Post Stroke Pain* (CPSP).

Some stroke victims with central pain notice it when the stroke hits, but for most victims, the pain strikes several months later. It may be a burning, throbbing, shooting, or stabbing pain. If you have central pain resulting from a stroke, you'll feel it in the part of the body affected by the stroke.

According to the Pain Relief Foundation, other characteristics include

- A loss of feeling in the affected part, such as not being able to tell the difference between hot and cold.
- Hypersensitivity to touch. In some patients, light touch, such as clothing brushing against the skin, causes severe pain. In some cases, a minor movement may cause severe pain (allodynia).
- For one in five people with CPSP, the pain gets better over a period of years. A third of these people will get better in the first year.

Strokes vary in the location and size of brain damage they cause, producing different symptoms for different people. For example, Lois may have severe chronic pain after her stroke, but her roommate, Roberta, is more fortunate and has none.

Chronic pain after a stroke is usually due to damage to cells or axons in the individual's pain pathway. We hear you sighing and asking: "Shouldn't damage to the pain pathway *get rid* of pain?" Well, it can, but, curiously, it can also cause chronic pain.

Spotting the signs of a stroke

If you have any stroke symptoms, seek immediate medical attention. Symptoms include the following, all of which come on suddenly:

- Numbness or weakness of face, arm, or leg — especially on one side of the body
- Confusion, trouble speaking or understanding
- Trouble seeing in one or both eyes
- Trouble walking, dizziness, loss of balance or coordination
- Severe headache with no known cause

If you've experienced any of these symptoms, you may have had a mini-stroke and are at risk for a larger stroke. Ask your doctor whether you can lower your risk for stroke by taking aspirin or using other means. (For more on prevention, see the section called "Stroke prevention," later in this chapter.)

Surviving Traumatic Brain Injury

A *traumatic brain injury* (TBI) is a blow, jolt, or penetrating injury that leads to damage to the head, disrupting brain function. Of course, not all blows or jolts to the head result in a TBI. But when they do, TBI may cause short or long-term problems with independent function.

Symptoms of a brain injury can be mild to severe, depending on the amount of damage. Some symptoms show up right away, while others may not appear until several days or weeks after the injury. Headaches are a common long- and short-term problem after a TBI.

According to the Brain Injury Association, other symptoms may include (but are not limited to):

- Spinal fluid (thin water-looking liquid) coming from the ears or nose
- Loss of consciousness
- Dilated or unequally sized pupils
- Vision changes (blurred vision or seeing double, inability to tolerate bright light, loss of eye movement, blindness)
- Dizziness, balance problems
- Respiratory failure (not breathing)
- *Coma* (not alert and unable to respond to others) or a semicomatose state
- Paralysis, difficulty moving body parts, weakness, poor coordination
- Slow pulse

- Slow breathing rate, with an increase in blood pressure
- Vomiting
- Lethargy (sluggish, sleepy, gets tired easily)
- Confusion
- Ringing in the ears or changes in ability to hear

Half of all brain injuries are due to transportation-related accidents, such as car, motorcycle, and bicycle accidents, as well as injuries to pedestrians. About 20 percent of brain injuries are caused by violence, including firearm use and child abuse. For people ages 75 years and older, brain injuries are most often caused by falls.

In addition, blasts are a leading cause of TBIs for active duty military personnel in war zones.

The chronic pain triggered by brain damage usually results in one of the following types of injuries:

- **Concussion:** A *concussion* is by far the most frequently occurring type of traumatic brain injury. Also called a mild traumatic brain injury, concussions cause a temporary loss of mental activity. Often the individual won't remember what happened immediately after the injury. Concussions can result from any blow to or jarring of the head, but generally don't involve bleeding or punctures.
- **Diffuse Axonal Injury:** *Diffuse Axonal Injury* (DAI) is the result of a TBI and whiplash. With this type of injury, axons throughout the brain are severely stretched or distorted by movement of the brain in the skull. And because axons are responsible for communication between brain cells, such an injury can disrupt important functions resulting in a coma. DAI is typically the underlying injury in shaken baby syndrome.
- **Contusion:** A *contusion* is bleeding in the brain. It basically describes a bruised brain!
- **Coup-Contrecoup Injury:** *Coup-Contrecoup Injury* refers to contusions occurring at the site of the injury as well as the opposite side of the brain. It is caused by the brain swinging back and forth against the skull. (Brains are not meant to swing back and forth.)

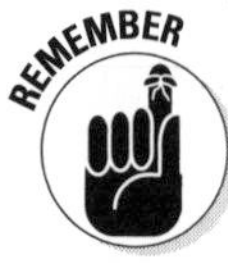

For all brain injuries, treatment should begin at the time of the injury. The first two goals are to stabilize the person and prevent further injury. About half of all severely injured people will require surgery. Recovery from a brain injury is a difficult and long process, often requiring physical therapy and retraining. The good news is that undamaged regions of the brain can often be trained to take over functions lost or reduced by damage to other parts of the brain.

Seeing the signs of a concussion

Immediate signs of concussion, seen within seconds or minutes of an injury, include loss of consciousness; impaired attention, such as a vacant stare, delayed responses, and inability to focus; slurred or incoherent speech; lack of coordination; disorientation; extreme emotional reactions; and memory problems.

The following symptoms can occur hours or even days or weeks after a concussion: persistent headache; dizziness/vertigo; poor attention and concentration; memory problems; nausea or vomiting; fatigue; irritability; intolerance of bright lights and/or loud noises; anxiety and/or depression; and disturbed sleep.

Preventing Spinal Cord and Brain Injuries

The bottom line in regard to injury to the spinal cord and brain — regardless of the cause — is that the resulting pain syndromes and related conditions can be severe and debilitating. Prevention for all these conditions is mostly common sense: practice safety to prevent spinal and brain injuries and practice a healthy lifestyle to prevent strokes. This section provides some tips on how to add these practices to your daily life. (Unfortunately, CRPS has no specific preventive measures.)

Spinal cord and traumatic brain injury prevention

The following tips to preventing spinal cord injuries are from the Centers for Disease Control and Prevention (CDC).

Motor vehicles

Motor vehicles are the leading cause of SCI in the United States for people under age 65. Here are some safety tips for driving and riding in motor vehicles.

- Always wear a seat belt.
- Secure or buckle children into age- and weight-appropriate child safety seats.
- Secure or buckle children under 12 years old in the back seat to avoid air bag injuries.
- Never drive under the influence of alcohol or drugs.
- Don’t ride in a car with a driver impaired by alcohol or drugs.

- Prevent others from driving while impaired by alcohol or drugs.
- Raise the headrest on the seats of the vehicle so that the headrest contacts the back of the head, not the neck.
- Avoid talking on cell phones while driving a motor vehicle.

Falls

Falls are the leading cause of SCI for people ages 65 and older. To prevent falls, take the following steps:

- Secure banisters and handrails at all stairwells.
- Use a step stool with a grab bar to reach objects on high shelves.
- Place nonslip mats on the bathtub and shower floor.
- Install grab bars in the shower and bathtub.
- Exercise regularly to keep muscle tone and balance.
- Wear sturdy nonslip shoes.
- When possible, reduce the use of sedatives or other medications that increase the risk of falling.
- Perform a home safety check and remove things that may be tripped over.
- Use safety gates at the bottom and top of stairs when young children are around.
- Install window guards in windows above the first floor.
- Consider installing a ramp to a porch rather than using stairs.

Sports and recreation

The majority of sports and recreation injuries occur among infants to adults age 29. Following are tips to help make sports and recreation activities safer.

- Wear a helmet when riding a bike, motorcycle, scooter, or skateboard; in-line skating and roller-skating; skiing or snowboarding; horseback riding; and during football, ice hockey, batting; and running the bases in baseball and softball.
- Make sure that the water is deep enough before you dive in head-first. If water is too shallow, you may be seriously injured. Entering feet-first is safer than diving.
- Wear appropriate safety gear when engaging in sports activities.
- Avoid head-first moves, such as tackling with the top of your head or sliding head-first into a base.
- Insist on spotters when performing activities that put you at risk, such as new gymnastics moves.

Firearms

Firearms are a leading cause of spinal cord injury. If you have firearms in your home, the following precautions can make your home safer:

- Keep firearms stored unloaded in a locked cabinet or safe.
- Store bullets secured in a separate location.

Stroke prevention

The following tips to preventing a stroke are adapted from the National Stroke Association.

- Know your blood pressure and have it checked at least annually. If it's elevated, work with your doctor to keep it under control. High blood pressure (hypertension) is a leading cause of stroke. If the higher number (your systolic blood pressure) is consistently above 120 or the lower number (your diastolic blood pressure) is consistently over 80, talk to your doctor.
- Find out whether you have *atrial fibrillation.* Atrial fibrillation (AF) is an irregular heartbeat that changes how your heart works and allows blood to collect in the chambers of your heart. This blood, which is not moving through your body, tends to clot. The beating of your heart can move a clot into the blood supply to part of your brain, causing a stroke. If you have AF, your doctor may prescribe medicines called blood thinners. Aspirin and warfarin (Coumadin) are the most commonly prescribed treatments.
- If you smoke, stop. Smoking doubles the risk for stroke.
- If you drink alcohol, use moderation. Studies show that drinking up to two alcoholic drinks per day can reduce your risk for stroke by about half. But *more* alcohol than this each day can increase your risk for stroke by three times and also lead to liver disease, accidents, and more. If you drink, limit yourself to two drinks each day.
- Find out whether you have high *cholesterol* (a soft, waxy fat/lipid in the bloodstream and all body cells). If your total cholesterol level is over 200, talk to your doctor. You may be at an increased risk for stroke.
- If you're diabetic, follow your doctor's advice carefully. Having diabetes puts you at an increased risk for stroke, but if you control your diabetes, you may lower your risk for stroke. Your doctor can prescribe lifestyle changes and medicine to help control your diabetes.
- Include exercise in your daily activities. A brisk walk for as little as 30 minutes a day may reduce your risk for stroke.

- Adopt a lower sodium (salt), lower fat diet. By cutting down on sodium and fat in your diet, you may lower your blood pressure and, most importantly, lower your risk for stroke.
- Ask your doctor whether you have vascular (blood circulation) problems that may increase your risk for stroke. For example, fatty deposits can block the arteries that carry blood from your heart to your brain. This kind of blockage, if untreated, can cause stroke.
- If you have blood problems such as sickle cell disease, severe *anemia* (lower than normal number of red blood cells), or other diseases, work with your doctor to manage these problems. Left untreated, these can cause stroke.

Resources for people with CNS and stroke injury

The following list covers important resources for people with stroke:

Brain Injury Association of America, 8201 Greensboro Dr., Suite 611, McLean, VA 22102; 703-761-0750, Family Helpline, 800-444-6443; www.biausa.org. The Brain Injury Association of America provides fact sheets on many safety topics and recommendations on how to prevent injuries. The association provides free online access to *Prevention Matters,* a newsletter that focuses on current brain injury prevention issues. It also provides a Family Helpline.

National Spinal Cord Injury Association, 6701 Democracy Blvd., Suite 300-9, Bethesda, MD 20817; Helpline: 800-962-9629; www.spinalcord.org. The National Spinal Cord Injury Association is dedicated to improving the quality of life for hundreds of thousands of Americans living with spinal cord injury and disease (SCI/D) and their families. Its Resource Center answers calls and e-mails and provides information and referral to individuals with new and existing SCI/D, their families, and their service providers. Its National Peer Support Network provides peer-support referrals to programs across the country, linking people with SCI/D to each other. The Christopher Reeve Paralysis Foundation recently funded the association to expand the program. NSCIA has 21 chapters and 19 support groups actively serving communities.

National Stroke Association, 9707 E. Easter Lane, Englewood, CO 80112-3747; 800-STROKES (787-6537); www.stroke.org. The National Stroke Association provides education, services, and community-based activities in prevention, treatment, rehabilitation, and recovery. The National Stroke Association serves the public and professional communities, people at risk, patients and their health-care providers, stroke survivors, and their families and caregivers.

National Institute of Neurological Disorders and Stroke (NINDS), NIH Neurological Institute, P.O. Box 5801, Bethesda, MD 20824; Voice: 800-352-9424 or 301-496-5751, TTY (for people using adaptive equipment): (301) 468-5981; www.ninds.nih.gov. The mission of NINDS is to reduce the burden of neurological disease and stroke. NINDS provides educational materials to consumers about neurological disease and stroke.

Chapter 8

Burn Pain

In This Chapter

- Understanding burn classifications
- Identifying when burns need treatment at burn centers
- Managing chronic health problems caused by burns
- Discovering how posttraumatic stress disorder (PTSD) is connected to chronic pain

Most people think of severe burns as acute injuries, so you may wonder why a book about chronic pain contains a chapter about burn pain. The truth is that burns are one of the most preventable *causes* of chronic pain.

Many serious burns ultimately lead to chronic pain. For example, researchers at the New England Medical Center in Boston, Massachusetts, studied 358 burn survivors. These survivors had burns over 59 percent of their bodies. Many were burned years ago — on average, they were studied 12 years from the time of the burn injury. Yet even though it had been more than a decade since their burns, over half of this group (52 percent) had constant and chronic pain as a direct result of their former burns.

In addition to the physical trauma of burns, the event that caused the injury can lead to a mental and emotional problem called posttraumatic stress disorder (PTSD). This form of anxiety develops after a terrifying and sometimes pain-inducing event. PTSD is sometimes thought to cause chronic pain, but its impact is often overlooked or misunderstood. Fortunately, treatments and resources described in the section called "Understanding the PTSD/Chronic Pain Connection," later in this chapter can help you deal with the problem.

Lamenting the Tragedy of Burns

Burn injuries in the United States result in more than 1 million emergency department visits and about 3,000 deaths a year. Children and the elderly have the toughest time recovering from their burns as well as from the horrific events that cause them. Tragically, children account for more than a third of all burn injuries in the United States. A surprising 75 percent of all burns are believed preventable.

While you're driving in traffic, or when you're home or with your children on the playground, you and your loved ones may risk burn injuries from a range of sources:

- **Fires:** Burns from fire, often referred to as *thermal fires,* can be caused by anything — flames, liquids, gases, and objects — if temperatures exceed 115º F (46°C), and the hot substance comes in contact with your skin. The higher the temperature, the faster the skin burns, and in only 3 1/2 minutes, the heat from a house fire can reach more than 1,100° F.
- **Chemical burns:** Chemical burns are caused by strong acids or alkalines touching your skin. Unfortunately, you can find these products stored under your bathroom sink and on the utility shelf in your garage. Dangerous chemicals used in the home include bleach, boric acid, paint thinner, and products used to clear drains. If you have children or grandchildren around, keep your cleaning supplies locked up! In addition, handle these chemicals gingerly yourself.
- **Radiation burns:** Radiation burns are most often the result of spending too much time in the sun or in a tanning bed. Excessive X-rays or nonsolar radiation can also cause this type of burn. Deep radiation burns from X-rays may not be visible for days or weeks after exposure.
- **Electric shock:** Electrical burns may be deceptive because often the only visible damage occurs at the point where the electrical current entered and exited the body. However, on its way through your body, the electrical current may seriously damage internal organs. Lightning strikes, high-voltage power lines, or faulty electrical equipment can all cause electrical burns. Next time you're at a summer picnic and a thunderstorm starts up, pack up and get out! The safest place is in your car and *not* under a tree!

Classifying Burns

Burns can cause serious damage to the victim's skin, harm the body's organs, and elicit horrific pain. The level of pain suffered depends on the dimensions of the injury. The deeper and wider the injury, the more excruciating the pain.

Burns are classified by how deep they go, as well as by the percentage of the body that they cover (see Figure 8-1):

- When burns are limited to the epidermis (the outer layer of the skin), they're **first-degree burns.** They cause pain, redness, swelling, and minor damage to the skin. The skin is dry, but blister-free.

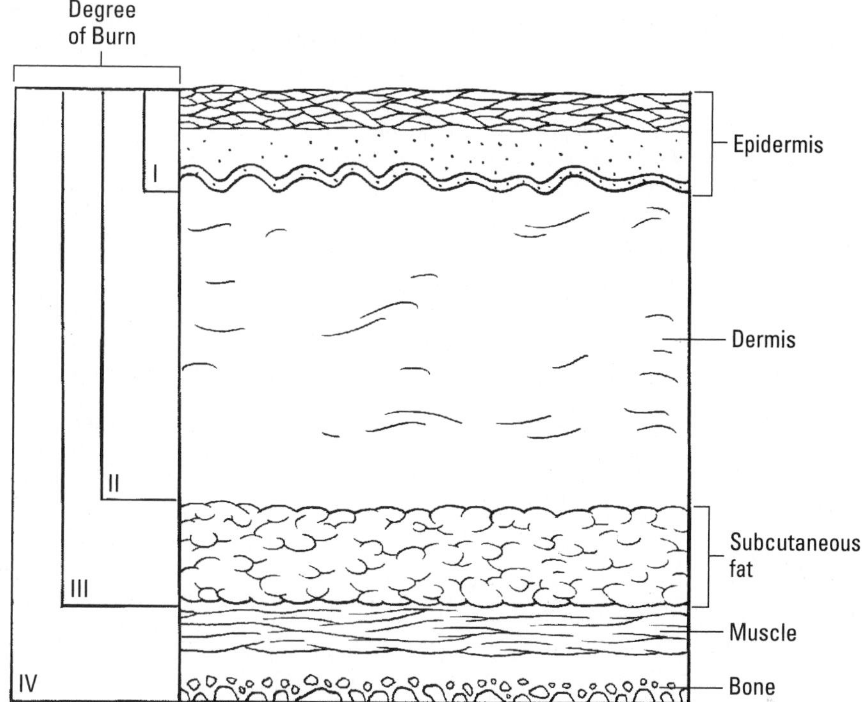

Figure 8-1: First- to fourth-degree burns.

- When damage from burns reaches the *dermis* (the next deeper layer of skin), these burns are **second-degree burns.** Second-degree burns are very painful and cause redness, swelling, and blistering. The skin is moist and weepy. They'll heal in a couple of weeks, but some second-degree burns require surgery and skin grafting.
- If burns reach the next layer, the site of the subcutaneous tissue, they're **third-degree burns.** In a third-degree burn, the skin layer is lost, and nerve endings may be destroyed, causing a loss of pain sensation in the area. However, the area of the third-degree burn is surrounded by second-degree burns, which cause severe pain.

  Charred veins and nerve endings are visible with third-degree burns. Remnants of skin are leathery. Third-degree burns cause scars and can result in loss of function. They won't heal without surgery, and they're the burns that can cause chronic pain, even though other sensations are lost.
- **Fourth-degree burns** — the most severe type of burn — involve damage and destruction to the underlying muscle, bone, ligaments, and tendons and will require skin grafting along with reconstructive surgery when possible. At times, amputation is needed for fourth-degree burns.

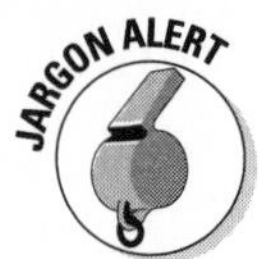

The percentage of the body that a burn covers is called *total body surface area* (TBSA).The more TBSA covered, the more serious the injury.

Preventing Chronic Pain

To prevent burn pain from becoming a chronic problem, you need to manage the pain immediately after the injury. Untreated pain can spin out of control and cause long-lasting problems and heightened anxiety.

Here's a good example of the physical processes that cause trouble later on when adequate pain management isn't administered after a burn injury:

- The burn causes a condition called *hypermetabolism,* which means that your body's energy output increases. In addition, the stress of the injury causes the release of *catecholamine neurotransmitters,* which further heighten your body's energy output. The increased hypermetabolsim (dare we say hyper-hyper-metabolism?) has the effect of decreasing blood flow to the area of the burn. But your body greatly *needs* that blood flow to heal back up again.
- At the same time that this decreased blood flow is happening, the excruciating pain of the burn can curb your immune system, which you need for healing and avoiding infections and other complications. The acute pain also derails blood flow. So, if the pain is not dealt with aggressively, the injury doesn't heal.

Treating Burns

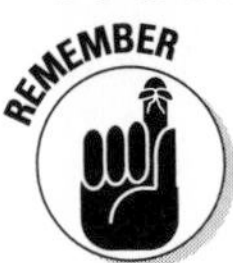

It's important to do everything possible to heal well and control pain in the days and weeks after a burn injury in order to prevent acute pain from morphing into chronic pain.

After the initial emergency of caring for burn victims, treating the injury means that the patient must endure a lot of painful procedures, including the removal of dead tissue, which is called *debridement.* The doctor or other medical professional must also clean the burn area, replace dressings, exercise burned limbs and joints, and possibly perform a skin graft. In addition, physical and occupational therapy begins as soon as possible to return function to the burn area. Many burn victims also require repeated surgeries.

Some long-term medical issues that occur for burn victims are

- **Scarring:** After the initial phase of a burn, your skin generates scar tissue. Getting appropriate treatment during the scarring process is extremely important to prevent chronic problems.

  If a burn injury doesn't heal on its own in a week to ten days, the doctor cuts away dead tissue and performs skin grafts. Without such treatment, the skin regenerated at this point is very thin and only marginally protective. In addition, the area heals with ugly protruding scars called *granulations* or *hypertrophic scarring,* which grow out of control. To prevent granulations, burn victims often wear garments that put pressure on the burn area.

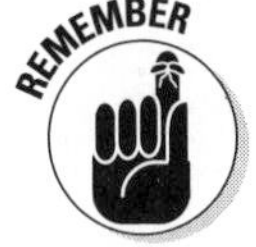

  If you or a loved one has suffered a severe burn, prevention of long-term scars is a serious challenge. The victim's face, hands, and so on may be extremely disfigured, causing serious adjustment problems. The good news is that treatments are being developed all the time, including facial transplants.

- **Contractures:** As scar tissue forms after a burn, the skin contracts, and joints can no longer move normally. To prevent muscles from shortening (called *contractures*), which can cause deformities, burn victims must go through extremely painful exercises of the involved joints. If these exercises are done repeatedly, they can prevent the problem. However, sometimes contractures have to be released surgically or are permanent.
- **Loss of the ability to sweat:** Sweat glands are destroyed in second- or third-degree burns and don't regenerate. Because sweating helps regulate body temperature, victims of extensive burns may not do well in hot, cold, or humid environments and often have to restrict exercise.
- **Skin problems:** Deep burns destroy glands in the skin so that the skin becomes very dry. In addition, new skin is weak and vulnerable and needs to be protected.

Understanding the PTSD/Chronic Pain Connection

Severe burns are caused by horrifying events, such as burning buildings, chemical explosions, or other frightening calamities. One of the most difficult health problems resulting from such events is *post-traumatic stress disorder* (PTSD), a chronic anxiety syndrome in which the burn victim keeps mentally re-experiencing the event. People with the disorder may have a difficult time healing, both physically and emotionally.

Praising burn centers

Severe burns should be treated at one of the 125 specialized burn centers located across the country. (Military personnel with burns are treated at the Brooke Army Medical Center in San Antonio, Texas.) Getting appropriate treatment can help victims avoid chronic pain and other health problems later.

Burn centers have specially trained staffs to treat people with extensive burn injuries. The American College of Surgeons has developed criteria for the types of burn injuries that should be treated in a specialized burn center:

- Burns that damage the first and second layers of skin *(partial thickness burns)* that are greater than 10 percent of the total body surface area (TBSA)
- Burns that involve the face, hands, feet, genitalia, the pelvic floor, or major joints
- Third-degree burns in any age group
- Electrical burns, including lightning injury
- Chemical burns
- Inhalation injury
- Burn injury in patients with preexisting medical problems such as cancer or heart disease that may complicate management, prolong recovery, or affect survival
- Any patients with burns and trauma (such as fractures), for whom the burn injury poses the greatest risk of morbidity or mortality
- Burned children in hospitals without qualified personnel or equipment for the care of children
- Burn injury in patients who require special social, emotional, or long-term rehabilitative intervention

PTSD may strike soon after the burn has occurred or months later. Symptoms of PTSD include

- Obsessively recalling the event over and over again, so much that it intrudes on other thoughts
- Avoiding things associated with the event
- Experiencing nightmares
- Feeling emotionally numb
- Being on guard, hyper-aroused, overly alert, or easily startled
- Experiencing flashbacks

PTSD is usually considered chronic if it lasts longer than three months. One of the unhappy results of the condition is that anxiety disorders and substance abuse are common for people with chronic PTSD.

The International Association for Traumatic Stress Studies (IATSS) has found that PTSD is linked to development of chronic pain. According to the IATSS, people with lasting PTSD symptoms frequently report high rates of health problems. The bottom line is that symptoms of PTSD overlap with those associated with chronic physical pain, such as that from burns.

According to another organization that studies PTSD, the PTSD Alliance, symptoms of PTSD include the following physical complaints, which may be accompanied by depression:

- Chronic pain with no medical basis (frequently gynecological problems in women)
- Chronic fatigue syndrome or fibromyalgia
- Stomach pain or other digestive problems, such as irritable bowel syndrome or alternating bouts of diarrhea and constipation
- Breathing problems or asthma
- Headaches
- Muscle cramps or aches such as low back pain
- Cardiovascular problems
- Sleep disorders

It's important to seek counseling for PTSD from a professional specifically trained to help people with the syndrome. For example, PTSD is such a huge problem for military victims that the VA has a specific program to assist soldiers with the disorder.

A therapeutic approach called *exposure therapy* is effective for many people with PTSD. The therapy involves talking about the event repeatedly with a counselor in order to get control over your thoughts and fears. Specific medications, including some antidepressants, also help.

Getting Help

Specialized groups help burn victims and their families, they can also help you cope with posttraumatic stress.

For burn recovery, try the following resources:

- **American Burn Association (ABA):** The ABA (www.ameriburn.org) works to improve the quality of care provided to burn patients. Activities include stimulating research in treating burn injuries, fostering prevention efforts, and providing continuing education courses, annual scientific meetings, and scientific publications.
- **Burn Recovery Center:** More than 100 specialized burn recovery hospitals treat an average of 200 burn patients a year. Physicians in these centers and their staffs specialize in the treatment of and recovery from burns. For a list of specialized burn centers, go to www.burn-recovery.org/burn-centers.htm.
- **Phoenix Society for Burn Survivors:** The name of the Phoenix Society for Burn Survivors (www.phoenix-society.org) is taken from the legendary bird that lived for 500 years and was consumed by flame, but rose again, reborn from its ashes. The organization offers peer support, education, and advocacy for burn survivors.

These organizations can offer help for PSTD:

- **Anxiety Disorders Association of America (ADAA):** The ADAA (www.adaa.org) promotes the treatment, prevention, and cure of anxiety disorders and improving the lives of people who suffer from them. The ADAA Web site is a resource for consumer information about PTSD, including a PTSD self-test, message boards, useful links, and a directory on where to find help.
- **International Society for Traumatic Stress Studies (ISTSS):** The ISTSS (www.istss.org) provides a forum for the sharing of research, clinical strategies, public policy concerns, and theoretical formulations on trauma in the United States and around the world. The ISTSS Web site provides videos of trauma survivors telling their stories of recovery.

Chapter 9

Digestive and Urinary Conditions

In This Chapter

- Discovering symptoms and major causes of chronic digestive pain
- Understanding your treatment options
- Weighing the risk of taking NSAIDs
- Analyzing chronic pain caused by chronic bladder diseases
- Finding a physician who specializes in digestive health

You may wonder what the common denominator is between digestion and urination, so here it is: When you eat food and drink liquids (which hopefully were tasty and nutritious), your digestion processes it all, pulling out the elements it needs. It then eliminates what it doesn't use. Urination is the end result of a similar process by the kidneys, which takes out what is needed by your body and eliminates the rest in the urine.

And usually life goes on with little disruption. However, if these body systems don't work well, the results can range from the nausea and bloating of dyspepsia to the severe pain of Crohn's disease in the digestive system. And in the urinary tract, urethritis and interstitial cystitis are two painful chronic diseases that may develop when things go awry.

Some of these chronic conditions are beyond your control. As with the color of your eyes, you inherit a predisposition to develop them from previous generations. However, many diseases are caused by — or worsened by — what and how much you eat, drink, or even smoke.

Looking at Your Digestive and Urinary Systems

Simply put, your digestive system breaks food down into nutrients so that your body can use them, and then it excretes the rest. From your mouth to your rectum, it consists of the organs labeled in Figure 9-1.

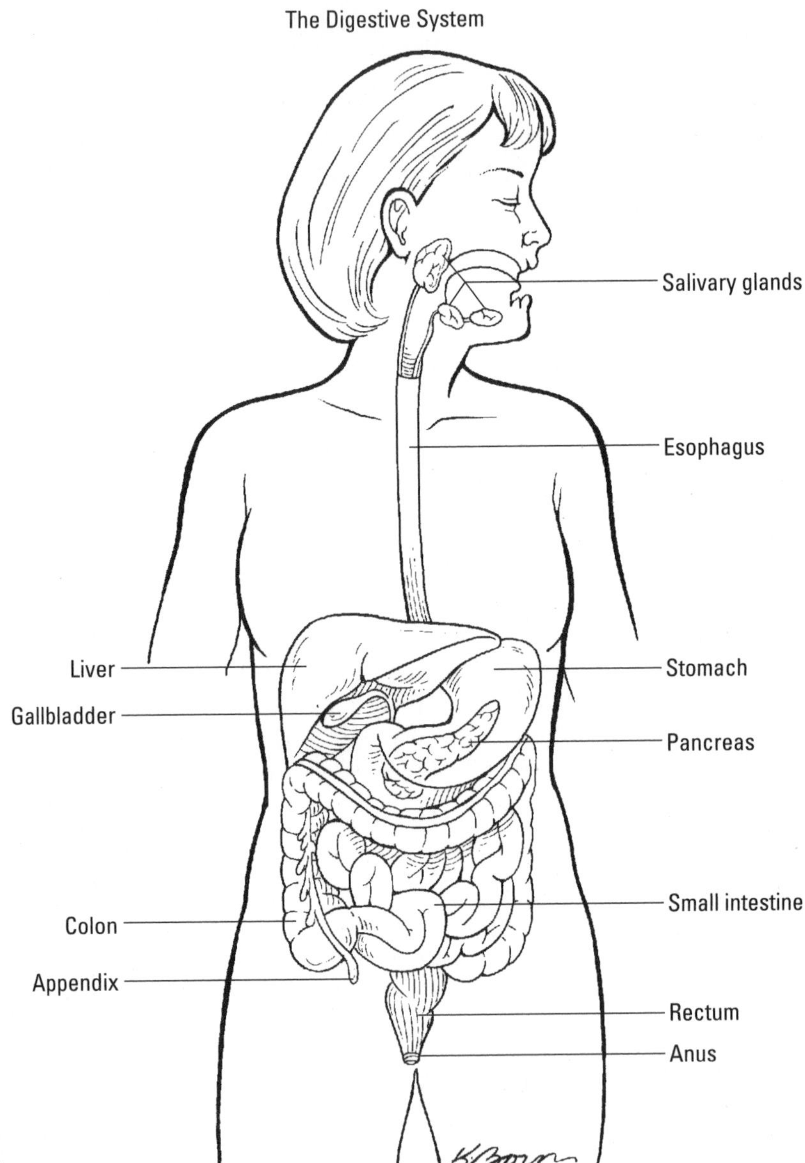

Figure 9-1: The digestive system.

Your kidneys and urinary tract get rid of the waste left over by your cells and organs after they've completed their jobs. These organs are shown in Figure 9-2.

Because many digestive and urinary conditions can cause relentless hurting, we can't possibly cover them all in one chapter. The following sections touch on major diseases and offer you resources to find out how to diagnose and treat them.

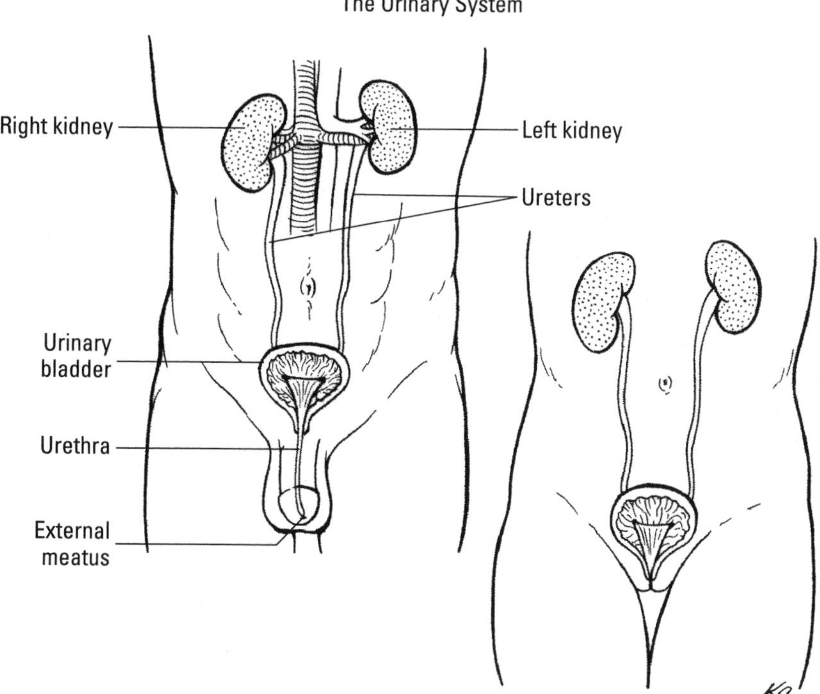

Figure 9-2: The urinary system.

Alcohol liver disease

The liver is the body's largest organ, with a startling 500 metabolic and regulatory functions. Drinking too much alcohol for too long can cause fatty liver, alcoholic hepatitis, and cirrhosis, three progressively worse liver diseases. Each one refers to harm done to the liver, a major organ that you can't live without. Of the three, cirrhosis is the most serious liver disease and can't be cured. The person with cirrhosis needs a liver transplant to survive.

Here are some facts about these diseases:

- **Fatty liver,** also called *steatosis,* is a buildup of fat in the liver cells. It has the dubious distinction of being the No. 1, alcohol-related health problem. (Fatty liver can sometimes be caused by obesity, in the absence of alcohol consumption.) Fatty liver doesn't cause pain, although some tenderness in the liver can occur.

- Regular binge drinking, or episodes of rapidly consuming five or more drinks for men or four or more drinks in women, can cause **alcoholic hepatitis,** which is often a precursor to the development of cirrhosis. Limit your alcohol consumption to one or two drinks only, once in awhile, and your liver will thank you! Alcoholic hepatitis can cause pain as well as fatigue, fever, and other symptoms.
- **Cirrhosis** is the most serious alcohol-related conditions. It's the massive loss of healthy liver cells and a buildup of scar tissue, which disturbs the blood flow. Cirrhosis causes pain and other symptoms, such as bleeding in the gastrointestinal (GI) tract.

The liver is enflamed and enlarged in all three conditions.

You can reverse fatty liver and alcoholic hepatitis by no longer consuming any alcohol. Cirrhosis isn't reversible, but can be arrested. (Read more about alcoholism in Chapter 14.)

Not all heavy drinkers develop alcohol liver disease, but it's impossible to tell who will get it and, for those who do, how severe the symptoms will be.

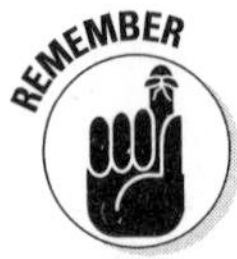

Sobriety (total abstinence from alcohol) is crucial to recovery from alcoholic liver disease. In addition, doctors usually prescribe nutritional fortification and vitamin supplementation, because many people with alcohol liver disease may have vitamin deficiencies. In addition, corticosteroids are prescribed to decrease inflammation.

Celiac disease

Celiac disease is the body's inability to absorb nutrients, which is related to its inability to digest gluten. (*Glutens* are proteins found in commonly eaten grains, including wheat, rye, oats, and barley.)

The condition may strike at any age, including infancy. Many people have celiac disease, but they don't know it. Most adults diagnosed with celiac disease have had it for ten years or longer before finally receiving an accurate diagnosis. (It's not that doctors are stupid, but rather that it's a tough disease to diagnose.)

Painful signs of celiac disease are chronic diarrhea, dyspepsia, gas, and a distended stomach. If you have celiac disease, you may be constantly exhausted, be depressed, and develop anemia or osteoporosis. Children with celiac disease may have a delayed puberty and even suffer from neurological symptoms, such as epilepsy. People of all ages who have celiac disease may develop a rash called *dermatitis herpetiformis* (DH). This skin condition is small clusters of red bumps that are extremely itchy. The clusters appear around the elbows, knees, scalp, buttocks, and back.

The good news is that removing gluten from your diet makes the condition go away and lets your aching intestines heal. The bad news is that getting rid of gluten isn't easy. Gluten hides in many products and restaurant foods. If you want to eliminate gluten altogether from your diet, you'll need to become a strict reader of food labels and an inquisitive customer in restaurants.

Crohn's disease

Crohn's disease is an inflammation of the wall of the intestine and causes chronic pain. Crohn's usually strikes during the teen years and early 20s. People who smoke have an increased risk for developing this disease. Crohn's is diagnosed by a colonoscopy, in which an optic tube with a tiny camera attached to it is inserted into the body through the rectum to examine the digestive tract.

Some common symptoms of Crohn's disease are

- Chronic diarrhea
- Bloody diarrhea
- Bleeding from the rectum
- Abdominal pain
- Fever
- Loss of appetite
- Dehydration
- Weight loss

As with other chronic inflammatory diseases, the symptoms of Crohn's disease may subside, but they come back again later. Crohn's can scar the wall of the intestines, leading to blockage and ulcers. Tunnels, called *fistulas,* can develop and interconnect an affected area of intestine with surrounding tissues, such as the bladder, vagina, or skin. Fistulas and cracks may also develop around the anus.

Treatment of Crohn's disease is focused on improving symptoms and controlling the disease process. People with Crohn's should never smoke cigarettes because smoking is a risk factor for Crohn's, and if you already have the disease, smoking increases the pain. Lactose intolerance is common for people with Crohn's, so dairy products should be limited in the diet if you're lactose-intolerant in addition to having Crohn's. (Read about lactose intolerance in the section called "Lactose intolerance," later in this chapter.)

The treatment for Crohn's depends on how severe the disease is and can include drug therapy, nutritional therapy, and surgery. Over half of those with Crohn's eventually require at least one surgical procedure.

Dyspepsia

Dyspepsia is discomfort in the upper abdomen. The condition can overlap with peptic ulcers and GERD. (Both conditions are covered in the "Peptic ulcers" and "GERD: Gastroesophageal reflux disease" sections later in this chapter.) Often the cause of dyspepsia is unknown.

This condition is very common, and at least one in four people have dyspepsia.

You may feel fullness in the top part of your stomach or feel full after eating just a small amount of food. You also may have bloating, burping, nausea, gagging, and/or vomiting. (It's bad enough that you're feeling the discomfort of dyspepsia, but if others notice you're burping and gagging, you may also feel embarrassed.)

If you have chronic dyspepsia, limit or eliminate alcohol, caffeine, and fatty foods from your diet. Keeping a food diary to identify symptoms is helpful. (See Chapter 18 for information on a food diary.) Your doctor may also prescribe medicines called antisecretory therapies or proton pump inhibitors.

GERD: Gastroesophageal reflux disease

After you swallow food, it travels down the esophagus and empties into your stomach. At the bottom of the esophagus is a muscle that acts as a door. When it becomes weak and doesn't close all the way, the acidic contents of your stomach may back up, sneaking through the door, entering the esophagus and irritating it. (This process is referred to as *reflux,* and the disease is called gastroesophageal reflux disease, sometimes also known as heartburn.)

People of all ages can have GERD, including babies whose esophageal muscle has not matured. One in five adults report that they have symptoms of GERD at least once a week. As many as one in ten have symptoms every day.

The most common symptoms of GERD are heartburn and indigestion. Other symptoms may include cough, hoarseness, and wheezing. When untreated, GERD can cause *esophagitis* (inflammation of the esophagus), narrowing of the esophagus, and a precancerous condition called *Barrett's esophagus.*

If you have GERD, you can control symptoms by following recommendations from the National Institutes of Health:

- Avoid alcohol and spicy, fatty, or acidic foods that trigger heartburn.
- Eat smaller meals.

- Don't eat within two hours of bedtime.
- Lose weight if needed.
- Wear loose-fitting clothes. Maybe you were a size 12 ten years ago, and now you're a size 16. Wear your actual size — until you get it back down to a size 14 (or 12) again.

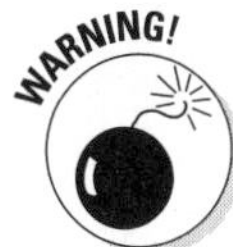

Many people find relief from GERD by taking over-the-counter antacids. But if you're popping antacids all day, every day, you have chronic GERD (or another serious problem), and you should see your doctor.

Additional techniques that can help are elevating the head of your bed by 6 inches, and staying away from caffeinated drinks, alcohol, and, sadly, chocolate. When you have GERD, you should also avoid grapefruit and orange juice, beans, cheese, onions, tomatoes, and cabbage.

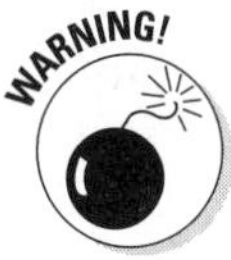

Some drugs, especially anticholinergics, can lead to GERD. Ask your doctor whether you can take a lower dosage of the drug.

Peptic ulcers

A *peptic ulcer* is a break in the lining (called the *mucosa*) of the stomach or *duodenum* (the first part of the small intestine). Peptic ulcers occur five times more commonly in the duodenum than the stomach. Ulcers range in size from a few millimeters to a few centimeters.

One in ten people develop peptic ulcers, and men are slightly more likely to have them than women. Contrary to myth, drinking alcohol, a bad diet, and excessive stress don't cause ulcers (although they can each make the pain from existing ulcers much worse).

Instead, the two major causes of peptic ulcers are

- ***Helicobacter pylori (H. pylori):*** *H. pylori* are bacteria that many people unknowingly carry around in their stomachs and duodenums. In fact, 50 percent of Americans over age 60 have the bacteria in their gastrointestinal systems, and most of them don't develop ulcers. Why they escape the pain of ulcers and others do not is unknown.
- **The heavy use of nonsteroidal anti-inflammatory drugs (NSAIDs).** You can find more information on these drugs in Chapter 14. People who take NSAIDs for a long time have a 10 to 20 percent chance that they'll develop ulcers in the stomach and a 1 to 2 percent chance that they will develop them in their duodenum. Incredibly, the risk of a gastric ulcer is 40 times higher if you take NSAIDs on a long-term basis compared to a person who doesn't take them. People who have *H. pylori* and also take NSAIDS are at an even greater risk for developing ulcers. (See Chapter 14 for information on NSAIDs.)

Pain and indigestion are the main signs of peptic ulcers. The symptoms are often relieved by eating.

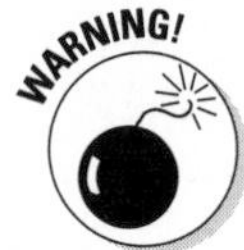

Ulcer pain comes and goes, often with eating cycles. If the pain is constant, it means that the ulcer has broken through the lining of the stomach or duodenum, which can cause the stomach or intestinal contents to flow into the abdominal cavity. In addition, it can cause inflammation of the lining of the stomach wall (peritonitis). Both problems can cause infection and are medical emergencies. See your doctor!

Treatment for peptic ulcers varies depending on the cause of the condition:

- ***H. pylori:*** The goal with treating ulcers caused by *H. pylori* is to relieve the painful symptoms, stop the infection, and heal the break. Your doctor will prescribe antibiotics to kill the bacteria and proton pump inhibitors to calm the stomach or small intestine. (*Proton pump inhibitors* are a group of drugs that reduce gastric acid production.)
- **NSAIDs:** If you must take NSAIDs to relieve pain and inflammation, treating your ulcers may be difficult. Your doctor may advise you to take a proton pump inhibitor on a daily basis as long as you continue to take NSAIDs.

Irritable bowel syndrome (IBS)

Irritable bowel syndrome (IBS) is a chronic problem of the large intestine that causes stomach pain and changes in bowel habits. Symptoms of IBS wax and wane, and sometimes it's not too bad and other times — bad!

The condition is common, and women are more likely to have IBS than men. Symptoms include constipation or diarrhea, and (this is truly maddening) some patients alternate between constipation and diarrhea. Bloating is also common.

The cause of IBS is not known, although hormones may play a role. Your doctor will probably run tests to make sure that you don't have another disease causing the symptoms.

If you have IBS, you can control your symptoms with diet, stress reduction, adjusting your medicines, and, when appropriate, taking specific drugs prescribed by your doctor. Symptom and food diaries are great tools for identifying food triggers. Trouble digesting dairy products (lactose intolerance) may also be a problem.

For many people with IBS, fatty foods and caffeine are the culprits triggering their symptoms. Other possible food triggers are fruit sugars, sorbitol (used in artificially sweetened foods), and foods that produce gas, such as brown beans and cabbage.

Lactose intolerance

People with lactose intolerance can't digest a sugar in dairy products that's called *lactose*. Their bodies don't produce enough *lactase*, an enzyme that digests lactose. That means no more ice cream, whipped cream, or milk. (However, sufferers may be able to consume a small amount of a product with lactose if they take an over-the-counter medication, such as Lactaid.)

The condition is common in people of non-European ancestry, particularly Asians, Native Americans, or African-Americans, and its incidence increases with age. Estimates are that 50 million people in the United States have partial to complete lactose intolerance. People with other conditions, such as Crohn's disease and a tropical disease called Sprue, may also develop lactose intolerance.

If you're lactose intolerant, you probably have some combination of chronic diarrhea, bloating, cramping, and gas if you regularly eat and/or drink dairy products. Quantity matters when it comes to lactose intolerance. Most people with lactose intolerance can drink one or two glasses of milk at different meals in one day, but if they exceed that amount, then they have symptoms.

If you have symptoms of lactose intolerance, your doctor will probably first recommend eliminating cow's milk from your diet to see whether they go away. If you give up cow's milk and your symptoms improve, but you would like additional confirmation, three types of tests are used most frequently: the lactose tolerance, hydrogen breath, and stool acidity tests.

Dairy products are so prominent in American diets that it's worth experimenting to find the amount of dairy you can actually eat or drink before symptoms begin. Always tell a new doctor that you're lactose-intolerant so that she can keep that in mind when prescribing drugs. (Lactose is used as a filler in many drugs, such as some brands of birth control pills and antacids, and certain antibiotics and other medications can inhibit lactose absorption.) Use the food diary, described in Chapter 18, to help you discover whether you may be lactose-intolerant. Your physician may order blood or breath tests to verify that you have a problem.

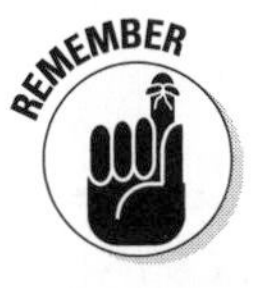

Foods high in lactose include milk, ice cream, and cottage cheese. (Who cares about the cottage cheese, but ice cream is tough to give up!) Aged cheeses, such as Parmesan, have a lower lactose content than fresher cheeses. Unpasteurized yogurt contains bacteria that produce lactase and, as a result is usually okay to eat if you're lactose-intolerant.

If you eliminate dairy from your diet, take calcium supplements to prevent osteoporosis.

You can find milk pretreated with lactase in most grocery stores. However, lactase-treated milk sometimes still has some lactose in it, so be cautious about how much you drink at one time. Lactase enzyme replacement is also available commercially (Lactaid).

Pancreatitis

Chronic pancreatitis is an inflammation of the pancreas that doesn't go away. A gland behind the stomach, the pancreas plays an important role in digesting food and metabolizing carbohydrates. Heavy drinkers of alcohol and/or people who smoke cigarettes are the most likely to develop pancreatitis.

If you have pancreatitis, you're likely to have pain, loss of appetite, nausea, vomiting, constipation, gas, and weight loss. During flares, you'll feel tenderness over the pancreas. Attacks can last as long as two weeks, but some pain may be constant.

If you have chronic pancreatitis, you must eat a low-fat diet and eliminate alcohol and narcotics. Doctors prescribe drugs that specifically treat the condition.

Interstitial cystitis (IC)

A chronically inflamed bladder that causes major pain is called *interstitial cystitis* (IC). This condition is also known as painful bladder syndrome (PBS).

Both men and women develop IC, but it's more common in women. The average age of people with IC is 40. IC may be caused by several diseases and is associated with allergies, irritable bowel syndrome, and inflammatory bowel disease.

IC causes pain when the bladder fills up and also causes the urgent need to urinate. IC may cause difficulty in controlling the flow of urine. The person with IC may constantly feel like she has a bladder infection. In fact, some doctors give antibiotics to people with such chronic bladder pain, but antibiotics don't help unless the person really does have an infection.

IC has no cure, but treatments are available to control symptoms. For example, if you have IC, you should avoid smoking cigarettes, drinking alcohol, and eating spicy foods. Medical treatment includes inflating the bladder and bathing the inside of the bladder with a medicine called dimethylsulfoxide (DMSO), which is approved by the FDA to treat this condition. Oral medications may also be used to control bladder spasms. Consult an urologist who specializes in IC if you think you may have this disorder.

Advanced treatments for IC include implanting a *sacral nerve stimulator device.* The device is a reversible treatment that sends mild electrical pulses to the *sacral nerve,* the nerve near the tailbone that influences bladder control muscles.

Urethritis

Chronic urethritis is an ongoing inflammation of the urethra that can strike both women and men. (The *urethra* is the canal that eliminates urine from the body.) It may be caused by injury, bacteria, a virus, or sensitivity to chemicals. People who are sexually active with many partners are particularly at risk for urethritis. Symptoms of chronic urethritis for men include a discharge from the penis, itching or pain when urinating, and blood in the urine. Women experience pain while urinating, an increased need to urinate, and a vaginal discharge. Antibiotics are frequently prescribed along with painkillers for chronic urethritis.

Practicing safe sex is extremely important to prevent spreading the infection and potentially causing urethritis in others. Often, your sexual partner must also be treated. If the condition is made worse by chemicals, such as spermicides, stop using them.

Chronic urethritis can cause permanent damage to the urethra and genitourinary organs in both sexes.

Diagnosing Digestive and Urinary Conditions

Each type of chronic digestive or urinary condition has its own set of diagnostic criteria. To diagnose and treat these problems, your primary care physician may refer you to a physician who specializes in digestive or urinary health. In addition, the following organizations can help you locate a specialist:

- **American College of Gastroenterology,** P.O. Box 342260, Bethesda, MD 20827-2260; phone 301-263-9000; Web site `www.acg.gi.org`. To locate a specialist in digestive health, use the American College of Gastroenterology's Physician Locater by clicking Patients and then GI Physician Locator.
- **American Urologist's Association,** 1000 Corporate Blvd., Linthicum, MD 21090; phone 1-866-RING (toll-free), `www.urologyhealth.org`. For urinary problems, use the American Urological Association's Urologist Locator_by clicking Find a Urologist.
- **National Digestive Diseases Information Clearinghouse,** 2 Information Way, Bethesda, MD 20892–3570; phone 800-891-5389; Web site `http://digestive.niddk.nih.gov`. The clearinghouse provides consumer information about digestive diseases.

Chapter 10

Reproductive Conditions

In This Chapter

- Understanding the parts of the male and female reproductive systems
- Looking at major female reproductive conditions that cause chronic pain
- Figuring out how the male prostate gland can cause chronic pain

The amazing reproductive systems of a man and woman together can create new life — what can be more remarkable than that? But from raging hormones to enlarged prostates, your reproductive system can also be the source of many chronic pain problems. In this chapter, we tell you what you need to know to understand the tie between chronic pain and the reproductive system.

Understanding Your Reproductive Systems

Most of the time, the reproductive system works fine. But sometimes something goes wrong, causing chronic pain for a man or woman. Fortunately, treatments are available for most chronic pain conditions in the reproductive system.

As you can see from Figure 10-1, the female reproductive system is much more complex than the male system. While the female reproductive system is deep inside the woman's body, most of the male reproductive system is external and accessible, such as the penis and the scrotum, the sac that contains the testicles. The result of these differences in anatomy means that reproductive conditions in women are much more difficult to diagnose and treat than those in men. For this reason, we spend much more time in this chapter discussing women's reproductive conditions than we do discussing men's problems.

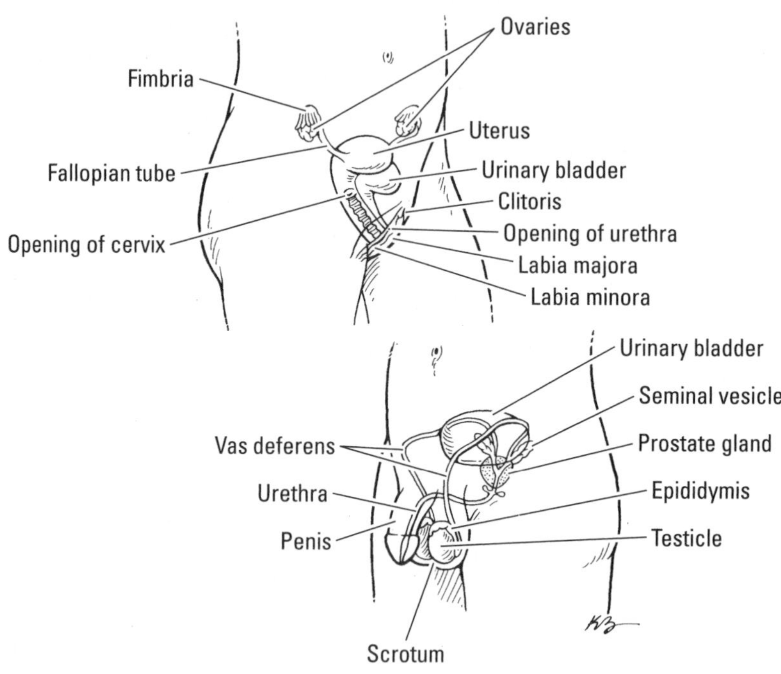

Figure 10-1: Female and male reproductive systems.

For Women Only: Problems in the Reproductive System

Women's reproductive systems give them a lot of practice with handling pain. Monthly cramps and, for many, childbirth, go together with being female. Unfortunately, some chronic pain conditions can also strike women. The most common chronic painful conditions of the female reproductive system are endometriosis, pelvic inflammatory disease (PID), and premenstrual syndrome. The onset and the early stages of menopause can cause considerable distress as well.

Endometriosis

The *endometrium* is the lining of the *uterus* (the part of the body that babies grow inside). About 12 times a year, the uterine lining builds up in preparation for a fetus, and then it sloughs off during menstruation when no pregnancy occurs. Most women refer to this monthly cycle as "my period."

Some unhappy women have a problem in which the rogue endometrium somehow escapes outside the uterus, hiding out in other parts of their bodies, such as the bladder or ovaries. This escapee tissue actually goes through the menstrual cycle in its new location, the same as it would have if it had remained where it was *supposed* to be, in the uterus. Stuck in its new location and with no way out, the endometrium becomes inflamed, and it can develop cysts and create other problems, a condition called *endometriosis.* Figure 10-2 shows common areas in the female anatomy where endometriosis occurs.

Endometriosis causes aching in the abdomen, lower back, and/or rectum. The pain may migrate to the vagina or upper legs. If you have this condition, you'll probably start to feel pain two to seven days before your period, and it will become increasingly severe until your period stops. You may also experience bleeding from the rectum. As the disease progresses, the pain may become constant and unremitting. Infertility is also common for women with endometriosis.

Six to 10 percent of women in the United States suffer from the chronic pain of endometriosis, and it's four or five times more likely to strike infertile than fertile women.

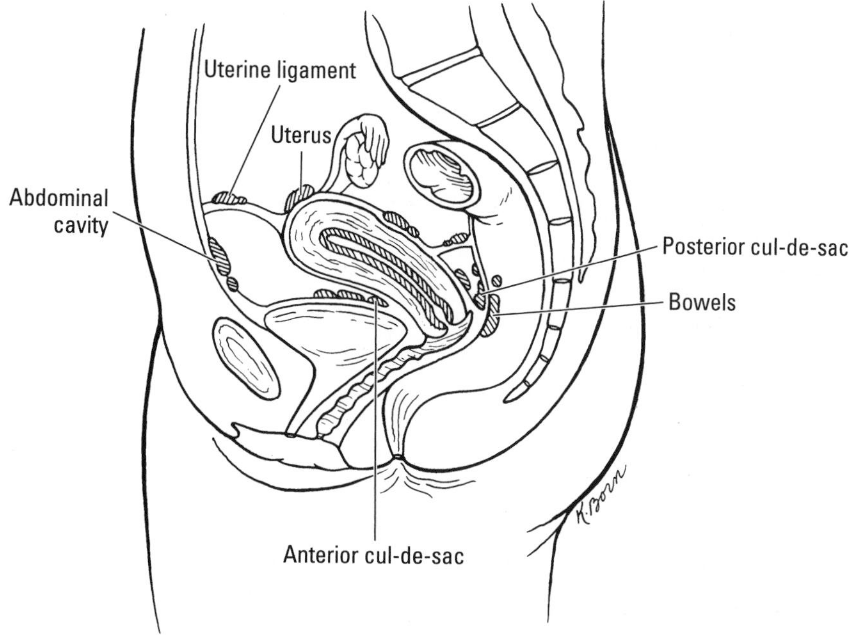

Figure 10-2: Endometrial tissue's common escape sites.

Treatment may include hormone therapy, prescribed painkillers, and, in severe cases, surgically removing affected tissues. For women who want to become pregnant, surgery can greatly improve their chances.

Pelvic inflammatory disease

Pelvic inflammatory disease (PID) is a painful infection of the upper genital tract that's caused by a variety of sexually transmitted organisms, including the ones that cause gonorrhea and chlamydia. It's a serious disease that can damage the fallopian tubes, causing infertility. PID can also become a chronic pain problem for some women. (PID is also called *salpingitis.*)

Pelvic inflammatory disease is most common among young, sexually active women who've never given birth and who have had multiple sexual partners. Nonwhite race, douching, and smoking are also factors associated with PID. The use of birth control pills or barrier contraceptives (such as the cervical cap or diaphragm) may protect against PID. However, use of an intrauterine device (IUD) is a risk factor *for* developing PID.

If you've had sex with a partner who may have a sexually transmitted disease (STD), see your doctor right away. She can help you treat most infections that you may be developing.

Symptoms of PID are lower abdominal pain, chills, fever, irregular periods, a yellow or green vaginal discharge, and pain during intercourse. On a scale of 1 to 10, many women will say that PID pain is about a 200.

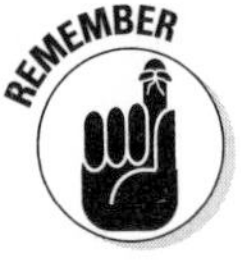

Early treatment with antibiotics is important for the person with PID and her sexual partner(s). Treatment with antibiotics in a hospital and/or surgery may be necessary.

Premenstrual Syndrome

Ask most women the definition of Premenstrual Syndrome (PMS), and they'll say, "That's easy. PMS is hell." Scientifically speaking, however, PMS is actually a group of painful physical and emotional symptoms that develop during the 7 to 14 days before the onset of a menstrual period and that go away when menstruation occurs.

PMS symptoms differ from woman to woman. Also, if you have PMS, your own symptoms may change with each period. Common problems are

- Bloating
- Acne
- Painful breasts

- Weight gain
- Skin disorders
- Irritability and/anger
- Depression
- Inability to concentrate
- Mood swings
- Lack of interest in sex
- Lethargy
- Cravings for carbohydrates

We know what you are thinking: "Sure! Every woman has some of these symptoms before a period." Well, if you have PMS, these symptoms are severe. You're not just a bit of a fuzz-head; you truly can't think straight! You're not just yawning a little; you take to bed at any opportunity. You get the idea!

The condition attacks about two in five women, which is a lot of women! For most women with PMS, the condition is a chronic pain problem.

Sadly, little research has been done on how to treat PMS. Many experts recommend that women participate in aerobic exercise, reduce their caffeine, salt, and alcohol intake, and eat complex carbohydrates, such as vegetables. Your doctor may also prescribe a diuretic to help with bloating and tender breasts and may order hormones to decrease breast pain and cramping. Nonsteroidal anti-inflammatory drugs (NSAIDs) can help ease painful cramps. Many women also find that taking a selective serotonin reuptake inhibitor (SSRI) antidepressant can stabilize the mood swings that PMS can cause.

Soaking in a warm bath can help ease painful cramps considerably.

Menopause

Menopause is the winding down of female reproduction. Your body produces less and less estrogen, and then menstruation finally ends altogether, either due to aging or the surgical removal of both ovaries. When periods have stopped for one year, menopause is officially diagnosed.

The average age at menopause is 51 years. If menopause occurs before age 40, it's considered premature.

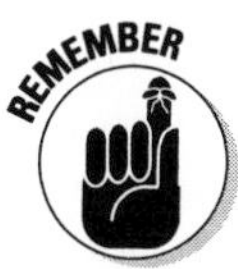

The process of menopause usually takes one to three years, with accompanying physical symptoms, but symptoms such as night sweats, hot flashes, and irritability can go on for many years.

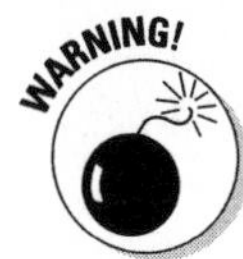

Vaginal bleeding that occurs after your periods have completely stopped for a year or more isn't normal. See your doctor to make sure that you don't have a medical problem.

Four in five menopausal women get *hot flashes* during menopause (feelings of intense heat, flushing and sweating). Hot flashes are particularly troublesome for women who have a surgical menopause. Other painful symptoms of menopause include

- Thinning and drying of the vagina
- Atrophy of the bladder
- Anxiety
- Mood swings
- Lethargy
- Osteoporosis

For many years, *hormone replacement therapy* (HRT) was frequently prescribed for menopause symptoms. However, taking hormones is now considered controversial and may even put you at risk for breast cancer. The decision for or against hormones is a personal one, and it's important to talk this issue over with your gynecologist.

Other treatments for menopause include estrogen creams for vaginal dryness, vaginal rings with estrogen, and antidepressants. Consuming estrogen-containing foods, such as pomegranates, rice, and barley, may help.

For Men Only: Problems in the Reproductive System

Reproductive problems for men are often linked to sexual activity or the aging process. Sometimes they're caused by infections, as with *prostatitis* (inflammation of the prostate).

For example, prostate problems are very common after age 50. And the older men get, the more likely they are to have such problems. Prostate cancer is diagnosed in many men, and, after lung cancer, it's the most commonly occurring form of cancer for men.

The *prostate* is a walnut-sized gland that is part of a man's reproductive system. The gland tends to expand with age and may squeeze the *urethra,* which carries urine away from your bladder. (The prostate surrounds the urethra.) Several prostate problems can develop:

- *Acute bacterial prostatitis* is an infection of the prostate caused by bacteria. Symptoms include chills, fever, and pain in the lower back and genital area. Problems with urination are also common. Bacterial prostatitis can become chronic.
- *Chronic prostatitis* is the most common type of prostatitis, and it's a common infection that can strike men of any age. The condition comes and goes and is difficult to treat.
- *Enlarged prostates,* or *benign prostatic hyperplasia* (BPH), are common in older men. Over time, an enlarged prostate may press against the urethra, making it hard to urinate. Dribbling and urgency can occur. A doctor does a rectal exam to check for BPH.

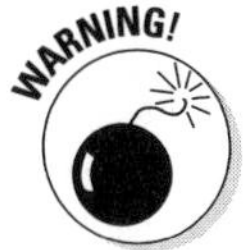

Many men try to avoid the rectal examination during their annual physical exam because it's so embarrassing. Don't be one of them! The rectal exam that your doctor performs can detect serious problems with the prostate, such as BPH, prostatitis, or even prostate cancer.

Antibiotics are used to treat acute bacterial prostatitis, but they will not help chronic prostatitis. For chronic prostatitis, doctors sometimes prescribe medicines to relax the gland. Other medicines used for BPH are alpha-blockers or finasteride, a medicine that lowers the testosterone level. However, taking finasteride can also dampen a man's libido and hamper his sexual performance. (Understandably, most men aren't very enthusiastic about these side effects.) Sometimes surgery is necessary to relieve BPH symptoms.

Diagnosing Pain Problems: Who Can Help

Each cause of reproductive pain has its own set of diagnostic criteria. To diagnose and treat these problems, your primary care physician may refer you to a physician who specializes in reproductive health. For women, this person is usually a gynecologist, and for men, it's usually an urologist.

For women:

American College of Obstetricians and Gynecologists, 409 12th St., S.W., P.O. Box 96920, Washington, DC 20090-6920; phone 202-638-5577; Web site `www.acog.org`. To locate a gynecologist, use the American College of Obstetricians and Gynecologists Physician Directory on its Web site.

American Society for Reproductive Medicine, 1209 Montgomery Highway, Birmingham, AL 35216-2809; phone 205-978-5000; Web site `www.asrm.org`. To locate a specialist in reproductive health, use the American Society of Reproductive Medicine's Physician Locater on its Web site.

The Society of Reproductive Surgeons, 1209 Montgomery Highway, Birmingham, AL 35216-2809; phone 205-978-5000; Web site `www.reprodsurgery.org`. To locate a reproductive surgeon, use the Society of Reproductive Surgeons' Surgeon Locater on its Web site.

For men:

American Urological Association, 1000 Corporate Blvd., Linthicum, MD 21090; phone: 866-746-4282 or 410-689-3700; Web site: `www.auanet.org`. To find an urologist, use the American Urological Association's Find an Urologist on its Web site.

Chapter 11

Following the Nerve Pathways: Neuralgias and Neuropathies

In This Chapter

- Understanding the basics of nerve pain
- Comprehending complex regional pain syndrome
- Coping with peripheral neuropathy
- Managing postherpetic neuralgia
- Dealing with trigeminal neuralgia

More than 15 million people in the United States suffer from nerve pain, called *neuralgias* and *neuropathies.* These conditions differ greatly in symptoms and treatments.

In this chapter, you find out more information about the different types of nerve conditions and chronic nerve pain.

Understanding Your Network of Nerves

Your body's network of nerves, called the *peripheral nervous system,* relays messages back and forth between your *central nervous system* (your brain and spinal cord) and the rest of your body. The network is stunningly intricate and complicated, which is probably because it has a really important job. It's responsible for everything from helping you move from point A to point B, to enabling you to feel sensations of pain and hot and cold temperatures, as well as the touch of a loved one's hand. It also helps maintain your heartbeat, digestion, and other vital body functions. (For more on the peripheral nervous system, see Chapter 2.)

You can injure the peripheral network and its nerve messengers in a number of ways — for example through an accident or as a result of diseases, such as diabetes and rheumatoid arthritis. Even treatments for some diseases — such as chemotherapy for cancer — can injure your nerves. If such damage occurs, some of your nerves may stop working altogether. Or they may go haywire on you and send mixed-up pain messages. For example, if you've damaged nerves, instead of feeling major pain when your neighbor's 120-pound dog leaps joyfully on your foot, you may feel merely a tingling sensation. On the other hand, nerve damage may make you so exquisitely sensitive to touch that even putting a cotton sock on your foot can cause excruciating pain.

The different types of nerve pain are associated with constant or recurring pain that doesn't get better. However, the type of pain that is experienced can vary. It can be a feeling that's like burning, numbness, tingling, a stabbing sensation, or feeling like pins and needles are pricking you, or feeling like you're receiving an electric shock.

Considering Complex Regional Pain Syndrome (CRPS)

Complex regional pain syndrome (CRPS) is a painful condition of the arm, hand, leg, or foot. The major symptom is intense pain out of all proportion to the type of injury that initially set it off. CRPS frequently develops in the hand, along with restriction of shoulder motion on that same side of the body (called *shoulder-hand syndrome*). (See Chapter 7 for more information about CRPS.)

CRPS causes burning pain, sweating, swelling, and disturbances of color and temperature in the affected area, which is often blotchy, purple, pale, or red. It also causes shiny and thin skin, stiffness in the affected joints, weakness and wasting of muscles, changes in the overlying skin and nails, and a limited range of motion. Not a pretty picture.

Unhappily, the pain and other symptoms of CRPS worsen over time. The sympathetic nervous system may be the culprit in maintaining the pain. (See Chapter 2 for information on the sympathetic nervous system.) Often, CRPS is set off by an injury, even a minor one. Mere bug bites can trigger the condition! Sometimes the cause isn't known.

CRPS may develop in three typical stages.

- **Stage I can last about three months.** You may feel a burning pain, stiffness in your joints, sweating, and warmth in the affected area. Other (rather odd) symptoms may include fast-growing nails and hair, thin and dry skin, and blotchy, purple, pale, or red skin color.
- **Stage II typically follows and can last for a year.** Swelling increases, and your skin in the affected area cools and becomes extremely sensitive to touch. Even the touch of a bed sheet can cause excruciating pain. The pain also typically becomes diffuse, and you may feel stiff.

- **Stage III is the last stage.** At this point, alas, the condition is permanent. The pain may cover your entire limb. Your joints may be very stiff.

If it's caught and treated in time, you can keep CRPS in a holding pattern and prevent it from ever advancing any further than Stage 1.

Physical therapy is the cornerstone of treatment for CRPS, and the priority is to restore your function and keep your body from becoming any weaker due to immobility. For tough cases, *prednisone,* a steroid medication, may help you considerably.

Sympathetic nerve blocks and a procedure called *spinal cord stimulation,* in which an electrode inside the spine elicits low-dosage impulses, also helps some people with CRPS.

Getting on Your Nerves: Peripheral Neuropathy

Peripheral neuropathy is well-named. *Peripheral* means beyond (in this case, away from the brain and the spinal cord and out into the body). *Neuro* means nerves, and *pathy* means disease. So, peripheral neuropathy describes conditions caused by damage to the nerves connecting the brain and spinal cord to the rest of the body (the peripheral nervous system).

Peripheral neuropathy has many causes. It occurs most commonly in people with diabetes mellitus and those who abuse or are dependent on alcohol.

Suffering the symptoms

The symptoms of peripheral neuropathy depend on which nerve or nerves are damaged. The following list of symptoms is adapted from information from the National Institutes of Health.

Sensation changes

Damage to sensory nerves can cause nerve pain, sensations of tingling or numbness, or an inability to determine your joint position, which, in turn, causes a lack of coordination. For many neuropathies, the symptoms begin in the feet and then move toward the center of the body.

Movement difficulties

Damage to motor nerves interferes with muscle control and can cause weakness, loss of muscle bulk, and loss of dexterity. Other muscle-related symptoms may include

- Cramps
- Lack of muscle control
- Difficulty or inability to move a part of the body (paralysis)
- Muscle atrophy
- Muscle twitching
- Difficulty breathing or swallowing
- Falling (from legs buckling or tripping over your own toes)
- Lack of dexterity (such as being unable to button a shirt)

Autonomic symptoms

The autonomic nerves control your involuntary or semivoluntary functions, such as the control of your internal organs and your blood pressure. Damage to autonomic nerves can cause many symptoms and signs, including

- Blurred vision
- Decreased ability to sweat
- Dizziness that occurs when standing up or fainting that's associated with a drop in blood pressure
- Heat intolerance with exertion (decreased ability to regulate body temperature)
- Nausea or vomiting after meals
- Stomach bloating
- Feeling full after eating a small amount (early satiety)
- Diarrhea or constipation
- Unintentional weight loss
- Urinary incontinence
- Feeling of incomplete bladder emptying
- Difficulty with starting to urinate (urinary hesitancy)
- Male impotence

Tagging the types

Peripheral neuropathies are common, especially among older people, and can cause both acute and chronic pain problems. More than a hundred different types of peripheral neuropathy exist, with many different causes. For example, *Bell's palsy* can be caused by a facial nerve becoming swollen or inflamed. It causes paralysis or weakness on one side of the face. Peripheral neuropathies are classified according to their symptoms and cause.

Anyone who suffers from nerve problems (or who loves someone who does) needs to know these two terms:

- **Polyneuropathies,** which are what most neuropathies are, occur when more than one peripheral nerve stops working or goes haywire at once, causing weakness and/or pain. Many conditions can cause polyneuropathies, including diabetes, cancer, and other diseases. Often, polyneuropathy affects the same nerves on both sides of the body, and frequently the problem begins in the legs. Polyneuropathy can affect the sensory, motor, and autonomic systems. Polyneuropathies in all these systems can occur together at one time. Polyneuropathies tend to progress slowly and become chronic over months and years.
- **Mononeuropathy** refers to damage to only one nerve. Individual nerves are injured or crowded out, compressed, or stretched by organs, discs, and other anatomic structures, especially if the nerve passes through a narrow space (called *entrapment neuropathy*). The symptoms that occur depend on the nerve that's involved. Mononeuropathies have many causes, including

    - Physical injury or trauma of a nerve caused by an accident
    - Long-lasting pressure on a nerve, caused by inactivity, such as when you're confined to a wheelchair or bed
    - Overuse of structures surrounding a nerve through such actions as typing, running a checkout stand, or other repetitive motions (for example, carpal tunnel syndrome, caused by compression of the nerve that extends through the wrist)
    - Damage to a disc in the spine, which causes pressure on a nerve

  Nerves come in different varieties, depending on whether they're motor, autonomic, sensory, or mixed nerves (with sensory, motor and autonomic components). A mononeuropathy can involve one or all of the following:

    - Damage to a nerve that controls muscle movement (motor nerves), causing reduction of strength and dexterity
    - Damage to a sensory nerve, which detects sensations, such as cold or pain
    - Damage to a nerve that affects the heart, blood vessels, bladder, intestines, or other internal organs *(autonomic neuropathy)*
    - *Mononeuropathy multiplex,* when several isolated nerves are injured at once

The Neuropathy Association

If you have neuropathic pain, the Neuropathy Association can be a great resource for information and emotional support. Here's a description of how to contact the organization and some of the key programs it has to offer:

The Neuropathy Association, 60 E. 42nd St., Suite 942, New York, NY 10165; phone: 212-692-0662; Web site `www.neuropathy.org`. The Neuropathy Association has 50,000 members, with approximately 120 support groups throughout the United States and abroad providing public awareness, patient support, education, and advocacy. At present, seven Neuropathy Centers are available at major university hospitals in the United States. The Web site offers a list of neurologists and support groups by state.

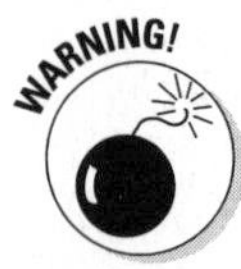

If you have peripheral neuropathy, you're at risk for additional nerve injury at your body's pressure points. Avoid putting weight on these areas for long periods of time; for example, don't lean on your elbows or sit in one position for lengthy periods.

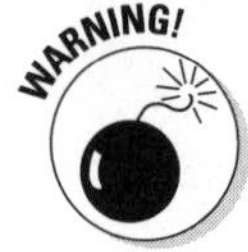

If you have chronic polyneuropathy, you can lose your ability to sense temperature and pain. As a result, you can severely burn yourself and not even know it. You can also develop open sores and calluses, especially on your feet, as the result of injury or prolonged pressure. Visually check your body, especially your feet, at least every day. Wear socks and don't go barefoot in or out of the house. Be sure to check between your toes. In addition, keep your feet clean and dry to prevent calluses and sores from developing. You should also look inside your shoes a few times each day to discover rocks or any other objects that may rub against your feet and cause sores.

To guard against burns, check the temperature of the water before you take a bath or shower. Measure the water temperature with a thermometer and make sure that the temperature setting of your hot-water heater is not set above 125° F (52°C). Also, use a part of your body that has normal sensation (such as your elbow) to check for hot surfaces.

Preventing peripheral neuropathies

Some causes of neuropathy are under your control. For example, if you have diabetes, controlling your blood sugar level is extremely important to prevent the death of nerve fibers. If you or a loved one drinks a lot of alcohol, do everything you can now to beat this dependence. Or, if you're being treated with chemotherapy, ask your doctor to prescribe one of the new medicines available to prevent nerve damage. Ask about one of the drugs presently being developed that includes neuroprotective and neurotrophic agents (also called nerve growth factors).

Eating a diet high in B vitamins (in meats, fish, eggs, low-fat dairy foods, and fortified cereals) is also preventive for neuropathy.

Major types of polyneuropathy

Many different types of polyneuropathies can cause chronic pain, including these key ones:

- **Diabetes-related polyneuropathy** has the dubious distinction of being the most common form of peripheral neuropathy. In this condition, high blood sugar levels of uncontrolled diabetes slowly destroy nerve cells. About 50 percent of people with diabetes develop peripheral neuropathy.
- **Nutritional polyneuropathy** is common among people who are malnourished or alcoholic. The cause is usually a lack of B vitamins, especially B1, B12, and folic acid. Poor diet, digestive problems, and long-term use of some medications can cause vitamin deficiencies. Alcoholism also depletes the body of B vitamins.
- **Rheumatoid arthritis** can cause a number of painful nerve conditions, such as entrapment neuropathies, which are caused by chronic compression of a nerve in a narrow space.
- **Alcoholic polyneuropathy** is caused by toxic effects of heavy long-term drinking. The condition can be hard to distinguish from nutrition-related neuropathies because of the loss of B vitamins that comes with heavy drinking. People who've been alcoholic for 10 years or more are at high risk for alcoholic polyneuropathy.
- **Polyneuropathy due to cancer and cancer treatments** strike many people. In fact, some chemotherapies used for cancer treatments can damage peripheral nerves.
- **Polyneuropathies caused by inherited disorders** are rare, but occur. Examples are: *Charcot-Marie-Tooth disease,* which is a group of disorders that affect peripheral nerves (named after the scientists who discovered it), and *amyloid polyneuropathy,* a progressive condition of the sensory and motor systems.
- **Toxic neuropathies** are caused by exposure to industrial agents or pesticides, such as acrylamide and carbon disulfide, or to metals, such as arsenic and lead. They can also be caused by drugs such as phenytoin (Dilantin), used for epilepsy, and isoniazid, used for tuberculosis.
- **Guillain-Barre syndrome** is caused by the body's immune system attacking nerves in the body. The condition can lead to paralysis.

In addition to these conditions, diseases of the kidneys, thyroid, and liver, as well as infections can cause polyneuropathies.

Treating peripheral neuropathies

Treatment for peripheral neuropathies begins with identifying and treating the condition causing the problem (such as rheumatoid arthritis or diabetes) or getting rid of the cause (such as consuming too much alcohol or overexposure to lead). If this first approach is successful, the neuropathy may get better, and painful symptoms may go away. If painful symptoms won't budge, the next steps are to relieve them as much as possible and prevent immobility and deconditioning. A number of treatment choices are available, and a combination of several approaches may be most successful.

You can use many types of medications to relieve the pain of peripheral neuropathy. You can treat milder pain with over-the-counter drugs, such as acetaminophen (Tylenol) or aspirin. Stronger pain may require prescription pain medications, such as codeine, Demerol, or morphine. For electric-like pain, doctors also prescribe anticonvulsants, such as carbamazepine (Tegretol) and gabapentin (Neurontin). Serotonin norepinephrine reuptake inhibitor (SNRI) antidepressants, such as duloxetine (Cymbalta), are also used. Some people find that capsaicin cream (Zostrix), the substance found in hot peppers, or the topical numbing cream, lidocaine, to be helpful. Lidocaine is also available in a prescribed patch (Lidoderm).

If you have peripheral neuropathy, you need to know that both physical and occupational therapy are important to build muscle strength and control, and prevent deconditioning. If the neuropathy is severe, wheelchairs, splints, and other assistive devices may be necessary to help you maintain your basic functions and carry out daily activities. Many people use special frames to keep their bedclothes from touching tender areas.

Pain in the Face: Trigeminal Neuralgia

Trigeminal neuralgia (TN) is nerve pain in the cheekbone area, where the trigeminal nerve is located. Your *trigeminal nerve* is responsible for sensations on your face, and it's the motor nerve controlling the muscles you use to chew. If you develop trigeminal neuralgia (also called *tic douloureux*), you'll experience episodes of sudden and sharp facial pain.

TN usually strikes near one side of the mouth and shoots toward the ear, eye, or nostril on the same side. Episodes last from two seconds to two minutes. Some people can have a hundred episodes a day. People with TN often describe the pain as intense and excruciating.

Unfortunately, TN episodes can worsen over time, and the time between the attacks shortens. In addition, a dull ache or burning may occur between episodes. Symptoms are confined to tissues innervated by the trigeminal nerve, running on one side of the face only.

The pain may be triggered by such seemingly innocuous things as a light touch on the skin, mild breezes (which most people enjoy), as well as by everyday acts, such as talking and eating. In order to prevent attacks, many people hold their faces as immobile and expressionless as possible while talking and eating. If you talk to someone with TN who seems emotionless, he is probably trying to prevent the pain by using inscrutable expressions.

Bouts of TN can stop for several months or longer. But the bad news is that they come back, sometimes with a vengeance.

TN most commonly occurs in middle and later life, but it can occur in all ages. TN affects women more often than men. Often the cause of TN is difficult to detect. Sometimes it's caused by multiple sclerosis, a tumor, or an aneurysm pressing on a nerve.

In the recent past, doctors tried to eliminate the pain of TN with techniques such as injecting the trigeminal nerve with alcohol or a procedure called *balloon rhizotomy,* which destroys the affected part of the nerve.

Recently, surgeons have successfully relieved pressure on the trigeminal nerve by separating blood vessels from it. However, if you or a loved one is elderly, a procedure called *radiofrequency rhizotomy* is still the preferred procedure because recovery is easier.

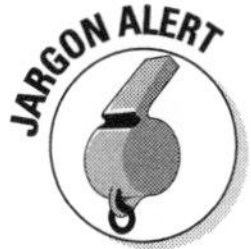

Gamma radiosurgery, a nonivasive procedure that uses beams of radiation to the trigeminal root, successfully treats TN in 4 out of 5 people.

Anticonvulsants, such as carbamazepine (Tegretol) and phenytoin (Dilantin), are used to treat TN. Other drugs used to treat TN include antidepressants, muscles relaxants, and opioids.

The Trigeminal Neuralgia Association

If you have Trigeminal Neuralgia, the Trigeminal Neuralgia Association can be a great resource for information and emotional support. Here's a description of how to contact the organization and some of the key programs it has to offer.

Trigeminal Neuralgia Association, 925 Northwest 56th Terrace, Suite C, Gainesville, FL 32605; e-mail `tnanational@tna-support.org`; phone 352-331-7009 or 800-923-3608; Web site `www.tna-support.org`. TNA provides one-on-one patient support through its toll-free telephone lines and its Web site and helps maintain more than 65 local support groups throughout the United States, Canada, Europe, and Australia.

Postherpetic Neuralgia

Until a vaccine for chicken pox first became available in 1995, most children suffered from the infection, which also made some of them vulnerable to developing a painful condition in adulthood called *shingles.* Now vaccinated children won't get shingles when they grow up. Unfortunately, everyone else who suffered through chicken pox before then — and that's most readers! — is at risk for developing shingles.

Shingles causes painful blisters in a band on the torso or around the nose and eyes. Both chicken pox and shingles are caused by an infection of one or more nerves with a virus called varicella-zoster. About 15 percent of patients who develop shingles go on to develop a painful condition called *postherpetic neuralgia* (PHN). If an initial bout of shingles is severe, it's even more likely to cause PHN. Both shingles and PHN primarily strike older people ages 65 and older.

PHN causes throbbing, aching, itching, and other painful symptoms that can last for years. The affected area can become so sensitive that even a slight touch can be excruciatingly painful.

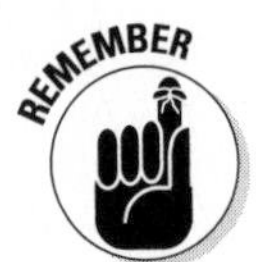

Getting immunized (even if you've had chicken pox) with the varicella vaccine may reduce the chances of getting shingles or PHN. In addition, taking oral acyclovir, used to treat outbreaks caused by the herpes viruses, may also be preventive. The faster you take these drugs, the more effective they'll be.

As with TN, the drugs used most frequently for treating PHN are anticonvulsants, such as carbamazepine (Tegretol) and phenytoin (Dilantin). Other drugs used to treat this condition are antidepressants, muscles relaxants, and opioids. Some people find capsaicin cream (Zostrix), the substance found in hot peppers, or the topical numbing cream, lidocaine, to be helpful. Lidocaine is also available in a patch, available by prescription (Lidoderm). Epidural steroid injections, which places the anti-inflammatory cortisone directly around spinal nerves, may also be helpful in bringing relief.

Chapter 12

Cancer Pain

In This Chapter

- Discovering who suffers from chronic cancer pain
- Understanding the World Health Organization's pain position
- Exploring helper analgesics for advanced cancer pain

Many people fear the pain that's caused by cancer more than anything else about the disease, including death. However, while pain management for people with cancer is still evolving, many alternatives for pain control are available to you and your loved ones with cancer. This chapter discusses the major types of medical treatment for cancer pain. Many people also find that complementary and alternative methods, such as biofeedback and acupuncture, are helpful for cancer pain. For more information on these methods, see Chapter 15.

Frightening and Shockingly Common: Cancer

Perhaps nothing is more frightening than hearing the words, "You have cancer." And it's incredible to think that men have a 1 in 2 chance of hearing these words from their doctor in their lifetime, and women have a 1 in 3 chance of getting this diagnosis.

More than 100 types of cancer can invade virtually every part of your body, from your skin and bones to your internal organs and your blood. All types of cancer are caused by abnormal runaway cells that, for some reason, begin to replicate wildly. These turncoat cells sometimes spread to other parts of your body and attack healthy tissue. It's this disease process, called *metastasis,* that makes cancer such a monster and that also can lead to severe, long-term pain.

The cruel truth is that chronic pain often accompanies cancer. According to the National Cancer Institute, 70 to 90 percent of people with advanced cancer have pain, and about a third of people with early cancers also have pain. Yet many types of cancer, such as leukemia and lymphoma, are not painful at all.

In general, the painful cancers are those that cause *tumors* (growths of tissue that group together in a mass).

Cancer pain has been described as aching, sharp, burning, and throbbing. It is usually caused by tumors that are growing and pressing in on nociceptors in healthy tissues, organs, and vessels. (For an explanation of nociceptors, see Chapter 2.) Bone pain is a common consequence of advanced cancer. It is the result of the disease moving to the spine, skull, or other parts of the skeleton. Bone pain is most common for patients with advanced cancers of the lung, bronchus, breast, rectum, prostate, colon, and kidney. Other types of cancer pain are caused by:

- Surgery to remove tumors
- A low blood supply due to blood vessels squeezed by tumors
- Inflammation due to the damage caused by growing tumors
- Musculoskeletal pain caused by immobility

Unfortunately, you can get hit with all these types of pain. In addition, the cancer may secrete chemicals in the region of the tumor that can cause pain. Treating the cancer can help relieve this pain.

If you or a loved one has cancer and you experience changes in your bowel and bladder function and/or a sharp pain in your back or neck, the cancer may have reached your spine. This metastasizing can cause paralysis and other problems, so get help right away. The tumor can be treated by radiation or surgery.

It's not a pleasant prospect, but *breakthrough pain,* or pain overlaying pain, is common for people with cancer. Breakthrough pain occurs when the individual has a continuous level of pain and then, despite using painkillers, even more pain breaks through, causing the pain level to soar. More than half of people with cancer report this type of severe pain. Breakthrough pain is often treated with opiates. A short-acting drug may be combined with a long-acting drug to combat breakthrough pain.

Shingles pain and cancer

Shingles, a painful re-outbreak of the chicken pox virus that you had as child, can strike people with cancer because their immune systems are so impaired. Shingles attacks can lead to post-herpetic neuralgia, which is extremely painful and difficult to treat. (For more information on post-herpetic neuralgia, see Chapter 11.) Treatment for shingles includes painkillers, as well as sedatives, antidepressants, and antiseizure medications.

If you have breakthrough pain at predictable intervals, head it off by taking a painkiller a half hour or so *before* the pain usually strikes.

The WHO? The World Health Organization

Yes, the WHO was a '70s rock group, but there's also the WHO as in the World Health Organization, an international group devoted to medical issues. According to WHO, about 90 percent of all cancer pain is treatable. In fact, WHO developed a *treatment ladder,* shown in Figure 12-1, which is widely used by physicians around the world as a guideline for treating cancer pain.

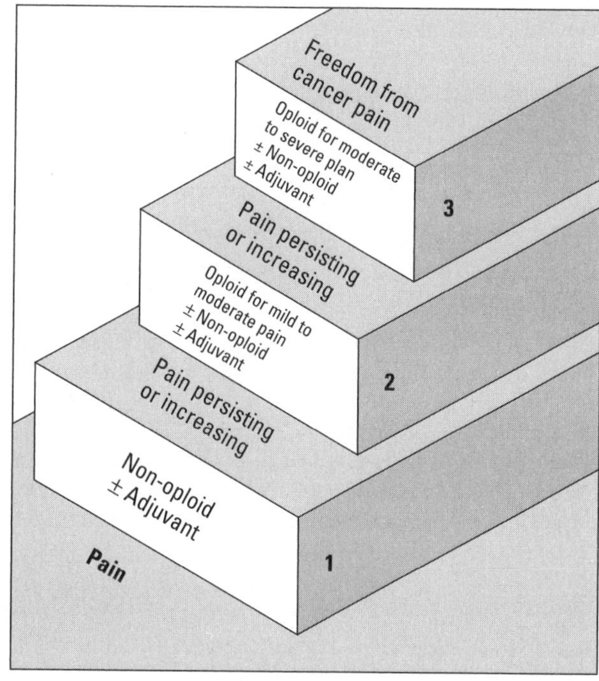

www.who.int/cancer/palliative/painladder/en/index.html

Figure 12-1: WHO analgesic ladder.

The American Cancer Society's position on pain medicines

Many people fear becoming addicted to pain medicines. But, in fact, the American Cancer Society's official position is the following: "People who take cancer pain medicines, as prescribed by the doctor, rarely become addicted to them: Addiction is a common fear of people taking pain medicine. Such fear may prevent people from taking the medicine."

The American Cancer Society also says that fear of possible addiction may cause family members to encourage a cancer patient to "hold off" as long as possible between doses. This is a bad idea! Instead, pain should be treated before it hits a peak. Otherwise, it's much harder to control it.

When opioids (also known as narcotics) — the strongest pain relievers available — are used for pain, they rarely cause addiction. When you're ready to stop taking opioids, the doctor gradually lowers the amount of medicine you're taking. By the time you stop using the drug, the body has had time to adjust. Talk to your doctor, nurse, or pharmacist about how to use pain medicines safely and discuss any concerns you have about addiction.

The analgesic ladder has three steps:

1. **Start with non-opioid analgesics for mild pain.**
2. **If non-opioids don't provide relief, move to weak opioids in addition to, or without, a non-opioid.**
3. **If the weaker opioids don't work, use stronger opioids for more severe pain or combine non-opioids with stronger opioids in this stage.**

In 2006, on the 20th anniversary of the launching of the WHO analgesic ladder, Dr. Kathleen Foley, former chair of the WHO Expert Committee on Cancer Pain Relief and Active Supportive Care, made important clarifications to the WHO analgesic ladder. Many of these suggestions are important to understand if you or a loved one has cancer pain.

- Your goals as a cancer patient and your doctor's goals should be to
  - Increase your hours of pain-free sleep
  - Relieve your pain when you're resting
  - Relieve your pain when you're standing or active
- Drugs alone can usually give you adequate relief from pain caused by cancer.
- The drug must be given in the right dose and at the right time.
- Taking all pain-killing drugs by mouth is preferred.

- Take your drugs by the clock for persistent pain. In other words, take painkillers according to directions at the prescribed times, not as needed or when you think of it.
- The right dose of an analgesic is the dose that relieves your pain. For example, the dose of oral morphine may range from as little as 5 mg to more than 1,000 mg depending on the patient's tolerance level.
- Adjuvant drugs should be prescribed as indicated. (For information about adjuvant drugs, check out the upcoming section "Checking Out Helper Drugs.")
- Pay attention to detail. Be sure to tell your doctor(s) whether the painkillers you're taking are working. Maybe you need a different drug. Your goal is to receive the maximum benefit with as few side effects as possible.

Educating Yourself about Opioids

If you or a loved one has extensive tumors, you may quickly progress to the third step on the WHO ladder. (See the section "The WHO? The World Health Organization," earlier in this chapter, for more on this ladder.) If so, opioids are the core treatment for your cancer pain. Different types of opioids help with different types of pain.

- **Short-acting opiods:** If pain strikes primarily when you're active, such as when you're shopping at the grocery store, visiting your grandchildren, or doing housework, then your doctor may prescribe a short-acting opioid to help you continue with these activities. Examples of short-acting opiods are oxycodone or hydromorphone.
- **Long-acting opiods:** If your pain is a constant companion, your doctor may prescribe long-acting opioids. Examples of long-acting opioids are MS Contin, OxyContin, Methadone, and Duragesic. You may also need a low dose of a short-acting opioid.

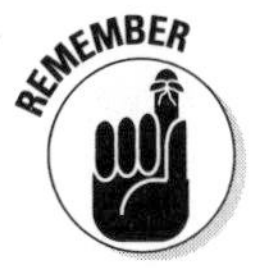

Unfortunately, most people who've been taking opioids for a long period of time develop a tolerance to the opioid that they're using for pain. Tolerance means that it takes increasing dosages to achieve the same level of comfort that you were getting from your opioid medication. (For more information on tolerance to opioids, see Chapter 14.) Your doctor may use several methods to help you if you develop tolerance, including rotating with another opioid and adding in another type of drug called an *NMDA antagonist,* which can reduce pain sensitization within the central nervous system.

If your cancer progresses, you may not be able to take medication by mouth because of nausea. Fentanyl is an opioid available in a skin patch. It skips the digestive system altogether and is one substitute option. (If you and your doctor are considering Fentanyl patches, be sure to see the warning about the patch in Chapter 14.)

Your medical providers can also give you opioids by other routes. Less invasive methods include injections or infusions in muscles, veins, or under your skin. More invasive methods include inserting tubes in the space around the spinal cord *(epidural catheters)* or in the spinal cord *(intrathecal catheters).*

In addition, *patient-controlled analgesic devices* (PCAs) offer you the flexibility to control the delivery of your pain medication when you need it (within a limit set by your doctor). PCAs are usually used for intravenous (IV) opioids, which means that the opioid goes into your vein through tubing.

The handy devices can even be carried in your pocket. When you feel pain, you push a button, and pain medicine is delivered through the tube. Because you're the one with the pain, only you push the button.

You may decide that you'd rather live with the pain of cancer than put up with the drowsiness, hallucinations, and other side effects that can occur with opioids. Obviously, this choice is up to you.

If the opioids you're taking make you feel drowsy and/or confused, your doctors may be able to prescribe other medications to help with these side effects, such as stimulants or helper pain drugs (called *adjuvants*). If this approach is successful, you may be able to lower the dose of the opioid you are taking.

Checking Out "Helper" Drugs

If you or a loved one has side effects from cancer medications and/or the drugs are not managing your pain, adding helper drugs, called *adjuvant analgesics* may work for you. (*Adjuvant* means something that helps or assists.)

Adjuvant analgesics don't relieve pain on their own, but instead can boost the relief given by analgesics when taken along with them. Your doctor may prescribe these medications for you along with opioids and NSAIDs. Adjuvants are often used for bone pain and may also be prescribed together, such as an antidepressant and a bisphosphonate.

The following list gives examples of frequently used helper drugs for cancer.

- **Antidepressants,** such as amitriptyline (Elavil) and nortriptyline (Pamelor), can provide nerve pain relief and help people sleep better. Side effects may include dizziness and gastrointestinal problems. The drugs usually take a couple of weeks to take effect.

Resources for people with cancer pain

If you or a loved one has cancer, you have access to a wide range of valuable services, including a Web page on pain management and support networks of people with the condition. Resources include

American Cancer Society (ACS); phone 800-ACS-2345, 866-228-4327 for TTY; Web site `www.cancer.org`. ACS provides a Web page about pain management for people with cancer: click Coping with Physical and Emotional Changes on the ACS site index. ACS also publishes the *American Cancer Society Guide to Pain Control*, Revised Edition, $15.95, available online at the society's bookstore.

Cancer*Care*, 275 Seventh Ave., Floor 22, New York, NY 10001; phone 800-813-HOPE (4673); Web site `www.cancercare.org`. Cancer*Care*'s programs include free counseling, education, and practical help provided by trained oncology social workers.

Cancer Hope Network, 2 North Road, Suite A, Chester, NJ 07930; phone 877-467-3638; Web site `www.cancerhopenetwork.org`. The Cancer Hope Network matches patients with trained volunteers who have gone through similar experiences.

The Wellness Community, 919 18th St. NW, Suite 54, Washington, DC 20006; phone 888-793-WELL; Web site `www.thewellness community.org`. The Wellness Community provides free, professionally led support groups, educational workshops, nutrition and exercise programs, and mind/body classes for people with cancer.

- **Anticonvulsants,** such as Neurontin (Gabapentin), were originally developed to help control seizures, but they can also relieve tingling or burning from nerve injury (neuropathic pain). (See Chapter 11 for information on neuropathic pain.) Like antidepressants, the benefits of anticonvulsants take awhile to kick in. If you're taking an anticonvulsant, your doctor will want to run drug tests frequently because these drugs can damage the liver and reduce the number of red and white cells in the blood.
- **Bisphosphonates,** such as Actonelor Fosamax, are drugs that help slow down bone loss. They're used to treat cancers that have metastasized to the bones. Cancer cells in the bones cause the breakdown of too much tissue, weakening bone and putting you at high risk for fractures. The breakdown of bone cells also causes pain. Bisphosphonates can reduce both the pain and fractures. On the down side, bisphosphonates may cause upper gastrointestinal disorders, such as esophagitis, esophageal ulcer, and gastric ulcer.
- **Radiopharmaceuticals** are targeted drugs injected into an individual's veins. They accumulate in cancerous bone tissue and give off radiation that kills the cancer cells and can significantly relieve pain. Strontium chloride Sr 89 (strontium-89) is the most common radiopharmaceutical used to treat bone cancer or cancer that has metastasized to the bone.

When Medicine Isn't Enough

The harsh reality is that medications don't always conquer cancer pain. If this situation is the case for you or your loved one, several other treatments can reduce pain by shrinking tumors. Radiation is often the first choice. In addition, nerve blocks or implanted pumps may help relieve pain. When a tumor presses on nerves or other body parts, surgery may also help. (See Chapter 16 for more information on nerve blocks, pain pumps, and surgery.)

Part III

Managing Your Pain Medically

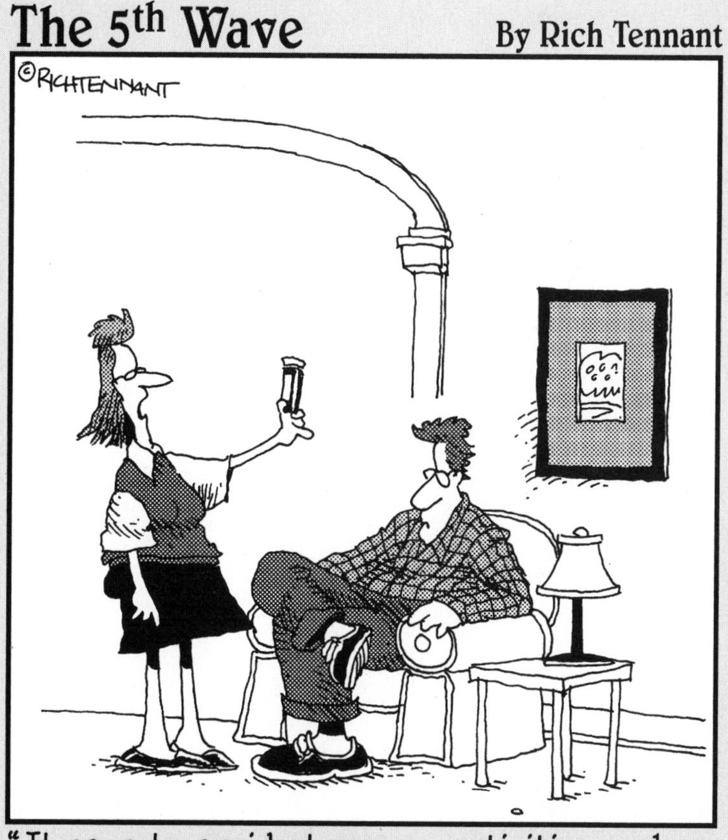

"It says to avoid strenuous activities such as wing walking, bear wrestling, or trying to find out if this medication is covered by your insurance company."

In this part . . .

This part gives you the information you need to start taking care of your chronic pain medically. We share information to help you put together an anti-pain team.

We cover the benefits and side effects of a wide range of drugs used against chronic pain. We also explore the potential benefits and risks of complementary and alternative medicine and help you separate the legit from the bogus. Finally, we give you an overview of the surgical options for chronic pain.

Chapter 13

Putting Together an Anti-Pain Team

In This Chapter

- Uncovering the right doctors
- Discovering the types of health-care providers available
- Checking out national resources and support groups
- Sharing information with your doctor

When you have a chronic pain condition, you need your own anti-pain team, but what on earth is that? Well, your treatment is likely to involve a number of medical professionals and paraprofessionals, such as a primary care physician (PCP), a medical specialist, a physical therapist, a massage therapist, a dietician, or others. Such experts are members of your anti-pain team.

Of course, you want a cracker-jack team to help tame your pain into a reasonable level of submission. To ensure the success of your team in combating your pain problem, enlist professionals with whom you're comfortable and who have the skills and experience to help you reduce your pain and actually enjoy your life. (Maybe you haven't had that experience for awhile!) Forming a team, though, doesn't just happen; it does require research on your part. To make your job easier, this chapter provides detailed information on what to look for in a doctor and questions to ask when assembling your team.

Understanding How a Team Helps You

If the word *team* scares you a little because you think you'll have to spend a lot of time managing the players, don't panic because the opposite is true.

Setting up an effective anti-pain team means that you'll spend less time with your doctors and other health providers and more time enjoying your life. With a skilled and efficient team, you won't have gaps in your care or treatment, which means you should have less pain. Also, the time you do spend with providers will be better spent, and you won't be going from health provider to health provider looking for relief that somehow never comes.

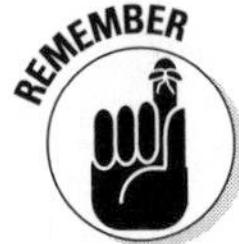

Once your team is assembled, be upfront with your care providers. The more the members of your team know about you and your chronic pain condition, the better they can do their jobs.

Assembling Your Team

You're the only one who knows what your pain feels like, so you're the only one who knows if and when your pain treatments are working. For these reasons, the person who should manage your anti-pain team is you.

An important responsibility of managing your team is to be informed about your condition or conditions so that you can communicate effectively with all the providers in your group. One way to educate yourself is to take advantage of resources available through national associations and support groups. (Read about these resources in the section "Educating Yourself as Much as Possible," later in this chapter.)

The first member on your team is your primary care physician (PCP), so you want to be extra careful when selecting this person. As the manager of your team, you'll be responsible, along with your PCP, for finding and recruiting the rest of the players.

An anti-pain team that works for someone else, even if that person is close to you, may not work well for you.

One of the first actions you should take as manager of your team is to make sure that you've lined up a qualified primary care physician who you feel respects and listens to you. A good primary care doctor will get to know you and your physical, psychological, and social situation. This big picture of you puts your doctor in a great position to help you take charge of your chronic pain. (The doctor acting in this capacity may also be a specialist such as a rheumatologist or pediatrician.)

What primary care physicians do

Primary care physicians hail back to the old-style family physician. In fact, your best choice for a primary care physician may be a family doctor whom you've been going to for many years.

The primary care physician looks at the whole person, not just one body part or disease state, which is particularly important because chronic pain affects all parts of your life. Many primary care physicians keep up to speed on treating pain and companion problems, such as depression and fatigue, and give you first-rate care. Often, they try to treat you before sending you to a specialist, such as a rheumatologist, cardiologist, or doctor who specializes in pain management.

Your primary care physician oversees all medical care. You see the doctor on a regular basis, and he conducts physicals to assess your overall health. He'll also order lab tests, refer you to and keep a list of the other doctors you see, and maintain records of your health conditions. In fact, the other doctors you see send a report back to your primary care physician every time you visit them. Your primary care physician also oversees all your medications, which helps prevent duplication, overmedication, and toxic drug reactions.

Your primary care physician may have taken care of you for years. In that case, use the following sections to assess her to make sure that continuing with this doctor is the right thing to do. If you're looking for someone new, use the guidelines in these sections to find the right person.

Primary care doctors come in different types with different backgrounds and skill sets, which may make a difference in your care.

- *General practitioners* or family doctors take care of the entire family. Their training enables them to diagnose and treat health problems of patients from childhood to older age. They're a great option if you prefer one doctor to get to know and take care of you and your whole family.
- *General internists* are trained in the wide range of adult health problems. As a general rule, they do not provide care for children.
- *Pediatricians* are internists who care for and treat children from birth through the teens. If your child has chronic pain, you'll want to find a pediatrician experienced in treating the condition causing the problem.
- *Geriatricians* are internists who care for and treat older adults. If you or a loved one is over age 65, geriatricians are a great choice because of their special training in taking care of age-related health problems. In addition, because chronic pain is common for older adults, geriatricians are usually quite knowledgeable about treating people who are hurting.

Resources for locating a PCP include these association Web sites where you can find lists of certified doctors who practice in every area of the country:

- **American Academy of Family Physicians:** `http://familydoctor.org`
- **American Board of Internal Medicine:** `www.abim.org`
- **American Academy of Pediatrics:** `www.aap.org`
- **American Geriatrics Society:** `www.americangeriatrics.org`

Searching for the Right Doctor

When looking for a PCP or any other doctor on your team, you need to know about their expertise level. In fact, you have the right to know this information. You also need to identify what's most important to you in your relationship with your doctors so that you can make the best choices. The following sections arm you with information to achieve both tasks.

Getting recommendations

How do you find the right doctors for your anti-pain team? If you have a good relationship with a physician — someone you respect and are comfortable with — you may want to start by talking to him. In addition, your family, friends, coworkers, and other health professionals can often help you.

Ask people you know these questions:

- What do you like about your primary care physician?
- Do you know any physicians who treat people with my condition?

You should collect several names because some physicians may not have some of the criteria that you'll want your doctor to meet. (For more on this topic, see the next section, "Figuring out what skills are important to you.") A doctor who is mentioned frequently may be a good one to check out.

If you need more help finding names of good doctors, your insurance provider may be a good resource. Also ask local doctors, local hospitals, or medical centers, medical societies, or medical schools in your community for the name of a doctor who treats your condition. You may even be able to call a county medical society.

In addition, if you belong to a managed-care plan, the plan's membership services office can give you a list of its approved doctors. We provide information on this topic in the sidebar called "Working within a managed-care plan" later on in this chapter.

Figuring out what skills are important to you

If you're like most people, you want your doctor to have great people skills. A 2005 survey of 2,267 adults by Harris Interactive Polls studied this issue. The researchers wanted to know what characteristics people look for when choosing a doctor. Eighty-five percent said it's extremely important for doctors to be respectful. They also wanted their doctors to carefully listen to their health concerns and questions (84 percent); be easy to talk to (84 percent); take their concerns seriously (83 percent); and be willing to spend enough time with them (81 percent). In the Harris survey, these people skills rated higher than good medical judgment (80 percent)!

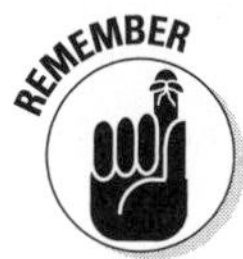

People skills are very important for doctors who treat patients with chronic pain because you can't measure hurting with blood tests or medical instruments. Pain is a subjective problem, and the only way the doctor can learn about it is through eye contact and conversation.

You also may have your own personal criteria for choosing a doctor. For example, many women prefer to go to female physicians, and some men prefer male doctors. Some people like to go to doctors who practice the same religion that they do. Some patients want to see only seasoned doctors who have been practicing for well over a decade. Others prefer that their doctors be in their early 30s because they feel that younger doctors are more aware of the latest treatments. Your personal criteria are important because they can affect your ability to relate to and trust your primary care physician. For example, if you're a woman who prefers female doctors, it may be because you don't feel comfortable taking your clothes off for a physical examination by a male doctor. Or, if you don't agree with your doctor's religious orientation, you may not trust her judgment when it comes to important medical decisions.

Don't talk yourself into a doctor who doesn't meet your criteria unless you are in a remote area and your options are very limited.

Checking out a doctor's qualifications

Not only is it important that your primary care doctor have great people skills and meet your personal criteria (see preceding section), but you'll also want your physician to be smart, up-to-date on new pain treatments and other important medical issues, and have great credentials.

When looking for a primary care physician, be prepared to do a little digging about her background and practice. A call to the doctor's office will probably give you the information you need. Doctors' staffs are usually trained to answer the following questions:

- **What are the doctor's professional credentials?** You want to know whether your doctor graduated from an accredited medical school. Ask the doctor's nurse or other staff where he went to medical school and then contact the Association of American Medical Colleges (AAMC) by calling 202-828-0400 or visiting its Web site at `www.aamc.org` to see whether the school is accredited.

  If the doctor graduated from a school in another country, the school won't be accredited by or listed on the AAMC Web site. However, you can check to see whether the country where the school is located uses U.S. standards to accredit its medical schools — 35 countries do so. The National Committee on Foreign Medical Education and Accreditation's Web site (`www.ed.gov`) lists these countries.
- **Is the doctor board certified?** One of the best ways to evaluate primary care physicians is to be sure that they're *board certified,* which means they had extra training after medical school in a field of medicine, such as family practice, internal medicine, or geriatrics, and passed a comprehensive examination in their specialty. To check out specific doctors, go to the American Board of Medical Specialties Web site at `www.abms.org` or call its hotline at 800-776-2378.
- **What are the doctor's professional affiliations?** Your doctor should have hospital privileges with a large, well-equipped hospital, which means he may admit patients to that hospital.

Evaluating whether a doctor fits your circumstances

Some doctors have great people skills or excellent medical qualifications, but other characteristics are deal breakers. For example, maybe you're interested in a particular doctor who is very successful at treating people with your condition, but the office isn't accessible by public transportation — and you don't drive or have a car.

Consider the following factors about a potential doctor's practice:

- **Type of health insurance:** Does the doctor accept your insurance? If not, it's a deal breaker. Keep looking.
- **Location of the office:** Is the office close by and convenient? Is parking easy to use? Is the office near public transportation?
- **Lab work:** Will you need to go to another location for blood tests? If so, how far away is it from the primary care physician's office? Is the lab that the doctor uses covered by your insurance?

- **Coverage:** Who will you see when the doctor isn't available? Are these doctors qualified? Do they see a lot of patients with your same health condition?
- **Hospital affiliation:** What hospital is the doctor affiliated with? Does it accept your insurance?
- **Physician extenders:** Do you feel comfortable in a practice that employs *physician extenders* (nurse practitioners or physician's assistants) that you may frequently see instead of the doctor?

Interviewing a doctor

If you've heard good things about a doctor who meets your needs (see preceding section), you're ready to interview him. Whenever possible, interview candidates for your anti-pain team in person before committing to a specific individual and a first medical appointment. An eye-to-eye meeting can tell you a lot about a doctor's people skills. Many doctors hold meet-and-greet appointments for this purpose so that you can sit and chat for 10 minutes or so and ask questions. The bad news is that the primary care physician may charge for this time, and your health insurance may not cover the costs of the appointment. But if you can swing the expense, it'll be worth it to help rule out doctors who aren't a good fit — and rule *in* physicians you like!

A major purpose of the interview is to discover the doctor's approach to managing pain. While many doctors are good at pain management, some primary care physicians don't focus on helping patients control pain, and they don't keep informed about new medications and techniques. When you go to your meet-and-greet meeting, ask the doctor or staff the following questions:

- **Do you have many patients with my type of chronic pain?** Of course, you should ask this question after you explain what your main problem is! The doctor doesn't have to give you an actual number, but should have a good idea what percentage of his practice has chronic pain. If he says less than 20 percent, proceed with caution. The doctor may not have as much experience as you'd like in treating patients with your condition.
- **How do you evaluate your patients' pain?** Hopefully, the doctor uses pain scales, a list of questions, or a similar technique to assess her patient's pain problem. (Read more about these evaluations in Chapter 17.) However, as long as the doctor makes a point to always discuss pain with her patients, this doctor still may be a great candidate.

- **What is your success rate in controlling my type of pain?** Of course, you'd love it if the doctor said, "100 percent!" but that number isn't realistic. However, the doctor saying something like, "Some people do well on XYZ, and others do well with ABC therapy," is a good sign that he's helping a number of people with a problem similar to yours, is willing to try different treatments to find the right one, and is having some success.
- **Do you have any special qualifications to treat my chronic pain?** Ideally, you'd like the doctor to have taken additional training in pain therapy, but a primary care physician with this type of qualification is hard to find; this issue should not be a deal breaker. If the doctor sees, diagnoses, and treats many patients with your condition, this hands-on experience may work well for you.
- **What is your approach to using medications to treat my type of chronic pain?** You're looking for a doctor willing to work with you to find the best medications for your chronic health problem.
- **What is your approach to using alternative or complementary medicine to treat my type of chronic pain?** You may prefer a doctor willing to try nontraditional approaches, such as acupuncture and biofeedback. If so, this question is important. If the doctor pooh-poohs these approaches, then he's not for you.
- **What is your approach to referring your patients to specialists, such as rheumatologists, cardiologists, or neurologists?** You want the doctor to be willing to refer you when your pain control needs are more specialized than treatments he can offer.
- **What pain treatments or therapies would you start with, and what would you do next if the first one doesn't work?** Your doctor should have a lot of experience with this issue. The answer should reflect this experience and be specific. If the doctor brushes off the question, proceed with caution.
- **What is your approach to treatments such as nerve blocks?** The answer to this question may be, "Only as a last resort." But the doctor should have some patients who have had these procedures. If not, he may not have enough experience treating patients with severe chronic pain.

Finding a specialist

A smoothly running anti-pain team addresses the major problems relating to your pain and makes you feel comfortable and safe, which often means including specialists who either focus on the condition itself or on pain management in general.

Condition specialists

Many people with chronic pain have a specialist on their team who helps them manage their particular condition and the pain it causes. For example, if you have migraines it's likely that a neurologist who specializes in caring for people with severe headaches is an important member of your team. Or, if you have cancer-related pain, it's a good bet that your oncologist is a central member of your team.

The following is a list of common pain problems and the specialists that treat them.

- **Arthritis:** Rheumatologists, orthopedic surgeons, physical medicine, and rehabilitation specialists
- **Asthma and allergies:** Allergists and otolaryngologists
- **Cancer-related pain:** Oncologists and anesthesiologists
- **Central pain syndrome:** Neurologists
- **Chest pain:** Cardiologists and pulmonologists
- **Colon and/or rectal pain:** Gastroenterologists and colon and rectal surgeons
- **Diabetes pain:** Endocrinologists
- **Digestive system problems:** Gastroenterologists
- **Ear, nose, throat, head or neck pain:** Otolaryngologists
- **Eye pain:** Ophthalmologists
- **Fibromyalgia:** Rheumatologists and immunologists
- **Headaches:** Neurologists and headache pain specialists with certificates of added qualification in headache management (see Chapter 6)
- **Inflammatory bowel problems:** Colon and rectal surgeons
- **Kidney pain:** Nephrologists
- **Lung pain:** Pulmonologist
- **Multiple sclerosis:** Neurologists
- **Neuropathic pain:** Neurologists
- **Occupational pain (chronic pain that is aggravated when at work):** Occupational medicine specialist
- **Pelvic floor pain (in woman):** Urogynecologists
- **Prostate pain in men:** Urologists

- **Skin conditions:** Dermatologists
- **Spinal cord and nervous system diseases:** Neurologists
- **Stomach pain:** Gastroenterologists and hepatologists
- **Stroke-related pain:** Neurologists
- **Urinary tract pain:** Urologists and nephrologists

You can read more about these pain-causing conditions in Part II.

Pain management specialists

If your pain is *intractable* (it won't go away or lessen), you may want to consider visiting a doctor who specializes in pain management. Pain specialists diagnose the cause of pain and then treat it. A pain specialist works closely with your primary care doctor to assess the cause of your pain and find an appropriate treatment option.

As with primary care doctors, pain specialists have different backgrounds and expertise:

- *Anesthesiologists* are traditionally known for making sure that patients are safe and pain-free during and after surgery or childbirth. In recent years, their role has expanded to include pain management outside the operating or delivery room.
- *Neurologists* diagnose and treat diseases of the nervous system, which processes pain signals throughout our bodies.
- *Neurosurgeons* perform surgery on the nervous system.
- *Psychiatrists* treat and diagnose mental health problems associated with chronic pain.
- *Physiatrists* specialize in physical medicine, a branch of medicine that deals with the treatment, prevention, and diagnosis of disease by physical means such as manipulation, massage, and exercise.

When looking for a pain specialist, make sure that you know the type of professional who you want to work with. For example, anesthesiologists are likely to prescribe medications for your pain. Neurologists or neurosurgeons are likely to suggest nerve blocks or surgeries if warranted. Physiatrists will do physical restoration and may prescribe medication, but do not perform surgery. And psychiatrists will conduct behavioral therapy or a similar approach.

For a comprehensive evaluation and approach to pain management, consider visiting a comprehensive pain clinic, which usually has all types of pain specialists on staff in addition to physical therapists and other professionals. Read about pain clinics in the upcoming "Locating a pain center" section.

The Web sites of these associations offer lists of pain specialists in every area of the country:

- **American Academy of Pain Management:** www.aapainmanage.org
- **American Academy of Pain Medicine:** www.painmed.org
- **National Pain Foundation:** www.nationalpainfoundation.org

Other pain professionals and paraprofessionals

Many types of professionals and paraprofessionals who aren't medical doctors can help you manage your pain. Some providers, such as physical therapists, are traditional members of health-care teams, while others are new to the mix. For example, more people than ever successfully use massage to help manage their pain; just a decade ago, massage therapy was regarded as a luxury.

The following are key health providers you may consider as members of your team:

- *Physical therapists* (PTs) may be among your best friends. Many people with chronic pain say that their PT is the one who makes them feel better day in and day out. (However, if you've ever had major orthopedic surgery, you probably encountered a PT who, at the peak of your post-surgical pain, made you get up and move around to get your lungs moving. Not a fun experience!)

  Physical therapists help their patients return function to injured or damaged parts of their bodies, improve the ability to move around, and relieve pain. They also use techniques that promote overall fitness and health, all of which contribute to pain reduction.

  Treatment by a PT can include electrical stimulation, hot packs, cold compresses, and ultrasound to relieve pain and reduce swelling. They may use traction or deep-tissue massage to relieve pain. Therapists also teach patients to use devices, such as crutches, prostheses (replacements for body parts), and wheelchairs. They also may show patients exercises to do at home to reduce pain and aid recovery.

  Some physical therapists treat a wide range of ailments; others specialize in areas such as pediatrics, geriatrics, orthopedics, sports medicine, neurology, and cardiopulmonary physical therapy.

PTs who are members of the American Physical Therapy Association are bound by its code of ethics and are licensed by the state in which they practice. You can find a list of credentialed PTs at its Web site (www.apta.org).

- *Occupational therapists* help people with chronic pain get along better in daily life and at work. They can help you learn or relearn how to carry out activities in new ways to lessen pain, such as using a computer or cooking in a different way than you've done before. If you have a permanent disability, such as a spinal cord injury or rheumatoid arthritis, they teach you how to use adaptive equipment, such as wheelchairs, *orthotics* (devises that help support a limb or other body part), and aids for eating and dressing. They can also design or make special equipment you may need at home or at work.

  To find a qualified occupational therapist, contact your state Occupational Therapy Association. All 50 states, the District of Columbia, and Puerto Rico have an association. Contact information for every state is on the American Occupational Therapy Association's Web site at www.aota.org.

- *Recreational therapists* use a variety of techniques, such as sports, dance, drama, and aqua-exercise, to help clients manage their pain. Often, you find them in hospitals and other facilities running beneficial exercise programs, such as warm water exercise for people with arthritis and other painful conditions or gentle sports programs for children with asthma. The National Council for Therapeutic Recreation Certification (www.nctrc.org/aboutnctrc.htm) is the nationally recognized credentialing organization for recreational therapists.

- *Dietitians* can help you plan special diets to better manage the condition causing your pain. They also help patients prevent and treat illnesses by promoting healthy eating habits and recommending dietary modifications, such as eating less salt for people with high blood pressure or consuming less sugar for people with diabetes. Look for a dietician who has received accreditation from the Commission on Accreditation for Dietetics Education at www.cdrnet.org.

- *Fitness instructors* can help people with pain enjoy exercise and get its benefits without causing new or further injury. Many organizations certify fitness instructors. One way to ensure that a certifying organization is reputable is to check whether it's accredited or seeking accreditation by the National Commission for Certifying Agencies (www.noca.org/ncca/accredorg.htm).

- *Massage therapists* use rubbing, stroking, and other manipulations on your soft tissues to improve your body's circulation and remove waste products from your knotted muscles. The treatment can loosen up and soothe a stiff and sore body.

Massage therapists can specialize in more than 80 different types of massage, such as Swedish massage (rubbing in the same direction as the flow of blood) and *acupressure* (applying pressure to key points on the skin). Talk with your primary care physician and/or physical therapist about the type of massage that would be most beneficial for you.

- *Orthotists and prosthetists (O and Ps)* help patients with disabling conditions of their arms, legs, or spine or with the loss of a limb by fitting and preparing orthopedic braces and prostheses. Materials originally developed for aerospace and new technologies have resulted in great advances in this industry. For example, people who have lost a foot can now purchase a special prosthesis for golf or tennis with custom muscle sensors and computer chips that enable them to comfortably enjoy their sport.

  If you need the services of these professionals, find a highly trained and competent provider because an ill-fitting devise can cause pain and loss of mobility. Look for a professional who is a member of the American Academy of Orthotists and Prosthetists (`www.opcareers.org`).

Educating Yourself as Much as Possible

Many other factors can influence the quality of your anti-pain team and the care it provides. For starters, the type of insurance you have can have wide-reaching effects on your care. For example, if you have fibromyalgia and the top fibro specialist in your town isn't covered by your insurance company, you may want to consider switching to a different plan.

Also, the type and quality of the hospital in which you're treated are keys to quality care. Recent studies have shown that patients at better hospitals have better results.

Last, roll up your sleeves and discover as much as possible about chronic pain and how to manage it. If you educate yourself, you'll make confident decisions.

Identifying a hospital

Depending on where you live, your health insurance, and other circumstances, you may not have a choice of hospitals available to you. However, hospitals differ greatly in staff competence, care quality, and success rates with different conditions. If you do have a choice, do a little detective work to find the best option for you. Here are some guidelines:

Working within a managed-care plan

If your insurance is through your employer or you are a Medicare beneficiary, you may be in a *managed-care plan*. These plans control the cost and delivery of health services by contracting with a network of doctors, hospitals, and other professionals.

Managed-care plans come in three major types:

- **Health Maintenance Organizations (HMOs)** contract with physicians, hospitals, and other providers who belong to their provider networks. Members select primary care physicians from the HMO's network, and that doctor oversees all aspects of the member's care. If you belong to an HMO, you can see a specialist or other "outside" providers, such as rheumatologists or physical therapists, only if your primary care physician authorizes it. If you visit a specialist on your own, your HMO won't pay for it.
- **Preferred Provider Organizations (PPOs)** are similar to HMOs, but provide more flexibility. They also contract with health-care providers to form provider networks. However, unlike HMOs, members don't have to have primary care providers, and they don't have to use one of the plan's contracted providers for their care. However, if you belong to a PPO, you pay less if you see the plan's doctors instead of someone outside the network, and you probably won't have to get a referral to see a specialist.
- **Point-Of-Service Plans (POSs)** are options in which members can choose to use an HMO or PPO each time they seek health care. Seeing a specialist depends on which alternative they choose.

It's important to understand how the plans operate because they often differ in how they work with primary care physicians and whether they allow referrals to pain and other specialists.

Two associations offer lists of managed-care plans for consumers in every area of the country. While they don't rate plans according to success in pain management, their evaluation measures show which plans are doing the best job of overall patient care:

- **The National Committee for Quality Assurance (NCQA)** evaluates and rates managed-care plans. NCQA's Health Plan Report Card (`http://hprc.ncqa.org`) is an interactive tool that can help consumers find health plans that fit their particular needs.
- **URAC,** which used to be called the Utilization Review Accreditation Commission until 1996 when its name was shortened, develops quality (accreditation) standards for managed-care plans. For a list of accredited managed-care programs, go to `http://webapps.urac.org/directory/dirsearch.asp`.

- Find out whether the hospital offers the full range of services needed to treat your condition and its expertise and success rate with it. For example, if you have rheumatoid arthritis and live in a rural area, your hospital may not have experience in treating your condition, and you may have to go out of your geographic area to find the care and pain control you need.

- Some government agencies or voluntary health organizations accredit or designate hospitals specializing in conditions, such as cancer, cardiac care, or rheumatology. Make sure that the hospital you're considering has received such an acknowledgment. To locate the appropriate contact information, check out the chapter in Part II that addresses your condition. For example, to find a hospital designated as a cancer care center, check with the National Cancer Institute or American Cancer Society. Its contact information is listed in Chapter 12.
- In some cases a hospital that conducts research into the cause and treatment of your condition is a good choice. To locate such hospitals, use the contact information provided in the chapter in Part II that relates to your condition.
- Find out whether the hospital has programs to improve patient safety and reduce medical errors. Most hospitals are now introducing such programs, and those that aren't are behind the times.
- Some states prepare reports showing outcomes for certain procedures, such as open-heart surgery. If your state publishes such information, find out the outcomes for the hospitals in your area.
- The Joint Commission on Accreditation of Healthcare Organizations (JCAHO) sets quality standards for hospitals. Reviews are done at least every three years. Most hospitals participate in this program, and it's a red flag when a facility doesn't follow JCAHO standards. To find hospitals in your area that adhere to JCAHO's quality standards, go to `www.jcaho.org`.

Locating a pain center

Being evaluated and treated at a pain center can be a lifesaver for people with relentless pain. Based on the understanding that chronic pain affects many areas of victims' lives, pain centers offer a broad range of evaluation and care. The staffs of pain centers typically include specialists from all medical disciplines, such as anesthesiologists, neurologists, neurosurgeons, physiatrists, psychiatrists, nurses, physical therapists, occupational therapists, counselors, nutritionists, and recreational therapists. Evaluation and treatment in pain centers can range from short-term and outpatient to extensive in-facility care.

The Commission on Accreditation of Rehabilitation Facilities (CARF) provides a listing of pain programs that meet its quality standards. Your health insurance may require that any program you visit be accredited by CARF (`www.carf.org`).

Exploring resources from condition-specific organizations

The old adage that information is power is particularly appropriate for managing chronic pain. The more you know about your health problem and the pain it causes, the better prepared you are to manage both. And, when you have up-to-date information about your condition and its treatments, you and your primary care physician can recruit a cracker-jack anti-pain team.

Be sure to look over the relevant chapter in Part II that addresses your pain condition and check out the resources listed there. In addition, the following Web sites offer information about managing pain and pain-causing conditions:

- **The National Pain Foundation:** `www.nationalpainfoundation.org`
- **The American Chronic Pain Association:** `www.theacpa.org`
- **The American Pain Foundation:** `www.painfoundation.org`

You can also find information specific to many pain-causing conditions on these Web sites:

- **The Cleveland Clinic:** `www.clevelandclinic.org`
- **Mayo Clinic:** `www.mayoclinic.com`
- **National Library of Medicine:** `www.nlm.nih.gov/medlineplus/healthtopics.html`

Joining a support group

The support and help of those who "have been there" and who also suffer from chronic pain can lessen your feelings of isolation, give comfort, and provide you with first-hand recommendations of providers and services. A first-rate support group focuses on positive ways to manage pain and doesn't wallow in the negatives of the condition. (In other words, support group meetings aren't pity parties.) Here are key resources for finding a group near you or on the Web:

- **The American Chronic Pain Association** (`www.theacpa.org`) has support groups across the country.
- **The American Pain Foundation's PainAid** (`http://painaid.painfoundation.org`) service is an interactive online community for

people with acute and chronic pain. It offers live chats, discussion boards, message boards, and Ask the Experts chat rooms.

- **The National Pain Foundation's My Community** (www.nationalpainfoundation.org/MyCommunity) offers a monitored online chat group and question and answer service.

Telling Your Doctors What They Need to Know

Incomplete and garbled information can result in a frustrating situation and a missed opportunity. If your doctors don't have complete and accurate information about you, their treatment of your health condition will likely be off target. When your health is at stake, being off target can have painful and serious consequences.

The following sections provide important topics to address so that your doctors have the information they need to give you first-class care.

Overcoming shyness

If you're like most people, your contacts with your doctors are one of the most intimate relationships you have. One of this book's authors, Dr. Kassan, puts it this way: "Some of my patients tell me things they don't tell anyone else. It's an honor." In fact, you, the patient, must tell your doctors the most intimate personal details about your health even if you've just met. Often, you'll also have to undress and allow the doctor to poke into private parts of your anatomy. Most people are uncomfortable with such exposure.

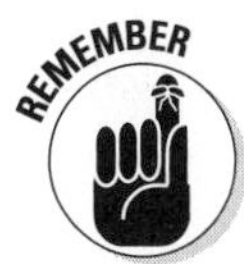

It's extremely important to override any feelings of discomfort and embarrassment you may have and to tell your doctor about all current and past health care problems that may be related to your condition.

Take Glenda, for example, who has had chronic pelvic floor pain for many years, but didn't make an appointment with her primary care doctor when she noticed blood in her urine. This situation went on for months until she finally had an annual physical, and lab tests revealed the problem. Glenda had avoided the conversation about her urine out of embarrassment, even though she knew that blood in urine is abnormal and one common symptom of bladder or kidney cancer. "I just didn't want to talk about it," says Glenda. Unfortunately, Glenda had bladder cancer. So far, she has beaten the cancer, but only after her bladder was removed, a life-changing outcome that complicated her pelvic floor pain. Glenda's story demonstrates the importance of telling your primary care doctor when health problems, signs, and symptoms occur.

Knowing what to tell your doctor

Be sure to share the following information during your exams with your primary care and other doctors:

- **All symptoms you're having:** Symptoms may include such problems as severe pain, rashes, shakiness, headaches, or stiffness.
- **Your health history:** Give the doctor a well-organized description of your present symptoms and any related personal history. For example, if your pain started soon after a car accident, tell the physician about the accident, even if the pain has moved to a different place in your body. Did your arthritis symptoms start after a tick bite? Mention it to your doctor. Many people find it helps to draw up lists to share with their doctors so that they don't forget anything. If you've created a personal health notebook, it's handy for such purposes.
- **Your pain diary:** Give the doctor the highlights from your pain diary if you have developed one.
- **A list of all medicines you're currently taking, including over-the-counter drugs:** Bring a list of your medications by name, how often you take them and at what times, and the strengths of the medicines. (You may want to copy and use the log we provide in Chapter 17.)
- **All side effects you have from your medicine(s):** Side effects are problems, such as sleepiness or rashes. Most medications and supplements have such reactions. However, each drug has its own particular set of side effects. Even aspirin can have side effects, and some painkillers have such harsh side effects that many people would rather put up with the pain than suffer through them.
- **All vitamins or supplements you take (particularly if you take them in high doses):** Vitamins and supplements can interact with any drugs you take or with each other and can be harmful in and of themselves. (See Chapter 15 for more information on how vitamins and supplements can be dangerous in certain combinations.)
- **Any relevant X-rays, tests results, or medical records:** These items may help your doctor diagnose and treat your condition.
- **Any emotional or mental health issues:** Let your doctor know whether you're depressed, anxious, or having other problems. Your doctor may be able to help with these issues, and she should know about them because they can affect your level of pain.

Chapter 14

Prescribing Medicines for Chronic Pain

In This Chapter

- Using OTC drugs to get pain relief
- Delving in to prescription medication
- Getting the right dose
- Avoiding drug and alcohol abuse

Many people turn to painkillers, both over the counter and prescribed, to alleviate or reduce their chronic pain. In this chapter, you read about the benefits and side effects of a wide range of drugs used against chronic pain. You may find that one of these medicines, either alone or in combination with another drug, works well for you.

Keep in mind that while they can reduce the severity of your chronic pain, even the most powerful medicines can't totally remove it forever. So while taking pain-killing drugs is central to the management of many types of chronic pain, you also need to try the other pain management techniques described in Parts III and IV.

Finding Pain Relief Over the Counter

If you have chronic pain, analgesics are probably an important part of your medical care. *Analgesia* means an absence of pain, but the word analgesic is used to describe drugs or treatments that lessen pain (but rarely eliminate it). Analgesics either reduce pain signals going to your brain, or they interfere with your brain's reaction to these signals.

Analgesics include over-the-counter (OTC) drugs, which you can buy without a prescription, and prescribed, nonsteroidal anti-inflammatory drugs (NSAIDs), as well as opioids.

Appreciating off-label use

All medications are officially approved by the Food and Drug Administration (FDA) for one or more medical problems. Based on their knowledge and experience, doctors sometimes practice *off-label use,* which is when they prescribe drugs for medical problems other than the originally intended use.

Most drugs have a variety of medical uses. For example, aspirin is effective against inflammation and pain, but it's also used as a blood thinner to prevent heart attacks. Similarly, many other drugs used for treating chronic pain were originally designed and marketed for other conditions, such as depression or heart rhythm problems.

Don't worry if your doctor is prescribing off label. It's accepted medical practice and perfectly legal for your doctor to use a medication off label. The only problem is that sometimes your insurer or health plan may object to paying for the particular use your doctor is recommending.

In addition, drugs that are often used for other purposes, such as antidepressants or antiseizure drugs, have been found to be beneficial (even though these other drugs aren't technically called analgesics).

OTC drugs come in many forms: tablets, patches, suppositories, sprays, creams, and ointments. OTC pain products include acetaminophen (Tylenol), aspirin (Bayer), naproxen sodium (Aleve), ketoprofen (Orudis KT), ibuprofen (Advil and Motrin), and combinations of these drugs. Less expensive generic versions of these OTC drugs are often available, sometimes from pharmacy chains.

Make sure that you know what's in the OTC drugs you're purchasing. Some pharmaceutical companies combine ingredients, such as a decongestant or antihistamine along with painkillers. Look for a drug's active ingredients, listed by generic name, on its product's label. The ingredients are listed in order of prominence on the label. One of the secondary ingredients may not agree with you. For example, Tylenol PM combines both acetaminophen and diphenhydramine hydrochloride (a drug used to treat hay fever, allergies, and the common cold). If you have trouble sleeping specifically because of your pain and you don't suffer from allergies, you could take regular Tylenol *without* the diphenhydramine hydrochloride to avoid feeling hung over and dried out the next day.

You may wonder what *extra strength* means on the labels of some painkillers. These drugs contain *more* of the main ingredient per dosage than the standard product sold by the same manufacturer. For example, regular strength Tylenol has 325 mg of acetaminophen in each tablet, and Extra Strength Tylenol has 500 mg of acetaminophen in each tablet.

Two categories of over-the-counter drugs are used to reduce pain:

- **Acetaminophen** is well known by its brand name, Tylenol. Scientists don't really know how acetaminophen works, but they know that it raises the *pain threshold.* In other words, if you take acetaminophen, you can tolerate a greater amount of pain before you feel it. Acetaminophen is used to relieve mild to moderate chronic pain and also reduces fever.
- **Nonsteroidal anti-inflammatory drugs** (NSAIDs) reduce pain, fever, and inflammation. (The term *nonsteroidal* is used to distinguish these drugs from steroids, which are also used for inflammation.) Aspirin and ibuprofen (Advil) are the best known NSAIDs. NSAIDs don't cause drowsiness, nor do they slow down breathing as some narcotics do. However, they're not problem-free. They can cause stomach ulcers and heartburn.

  While you can purchase most NSAIDs over the counter, some are available only by prescription. See the next section, "Seeking Pain Relief with Prescription Drugs," about these drugs.

OTC painkillers can be dangerous in some situations. For example, heavy drinkers should be wary of taking acetaminophen (the ingredient in Tylenol and many other OTC pain and cold remedies). Your liver will thank you if you're careful, because acetaminophen can actually be toxic to it. Of course, it's also a good idea to give up heavy drinking, which can cause many medical problems. Taking ibuprofen and drinking alcohol is also a no-no. Alcohol increases the risk of bleeding in the stomach and intestines, which is a side effect of this medication.

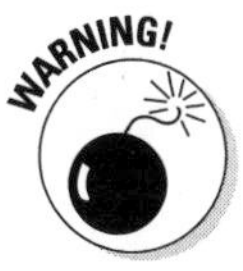

The maximum recommended dose for acetaminophen is 4 grams or 8 extra strength (500 mg) tablets in 24 hours. However, the maximum recommended dose for heavy drinkers is *half* that, or 2 grams or 4 extra-strength tablets in 24 hours. If you have liver disease, talk to your doctor before using acetaminophen at all.

Seeking Pain Relief with Prescription Drugs

Prescription drugs include some old standards like opioids, NSAIDS, and topical products. They also include drugs that you may not realize are effective against pain, including antidepressants, anti-epileptics, sodium channel blockers, anti-arrhymthic drugs, sedatives, anti-anxiety drugs, muscle relaxants, antihypertensives, and botulinum toxin.

Understanding generics and nongenerics

You can save precious dollars by buying generic prescriptions, when available. Generic and brand-name medicines act the same way in your body and contain the same active ingredients. Although generic drugs are chemically identical to their branded counterparts, they're typically sold at substantial discounts from the branded price. According to the Congressional Budget Office, generic drugs save consumers $8 to $10 billion a year. Medications can be pricey! Ask your doctor to prescribe generic drugs if available.

Cyclooxygenase (COX)-2 inhibitors are prescribed NSAIDs that have fewer gastrointestinal side effects with short-term use. As of this writing, celecoxib (Celebrex) is the only COX-2 inhibitor available. However, you can still develop ulcers with this drug. While COX-2 inhibitors are associated with heart risks, evidence is mounting that other NSAIDs may have similar risks. Some people claim that they gained significant pain relief with COX-2 inhibitors and were upset when most were removed from the market.

Opioids

Opioids are narcotics naturally derived from opium or synthetically derived and chemically similar to opium. They're controlled by the federal government, and your doctor must follow special rules when prescribing them; for example, the more potent opioids can't routinely be called in to the pharmacy by the doctor, and instead, a written prescription must be given to the patient. It can't be refilled.

Opioids are extremely effective in reducing pain. They're the foundation of medical treatment for chronic pain due to cancer and other conditions causing severe pain.

In some cases, opioids have less severe long-term side effects than anti-inflammatories. However, opioids have many side effects, including drowsiness, constipation, nausea, disorientation, and retention of urine. We're not talking regular constipation here. We're talking you-can't-go-for-days constipation. (Stimulant laxatives and increased fluids can help.) Taking too much of an opioid can cause other serious side effects, including a dangerous slowing of breathing and even coma. A drug called naloxone, given intravenously, can reverse these effects.

Some people taking opioids for long periods of time develop a *tolerance* to the drug, which means that they need higher doses to receive the pain-killing benefits. However, increased tolerance doesn't always occur. For some people, the same dose is effective for a long time. No one knows why this is true.

Opioids and addiction

Most people believe all narcotics — which are also called opioids — are addictive, and they think that if they take them, it's only a matter of time before they become junkies ready to sell their children for drugs. It's true that people with past addiction problems should be very careful with opioids. But most people who take narcotics to manage pain carefully follow their doctor's orders and rarely become drug addicts. (Read more about drug dependence in the section "Facing Prescription Drug Abuse" at the end of this chapter.)

The medical community is now behind effective prescribing of opioids for treating chronic pain. In 1996, the American Pain Society and the American Academy of Pain Medicine issued a joint consensus statement supporting cautious use of opioids for people with severe pain problems. *Cautious use* means patients and doctors discuss the risks and benefits of opioids. Doctors must maintain good records and careful follow-up so that they can determine whether the drugs are improving the condition and not causing other problems. (You may also want to look at Chapter 12 for information about the American Cancer Society's position on prescribing opioids for cancer pain. The society's position essentially agrees with the consensus statement by the American Pain Society and the American Academy of Pain Medicine.)

Many doctors today are concerned that their patients live with considerable pain because of unfounded fears of addiction.

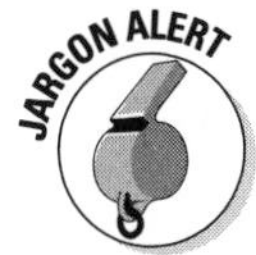

According to the National Institute of Drug Abuse, *addiction* is a chronic, relapsing brain disease characterized by compulsive drug seeking and use, despite harmful consequences.

When opioids are used regularly for a long time, your nervous system adapts by increasing the activity of transmitters that increase pain. The result is that you often experience withdrawal symptoms (including pain) if the drug is stopped suddenly. If you stop taking opioids after long-term use, taper off gradually (under your doctor's orders) to keep symptoms under control.

Opioids are taken by mouth, given by injection, absorbed through the lining of the cheek or gums, or applied through the skin in a patch. They can also be administered through special internal pumps for people with extremely severe chronic pain. If you receive good pain relief from opioids but can't tolerate their side effects, they can be injected directly into the space around your spinal cord.

Opioids administered through injections act faster than oral forms, but the pain relief doesn't last as long. One opioid, Fentanyl, is available as a transdermal skin patch and provides pain relief for up to 72 hours.

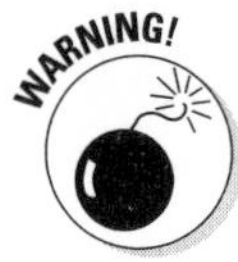

In 2005, the Food and Drug Administration (FDA) issued a public health advisory about reports of death and other serious side effects from patients who overdosed while using Fentanyl transdermal patches. Deaths and overdoses have occurred in patients using both the brand-name Duragesic and the generic form of the drug. Some health-care providers and consumers may not be fully aware of the dangers of this drug. The directions for using the Fentanyl skin patch must be followed exactly to prevent serious side effects from overdose.

Other prescription drugs used for pain management

A variety of other prescription drugs are successfully used to manage pain. The following list covers the pros and cons of these medications:

- **Tramadol** (Ultram) and **tramadol combined with acetaminophen** (Ultracet(tm)) are prescription pain medications for managing moderate to moderately severe pain. The combination of tramadol and acetaminophen is much more powerful than either drug alone. Tramadol is considered a weak opioid analgesic. Tramadol doesn't reduce inflammation. Avoid taking more than 400 mg (300 mg in the elderly) of tramadol a day.

  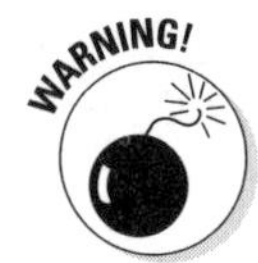

  If you're thinking about taking tramadol, use caution if you also take any medications that are monoamine oxidase inhibitors (MAOIs) or selective serotonin reuptake inhibitors (SSRIs). Also, watch out if you're taking some antipsychotic medications, such as Thorazine and Compazine. Sometimes the combination of these drugs with tramadol can cause problems. If you take any of these drugs, make sure that your doctor is aware of it before she writes a prescription for tramadol.

- **Propoxyphene** is a mild opioid analgesic used for the relief of mild to moderate pain. Darvocet-N 50, Darvocet-N 100, and more recently Darvocet A500 tablets contain propoxyphene with acetaminophen. The combination of propoxyphene and acetaminophen produces greater pain relief than produced by either drug alone. Propoxyphene is on the don't-take list of drugs for the elderly. (See Chapter 24 for other drugs older people should avoid.)

- **Fiorinal** is a strong, non-opioid pain reliever and muscle relaxant. It's used for the relief of tension headaches caused by stress or muscle contraction in the head, neck, and shoulder area. It combines a barbiturate (butalbital) with a pain reliever (aspirin) and a stimulant (caffeine). Another option for those who want to avoid aspirin is Fiorcet, which combines fiorinal with acetaminophen and caffeine.

- **Flavocoxid** (Limbrel) is a prescription-only product for the management of osteoarthritis. It's made from a combination of root and bark extracts from plants. The plant extracts contain a substance called *flavonoids*. Some of these same flavonoids are found in green tea. The flavonoid extracts, which are compounds found in fruits, vegetables, and certain beverages, in Limbrel appear to help by halting the production of an enzyme that causes inflammation. The FDA classifies Limbrel as a "medical food." It's given as a prescription, but the foods have been "generally recognized as safe" by the FDA.

  Limbrel has the same side-effects that NSAIDs have, including an increased risk of stomach ulcers. At this writing, no studies show whether flavocoxid is as effective as NSAIDs are for pain relief. Using NSAIDs and flavocoxid together may increase the risk of stomach irritation.

Antidepressants and anti-epileptics

Some antidepressants and antiepileptic drugs are helpful in managing chronic pain, especially *neuropathic pain* (chronic pain caused by injury to the peripheral nervous system). The pain-killing effect of these drugs is independent of their effect on depression.

Antidepressants and anti-epileptic drugs are about equally effective for neuropathic pain. Duloxetine (Cymbalta), an antidepressant, and pregabalin (Lyrica), an antiseizure drug, are modestly successful against fibromyalgia pain. However, they differ in their costs, safety, and side effects. Tricyclic antidepressants may also help reduce pain.

A few of the many antiepileptic drugs that are effective in the treatment of neuropathic pain include carbamazepine (Tegretol), phenytoin (Dilantin), gabapentin (Neurontin), and pregabalin (Lyrica).

If you take medicine for migraines and antidepressants, be sure to read Chapter 6 about the dangers of combining some drugs.

Antidepressants are particularly helpful in managing certain types of pain. Note that using antidepressants doesn't mean that the pain is "all in your head" and that you're really depressed *instead of* being in pain. The pain is real, but the limitations it imposes on you can be depressing. Some transmitters released during depression increase pain, and people are more active and effective in counteracting the pain if not depressed.

Some pain states that may respond well to antidepressants include the following:

- Central pain
- Rheumatoid arthritis
- Chemotherapy-induced peripheral neuropathy
- Complex Regional Pain Syndrome (CRPS), also known as Reflex Sympathetic Dystrophy Syndrome (RSDS)
- Diabetic neuropathy
- Fibromyalgia
- Irritable bowel syndrome
- Migraine and tension headache
- Neuropathic pain
- Phantom limb pain
- Phantom limb/neuroma pain
- Postherpetic neuralgia
- Sympathetic dystrophy

Sodium channel blocking and oral anti-arrhythmic agents

Injuries to the peripheral or central nervous system can cause spontaneous activity of neurons in pain pathways. (See Chapter 2 for an explanation of neurons and pain pathways.) Reducing this unwanted, ongoing activity can reduce pain, which is why anti-epileptic drugs can be helpful. (Epileptic seizures result from high levels of spontaneous activity in other regions of the CNS.)

Other drugs called antirhythmics also have quieting effects on CNS neurons. They're prescribed to prevent disturbances in heart rhythm, but they're also used for treating chronic pain. Just as they stop the premature firing of heart fibers, they also reduce pain signals. Two antiarrhythmics are used occasionally for chronic pain: mexiletine (Mexitil) and flecainide (Tambocor). These medications reduce the pain of diabetic neuropathy, post-stroke pain, CRPS/RDS, and traumatic nerve injury. Lidocaine, a local anesthetic, can reduce spontaneous activity in the CNS and is given intravenously for chronic pain.

Topical pain relievers

While no scientific evidence supports the use of OTC topical ointments (liniments), such as Ben-Gay or Tiger Balm, many people believe that stimulating their sore areas with these ointments relieves their hurting.

Most topical pain relievers are available over the counter. An exception is Lidoderm, which is a prescribed, transdermal skin patch.

Although side effects of liniments are usually considered minimal, don't overuse them. An unusual death of a teenage athlete occurred in 2007 because she used too many liniments, all of which contained methylsalicylates (aspirin). In fact, a variety of liniments contain the same active ingredient that's in aspirin. In addition to methylsalicylate, other types of topical pain relievers include such ingredients as menthol, camphor, eucalyptus oil, turpentine oil, and histamine dihydrochloride. Methyl nicotinate is used in neuropathic pain conditions and CRPS. Capsaicin, the active ingredient in hot peppers, is a topical treatment for neuropathic pain.

Some topical remedies include aspirin in chloroform or ethyl ether, capsaicin (Zostrix, Zostrix-HP), and EMLA (a mixture of local anesthetics) cream. Local anesthetics, such as the lidocaine patch 5% (Lidoderm), are topical treatments for neuropathic pain.

Lidoderm 5% (lidocaine) patches have been approved by the FDA to treat postherpetic neuralgia (PHN). Some people use Lidoderm in an off-label use for arthritic pain.

Other medications

Other medications are sometimes used to treat chronic pain. They include

- **Anti-hypertensive medications:** Some medications for high blood pressure (hypertension) can also relieve chronic pain; for example, clonidine (Catapres, Catapres-TTS patch) relieves the symptoms of complex regional pain syndrome /reflex sympathetic dystrophy.
- **Botulinum toxin:** Botox is a popular wrinkle reducer that acts by temporarily paralyzing muscles. You may have heard of this drug as something celebrities take to get rid of their facial wrinkles in their attempts to attain endless youth, but that's not its only use! This effect can also work for pain control. Botulinum toxin (Botox and Myobloc) can calm overactive muscles and can soothe chronic headaches and muscle pain. Side effects are rare. Botulinum also has direct effects in reducing skin neurotransmitters that transmit pain.

- **Implanted drug-delivery systems:** Some pain relievers such as Ziconotide (Prialt) are administered directly to the area around the spinal cord and to nerve roots. This method can have benefits such as reduced dosages and fewer side effects. For some people with severe injuries, this system is the best way they can take pain medications.
- **NMDA inhibitors:** Drugs called NMDA (N-methyl-D-aspartate) inhibitors are now being tested to relieve neuropathic pain. The hope is that they can stop acute pain from turning into chronic pain by arresting central sensitization (see Chapter 2).

Working with Your Doctor to Find the Right Medication Combo

All medications — including over-the-counter drugs or nutritional and herbal supplements — can act together and cause harmful side effects. It's very important to tell your doctor about everything you're taking, both for your pain and for other medical conditions, even if you don't regard them as medication. See Chapter 17 for a personal medication log that you can copy and use to make a comprehensive list. Your list should include supplements and vitamins you purchase without a prescription, caffeine, alcohol, tobacco, marijuana, and recreational drugs.

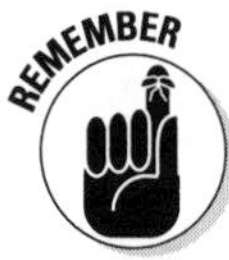

Take all your current medication bottles (or a complete list) with you to all doctor appointments and be honest about any other substances you're using. Even over-the-counter and herbal medications can have serious interactions with your prescription medications and with each other.

Medications differ in how they work and how you should take them. It's important to stay on top of the following pointers, adapted in part, from the National Institutes of Health:

- What type of medication has your doctor prescribed (for example is it a painkiller, an NSAID, an antidepressant, an anti-epileptic, or other type of drug)?
- What's the dosage of the medication?
- How often should you take it (or do you take it "as needed")?
- Should you take the medication at bedtime?
- Should you avoid eating anything when taking the medicine, or should you take it before, with, or after meals?
- Under what conditions should you stop taking the medicine?

- What should you do if you forget to take the medicine?
- What side effects may you expect, and what should you do if you have a problem?

Your doctor will take into account the following when she prescribes your medications:

- Your medical condition
- Your weight
- Your age
- Other medications you take

Check out Chapter 13 for a list of information you should always have with you when you see your doctor — including information about your medicines.

Avoiding serotonin syndrome

Many medicines that people with chronic pain take include *serotonin,* a brain chemical that affects both depression and appetite. Not enough serotonin causes depression, while too much can cause problems such as confusion, restlessness, hallucinations, extreme agitation, fluctuations in blood pressure, increased heart rate, nausea and vomiting, fever, seizures, and even coma.

More than 50 frequently used medicines now on the market can increase your serotonin levels. The following is a list of drugs that can add to your serotonin load. Watch for serotonin symptoms when you increase your dose of any of these medicines. This list was developed by the American Chronic Pain Association:

Antidepressants and anti-anxiety, and certain sleep medicines, including fluoxetine (Prozac, Sarafem), paroxetine (Paxil), sertraline (Zoloft), citalopram (Celexa), escitalopram (Lexapro), trazodone (Desyrel), venlafaxine (Effexor), duloxetine (Cymbalta) clomipramine (Anafranil), buspirone (BuSpar), mirtazapine (Remeron), lithium, St. John's Wort, phenelzine (Nardil), tranylcypromine (Parnate), or isocarboxazid (Marplan)

Antimigraine medicines in either the triptan or ergot groups, including sumatriptan (Imitrex), almotriptan (AxertTM), eletriptan (Relpax), frovatriptan (Frova), naratriptan (Amerge), rizatriptan (Maxalt), zolmitriptan (Zomig), ergotamine/caffeine (Cafergot), or dihydroergotamine (DHE 45, Migranal)

Diet pills, specifically L-tryptophan (5-HTP), sibutramine (Meridia), or phentermine

Certain pain medicines, including tramadol (Ultram), fentanyl (Duragesic patch), pentazocine (Talwin), duloxetine (Cymbalta), or meperidine (Demerol)

Certain drugs for nausea, specifically ondansetron (Zofran), granisetron (Kytril), or metoclopramide (Reglan)

Cough syrups or cold medicines if they contain the anti-cough ingredient dextromethorphan (DM) or linezolid (ZyvoxTM), an antibiotic for *staphylococcus* or *enterococcus* infections

Using Medicines Safely

Your pharmacist can answer many questions you have about your medicine. A good general rule is to try to have all your prescriptions filled at the same pharmacy so that your records are in one place. Your pharmacist can keep track of all your medications and tell you whether a new drug may cause problems. If you're not able to use just one pharmacy, keep a record and show all your pharmacists your list of medicines and over-the-counter drugs. (See Chapter24 for information on running your list of prescriptions through a drug interaction database.)

Here are some safety tips for taking pain medications:

- Read and understand the name of the medicine and the directions on the container. If the label is hard to read, ask your pharmacist to use larger type.
- Check that you can open the container; if not, ask the pharmacist to put your medicines in bottles that are easier to open.
- If you have trouble swallowing pills, ask your pharmacist whether a liquid medicine is available.
- Don't chew, break, or crush tablets. The drug may not be effective (because the active ingredients may not be evenly distributed in the pill) or can cause an overdose when crushed or chewed.
- Ask whether the pharmacy has instructions on where to store a medicine.
- Make a list of all medicines you take. Keep a copy in your wallet. The list should include the name of each medicine, the doctor who prescribed it, the reason prescribed, the amount you take, and time(s) you take it.
- Read and save all written information that comes with the medicine.
- Take your medicine in the exact amount and at the time your doctor prescribes.
- Take your medicine until it's finished or until your doctor says it's okay to stop.
- Call your doctor right away if you have any problems with your medicine.
- Do not skip doses of medication or take half doses unless specified by your prescription.
- Find out whether drinking alcohol while taking your medicines is okay. Some medicines don't mix well with alcohol and can make you sick. Anyone taking opioids or antianxiety drugs should not drink alcohol at all.

- Don't take other people's medicines or give yours to anyone else.
- Throw away outdated medicines.
- Make sure that medicines and supplements are out of the reach of children as well as adults with dementia problems.
- If you have prescribed narcotics, keep the main supply in a lockbox or safe.

Buying Drugs from the Internet

The Internet is home to many legitimate pharmacies, but it's also a site for a growing number of businesses that sell drugs to anyone with a credit card, regardless of whether he has a prescription.

No accurate figures exist on how many people buy medicines over the Net without a prescription. But with more sites appearing every week, its fair to say that online pharmacies are a growing market. Buying medicines over the Internet doesn't guarantee a quality product unless you follow certain guidelines to protect yourself.

If you decide you want to buy meds through the Internet, take these precautions:

- Talk with your doctor and have a physical exam before you get any new medicine for the first time.
- Use only medicine prescribed by your doctor or another trusted professional licensed in the United States to write prescriptions for medicine.
- Know your source to make sure that ordering from them is safe. Your state board of pharmacy can tell you whether a Web site is a state-licensed pharmacy, is in good standing, and is located in the United States. Find a list of state boards of pharmacy on the National Association of Boards of pharmacy (NABP) Web site at `www.nabp.info`. Internet Web sites that display the NABP seal have been checked to ensure that they meet state and federal rules.

Using Alcohol and Recreational Drugs

Alcohol is a recreational drug, but it's still a drug. Some people use alcohol to relieve chronic pain, which can be very dangerous and boost the effect of some prescription drugs. Chronic alcoholism frequently causes permanent and serious damage to the liver, greatly complicating the treatment of chronic pain. Many medications can't be given to people with damaged livers.

Marijuana is also a drug. Using marijuana for chronic pain relief is controversial. Some states allow the legal use of marijuana for people in pain. But the federal government continues to threaten physicians with prosecution for prescribing it (although it has yet to do it). If you drink alcohol, smoke marijuana, or take recreational drugs, tell your doctor.

If you live with chronic pain, you may find it easy to fall into medicating your pain with beer, wine, or hard alcohol. Using alcohol as a pain reliever isn't a new phenomenon. Through the generations, people have medicated their physical and emotional pain with alcohol.

Of course, many people who drink alcohol don't have a drinking problem, but for some, drinking to reduce pain can get out of control.

According to the National Institute on Alcohol Abuse and Alcoholism (NIAAA), the following four symptoms indicate an abuse problem has developed into an *addiction* (also known as *dependence*) to alcohol:

- **Craving:** A strong need, or urge, to drink
- **Loss of control:** Not being able to stop drinking once drinking has begun
- **Physical dependence:** Withdrawal symptoms, such as nausea, sweating, shakiness, and anxiety after stopping drinking
- **Tolerance:** The need to drink greater amounts of alcohol to get high

Getting someone to admit he has a problem with alcohol is usually hard. Denial of the disease among alcoholics is the norm. Doctors use a variety of techniques to uncover problem drinking, including:

- Questionnaires (such as the Short Michigan Alcoholism Screening Test)
- Blood tests measuring red blood cell size
- Blood tests measuring a protein called carbohydrate-deficient transferrin
- Tests showing liver damage
- Tests showing decreased testosterone in men

If you have an alcohol-related problem, draw upon the many national and local resources available. The National Drug and Alcohol Treatment Referral Routing Service offers advice via a toll-free telephone number, 800-662-HELP (4357). You or your loved one can speak directly to a representative about treatment, request printed material on alcohol or other drugs, or get information about programs in your state.

Many people find help through Alcoholics Anonymous (AA) support groups. AA groups meet in almost every community. Contact a nearby central office to find times and places of local meetings. Their phone numbers and addresses are listed in local phone directories or go to `www.alcoholics-anonymous.org`.

Facing Prescription Drug Abuse

Prescription painkillers can be effective when supervised by a physician to manage pain. On occasion, though, they can lead to an addiction if they're not managed appropriately by your doctor.

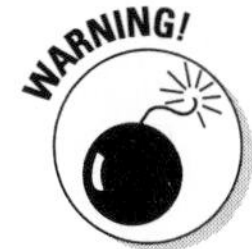

Never take more medications than your doctor ordered. Don't assume that if one pain pill helps, then two (or more!) would be even better. Not true! This dangerous belief can lead to bad side effects and a drug dependence. If your pain isn't sufficiently relieved by the dosage your doctor ordered, call her. Maybe you need a different medication.

Prescription drug abuse is a major problem in the United States. According to the 2005 National Survey on Drug Use and Health, 6.4 million Americans aged 12 and older used prescription medications for nonmedical purposes in the prior 30 days. Of these individuals, an estimated 4.7 million used pain relievers, 1.8 million used tranquilizers, 1.1 million used stimulants, and 272,000 used sedatives.

Based on a survey of hospital emergency rooms, the Drug Abuse Warning Network (DAWN) reports that two of the most frequently abused types of prescription medications are benzodiazepines (anti-anxiety drugs such as Valium, Xanax, Klonopin, and Ativan) and opioid pain relievers (such as oxycodone, hydrocodone, morphine, methadone, and combinations including these drugs). Stimulants such as methamphetamine, Ritalin, or Adderall represent another class of commonly abused medications.

Many people with chronic pain use their medications responsibly and don't become addicted to them. Those who do become addicted to drugs are usually either seeking a euphoric high or to blot out awareness of their problems or responsibilities. In other words, they're not taking drugs for pain, but for other reasons. In reality, strong painkillers are sometimes needed for severe pain, and as long as you work with a good doctor who manages your medications, you usually don't have to worry about becoming a drug addict.

In order to provide appropriate and legitimate monitoring of patients taking opioids, many physicians perform random urine drug tests on their patients to make sure that they're taking the narcotic as prescribed.

Chapter 15

Taking an Alternative Approach to Pain Management

In This Chapter

- Discovering the difference between complementary and conventional medicine
- Checking out the major CAM (complementary and alternative) therapies
- Distinguishing between CAMs that are proven or unproven
- Exploring how to detect unproven remedies

CAM is hot. In the United States, more than a third of all adults use some form of complementary and alternative medicine (CAM). When megavitamin therapy and prayer practiced specifically for health reasons are included in the definition of CAM, the percentage rises to a startling 62 percent. That's nearly two-thirds of the adults in America.

Exploring CAM

CAM is an umbrella term for health practices outside conventional medicine. (*Conventional medicine* is the discipline practiced by medical doctors or doctors of osteopathy and related health professionals, such as physical therapists, occupational therapists, psychologists, and registered nurses.)

Complementary medicine is often used alongside conventional medicine. For example, if you have chronic pain from arthritis, you may use two complementary therapies (massage and exercise) along with physical therapy and nonsteroidal anti-inflammatory drugs (NSAIDs) prescribed by a doctor to treat arthritis pain. And scientists have found that the vitamin folic acid prevents certain birth defects. In addition, a regimen of vitamins and zinc can slow the progression of the eye disease age-related macular degeneration.

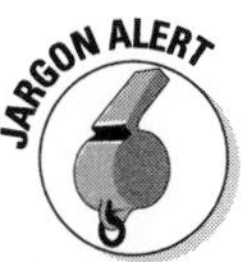

Some health-care providers practice *integrative medicine* (or integrated medicine), which is simply both CAM and conventional medicine.

Does CAM really work?

Medical professionals in pain management have become increasingly interested in CAM. For example, when talking about acupuncture, one of your authors, Dr. Kassan, has treated people with chronic pain for years, and he says of CAM, "It's almost mainstream now. As a result, CAM is safe when done properly and can be very helpful for pain."

Another of your authors, Dr. Vierck, has spent 40-plus years as a scientist studying pain. He swears by magnets (for giving him relief for the arthritis in his wrist, even though the relief he experiences may be a *placebo effect.* A placebo effect is when a useless remedy works because you think it'll work. Actually, it does nothing.)

Finally, your third author, Dr. Vierck's sister, Elizabeth Vierck, an experienced information specialist and health writer, says, "My brother's caught up in wishful thinking because he doesn't want to give up golf. Magnets are a lot of hooey."

But, and this is a big but, Ms. Vierck herself takes a dietary supplement twice a day, hoping it'll help her arthritis. So who's thinking wishfully?

Of course, you can make up your own mind about CAM. In many cases, the only harm it can do is to your pocket book, as long as you're well informed and avoid any approaches that may be harmful.

However, one big concern with CAM is that many of its techniques have not been researched and, therefore, don't have science-based credibility. As a consequence, many practitioners of conventional medicine are dubious about using CAM to treat diseases and pain.

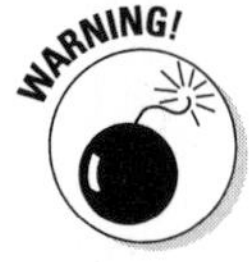

Sometimes people use alternative medicine instead of conventional medicine, which can be a very perilous choice. An example of such danger is using nutritional supplements to treat cancer instead of undergoing the surgery, radiation, or chemotherapy your doctor recommends. This idea is bad because it can kill you! Check out Chapter 26, which covers bogus "cures."

Using Dietary and Herbal Supplements

Many people who suffer from relentless pain take dietary supplements to boost their general health and feel better. *Supplements* are highly refined chemicals or plant extracts just like medicines, but supplements haven't been tested for long-term or short-term side effects, interactions with other medications or other supplements, or safety in people with serious medical conditions, such as cancer, heart disease, and liver or kidney failure.

Dietary supplements are sold in grocery, health-food, drug, and discount stores, as well as through mail-order catalogs, TV programs, the Internet, and direct sales.

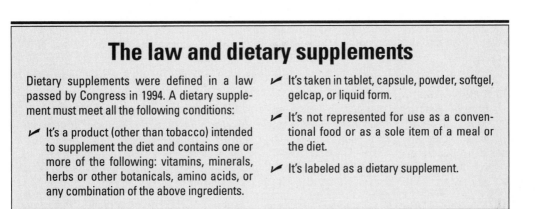

The law and dietary supplements

Dietary supplements were defined in a law passed by Congress in 1994. A dietary supplement must meet all the following conditions:

- It's a product (other than tobacco) intended to supplement the diet and contains one or more of the following: vitamins, minerals, herbs or other botanicals, amino acids, or any combination of the above ingredients.
- It's taken in tablet, capsule, powder, softgel, gelcap, or liquid form.
- It's not represented for use as a conventional food or as a sole item of a meal or the diet.
- It's labeled as a dietary supplement.

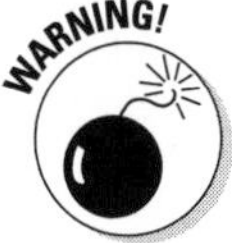

Some supplements act like medicines and can be harmful, depending on what other supplements you take, how much of the supplement you take, and how often you take it. In fact, 17 known supplements cause kidney dysfunction or failure, and several other dietary substances are known to cause toxicity to genes and possibly produce cancer, but lack of regulation prevents labeling of these supplements. In addition, if you take prescribed medicines, too, these drugs should be taken into account before you add any supplements to your anti-pain regimen.

Staying safe with dietary supplements

Keep the following safety points about dietary supplements in mind. They were adapted from information provided by the National Center for Complementary and Alternative Medicine (NCCAM).

- Some ingredients of supplements, including nutrients and plant components, can be toxic. Don't substitute a dietary supplement for a prescription medicine or therapy without talking such a change over with your doctor.
- Tell your health-care providers about complementary and alternative practices you use so that they have a full picture of how you try to manage your health. Better yet, tell them before you start using any supplements.
- Don't take a higher dose of a supplement than listed on the label, unless your health-care provider advises you to do so.
- If you experience any side effects that concern you, stop taking the supplement and contact your doctor. You can also report your experience to the FDA's MedWatch program (`www.fda.gov/medwatch`), which tracks consumer safety reports on supplements.

It's especially important to talk to your provider if you're using supplements and meet any of these conditions:

- You're thinking about replacing your regular medical care with one or more supplements.
- You're taking any medications (whether prescription or over the counter). Some supplements interact with medications.
- You have a chronic medical condition, such as diabetes or arthritis.
- You plan to have surgery. Certain supplements may increase the risk of bleeding or affect anesthetics and painkillers.
- You're pregnant or nursing, or you're considering giving a child a dietary supplement. Supplements can act like drugs, and many have not been tested in pregnant women, nursing mothers, or children.

Understanding how dietary supplements are regulated

The federal government regulates supplements through the Food and Drug Administration (FDA). Currently, the FDA regulates supplements as foods rather than drugs. In general, the laws about putting foods (including supplements) on the market and keeping them on the market are less strict than the laws for drugs.

However, in 2007 the FDA printed a rule requiring manufacturers to evaluate the identity, purity, strength, and composition of their dietary supplements. If dietary supplements contain contaminants or do not contain the dietary ingredient they are represented to contain, FDA would consider those products to be adulterated or misbranded. This is a step — albeit a small one — in the right direction for consumers.

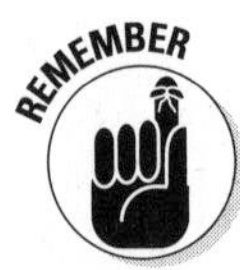

Research to prove a supplement's safety for human consumption is not required before the supplement is marketed, as it is with over-the-counter or prescribed drugs. In addition, the supplement manufacturer doesn't have to prove the product is effective, nor must he prove supplement quality. For example, one study that analyzed 59 preparations of Echinacea found that about half did not contain the items listed on the label.

Glucosamine and chondroitin

Glucosamine and chondroitin sulfate are popular (and controversial) supplements heavily marketed as effective at preventing and treating the damage that arthritis and sports injuries can do to your joints.

Mixing supplements and herbs with medications

Some supplements and herbs can cause serious harm when combined with prescription drugs or other substances. For example, St. John's Wort can increase the effects of some prescription drugs used to treat depression or cause side effects when used with other antidepressants. It can also interfere with drugs used to treat HIV infection or cancer. But you won't have to worry as long as you tell your doctor about the herbs and supplements that you take — or plan to take.

Ginseng is an herb that can increase the stimulant effects of caffeine (as in coffee, tea, and cola). It can also lower your blood sugar levels, creating the possibility of problems when used alongside diabetes drugs.

Ginkgo biloba, another herb, should never be taken with anticoagulant or antiplatelet drugs because it can increase the risk of bleeding. Ginkgo may also interact with some psychiatric drugs and with drugs that affect blood sugar levels.

Both substances are naturally present in your body. Glucosamine is a form of an amino sugar, and chondroitin is part of a protein. They're the building blocks that your body uses to build cartilage. The theory behind using the supplement is that the more building blocks you have, the more cartilage you'll maintain.

The glucosamine you buy in supplements comes from seashells, while chondroitin is derived from animal cartilage. These two supplements are packaged as individual supplements or combined with each other. They're also available in other combinations including MSM (methylsulfonylmethane) as a third ingredient.

A large study by researchers at the National Institutes of Health looked at the effectiveness of glucosamine and chondroitin, the COX-2 inhibitor, Celexecob, and a placebo. (See Chapter 14 for information on COX-2 inhibitors.) The result was that the group of participants as a whole showed no significant differences between any of them. However, for a small group of participants with moderate to severe (rather than mild) pain, glucosamine combined with chondroitin sulfate provided significant pain relief compared with a placebo.

But don't get too enthusiastic about glucosamine and chondroitin. Researchers warn that because of the small size of the group that received the benefit, these results must be backed up by more research.

What's the downside of these supplements? They both may cause gas and diarrhea.

SAMe

The supplement S-adenosyl- L-methionine (SAMe, for short, pronounced "Sammy') is almost as popular as glucosamine and chondroitin, described in the preceding section. This substance is naturally found in all the cells of your body, and it affects cartilage building and other physical processes. Supplemental SAMe is marketed as a pain reliever and an antidepressant. Research supports a possible benefit for depression and pain relief of osteoarthritis.

SAMe appears to be safe and may have fewer side effects than other pain relievers. But, long-term side effects and toxicity studies have not been conducted. In high doses, it may cause mild diarrhea, nausea, gas, and anxiety.

Omega-3 fatty acids

Omega-3 fatty acids are best known for preventing heart disease. However, one way in which they benefit your heart is through their important role as an inflammation fighter. As they reduce inflammation, they also reduce pain associated with it. Several studies demonstrate reductions in joint pain when taking omega 3-fatty acids.

Omega-3 fatty acids are found naturally in fatty, cold-water fish, dark green leafy vegetables, flaxseed oils, and some vegetable oils. Many types of supplements with omega-3 fatty acids are available in pill or capsule form. Fish oil is more beneficial than flaxseed oil.

High dosages of fish oil can cause thinning of the blood, and you can also have burps that taste like fish oil. Not a pleasant experience.

Herbal supplements

Herbal supplements are a type of dietary supplement. They're made up of a single herb or a mixture of herbs. An *herb* (also called a botanical) is a plant or plant part used for its scent, flavor, and/or therapeutic properties. Many herbs have a long history of use and of claimed health benefits.

Just because an herbal supplement is labeled *natural* doesn't mean it's good for you or safe to use. Herbal supplements can act the same way as drugs. After all, poison ivy is natural, too! Herbal remedies can cause medical problems if used incorrectly or taken in large amounts. Because there is rarely any quality assurance testing done on these products, knowing the content of these supplements is impossible. In general, it's safer to utilize products from major manufacturers and to avoid products made in China due to contamination with lead and mercury.

If you look for supplements to ease your chronic pain, there's a good chance that you'll also run into advertising for the following herbs. Marketers may claim they can cure your arthritis or prevent your headaches. Here's the real deal on many popular herbal supplements.

- **Aloe vera:** This plant is used for conditions such as asthma and arthritis. It's sold as ointments, lotions, and pills. Studies show that topical aloe gel may help heal burns and abrasions. Not enough scientific evidence supports aloe vera for any other use.

  Aloe vera used topically (on the skin) doesn't have side effects. Taken orally, however, aloe vera can cause diarrhea and cramping. Also, if you have diabetes, check with your doctor before taking aloe vera because it may decrease blood glucose levels.
- **Black cohosh:** Black cohosh purportedly treats arthritis, muscle pain, menstrual problems, and menopausal symptoms. No scientific studies have found that taking black cohosh is beneficial for any medical use. Side effects can include headaches, stomach discomfort, pain, and serious liver damage.
- **Cat's claw:** Cat's claw is used to treat cancer, arthritis, and other conditions. No scientific studies have found that taking cat's claw is beneficial for any medical use. If you have a compromised immune system or you may become pregnant (or you are pregnant), stay away from cat's claw.
- **Evening primrose oil (EPO):** Evening primrose oil is a fatty acid used for chronic skin conditions and a variety of other health problems, including rheumatoid arthritis. Evening primrose oil may have some benefits for skin conditions. However, no scientific studies have found that taking EPO is beneficial for any other medical use. Side effects are mild and can include stomach problems and headaches.
- **Feverfew:** Feverfew is purported to help with fevers, headaches, and rheumatoid arthritis. This herb may help prevent headaches, although more research is needed. However, insufficient scientific evidence makes it impossible to say that feverfew is helpful for any other medical condition. Feverfew can cause a variety of unpleasant side effects in your mouth, such as inflammation and canker sores. If you may become pregnant (or *are* pregnant) avoid feverfew, as it can cause miscarriage.
- **Ginger:** Ginger is used to treat stomachaches, nausea, and diarrhea, as well as arthritis-related conditions. It may also help relieve nausea. (An old remedy for upset stomach used to be ginger ale — when it actually had ginger in it!) Not enough research has been done to determine whether ginger is effective in treating other health conditions. No serious side effects for ginger have been found. Consuming too much, however, can cause indigestion. Animal studies have shown ginger to be protective against liver toxicity produced by acetaminophen, a commonly used pain medicine.

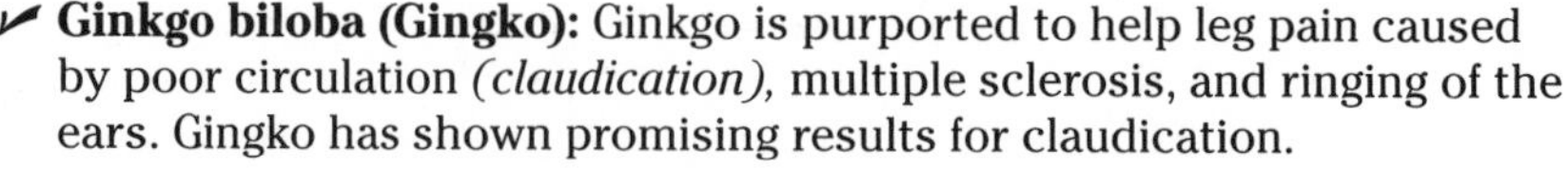

- **Ginkgo biloba (Gingko):** Ginkgo is purported to help leg pain caused by poor circulation *(claudication),* multiple sclerosis, and ringing of the ears. Gingko has shown promising results for claudication.

  The flip side of its benefit for claudication is that ginkgo has also been associated with bleeding problems, headaches, skin reactions, and other problems.

- **Kava Kava (Kava):** Kava contains kavalactones, which have calming and sedative effects. Many people with pain have tried kava for anxiety and/or sleep problems.

  The U.S. and foreign regulatory agencies have warned that kava can cause serious liver damage. Stay away from it.

- **Peppermint oil:** Peppermint oil allegedly helps indigestion, irritable bowel syndrome, and muscle and nerve pain. Peppermint oil may help with the symptoms of irritable bowel syndrome, but no scientific evidence suggests that it's beneficial for other health problems. Peppermint oil should be used in small dosages. It can cause heartburn.

- **St. John's Wort:** St. John's Wort allegedly helps with depression, nerve pain, and sleep problems. Depression and sleep problems often result from chronic pain. Some scientific evidence suggests that St. John's Wort can help people with mild to moderate depression. However, two large studies showed that the herb wasn't effective in treating major depression.

  St. John's Wort has a number of serious side effects and should be used only with caution and under a doctor's supervision. It may cause sensitivity to sunlight, anxiety, dry mouth, dizziness, gastrointestinal symptoms, fatigue, headache, or sexual dysfunction. St. John's Wort can also interact with other drugs. When combined with certain antidepressants, St. John's Wort may increase side effects, such as nausea, anxiety, headache, and confusion. According to the NCCAM, other drugs that can be adversely affected by St. John's Wort include

  - Indinavir and possibly other drugs used to control HIV infection
  - Irinotecan and possibly other drugs used to treat cancer
  - Cyclosporine, which prevents the body from rejecting transplanted organs
  - Digoxin, which strengthens heart muscle contractions
  - Warfarin and related anticoagulants
  - Birth control pills
  - Some antidepressants

- **Turmeric (Indian saffron):** Turmeric purportedly helps a range of diverse conditions, such as indigestion, liver disease, cancer, and inflammation. It's sometimes tried as a painkiller and as a topical remedy for eczema and wounds. Very little scientific research on turmeric has been done. However, turmeric is considered safe for most adults. It has been demonstrated to be ineffective in irritable bowel syndrome.
- **Valerian:** Although valerian is sold as a sleep aid, research has not shown it to effective for this use. And not enough research has been done to know whether it works for headaches, anxiety, or other conditions. Valerian can cause mild side effects, such as a hungover feeling the day after taking it.

Getting Back to Nature: Naturopathic Medicine

The premise behind *naturopathy* is that your body has natural healing power that establishes, maintains, and restores health. Practitioners work with you to support this power through treatments (such as nutrition and lifestyle counseling), dietary supplements, medicinal plants, exercise, and homeopathy.

Naturopathic physicians are trained in clinical nutrition, botanical medicine, homeopathic medicine, *physical medicine* (therapeutic manipulation of muscles, bones, and spine), *Oriental medicine* (acupuncture), natural childbirth care, psychological medicine, and minor surgery.

Naturopathy appears safe, especially if used as complementary medicine, but the National Center for Complementary and Alternative Medicine (NCCAM) offers several important qualifying points:

- Naturopathy isn't a complete substitute for conventional medical care.
- Some therapies used in naturopathy, may be harmful if they're not used properly or under the direction of a trained practitioner. For example, restrictive or other unconventional diets can be unsafe for some people.
- Some practitioners of naturopathy don't recommend using all or some of the childhood vaccinations that are standard practice in conventional medicine.
- The education and training of practitioners of naturopathy vary widely. Naturopathic physicians may not be licensed to practice in all states, and in some states, the profession is completely unregulated.

- Naturopathy as a whole medical system is challenging to study. Rigorous research on this whole medical system is taking place, but it's at an early stage.
- Naturopathic physicians are trained to know that herbs and some dietary supplements can potentially interact with drugs and to avoid those combinations. To do so, they need to be informed of all drugs (whether prescription or over the counter) and supplements that you are taking.

The American Association of Naturopathic Physicians (`www.naturopathic.org`) has a searchable database for finding naturopathic doctors in your area.

Curing Like with Like: Homeopathy

Homeopathic medicine is built around the belief that "like cures like." Practitioners mix small, highly diluted amounts of substances to cure symptoms. If these substances were given at higher or more concentrated doses, they would actually cause those same symptoms.

The term *homeopathy* was coined by the German physician Christian Friedrich Samuel Hahnemann in 1807. Despite being derided by scientists from the 19th century to the present, homeopathy has become increasingly popular in recent years. Almost a fourth of all allergy/cold medicines launched in the United States in recent years have been homeopathic remedies.

Homeopathic medicines widely used for pain include arnica (mountain daisy, hypericum (St. John's Wort), urtica urens (stinging nettle), ledum (marsh tea) rhus tox (poison ivy) ruta (rue) symphytum (comfrey), and calendula (marigold).

The FDA says homeopathic products are safe because they have little or no pharmacologically active ingredients.

Homeopathic substances contain no detectable ingredients apart from the water or other liquid used to dilute them. Therefore, critics believe that there's no known basis for them to heal. Although some patients report benefits from homeopathic preparations, the large majority of scientists attribute this to the placebo effect. This view was supported by a large review published in the British medical journal *The Lancet* in August 2005.

Assessing Complementary and Alternative Treatments

CAM covers a broad range of medical practices from acupuncture to magnets. We can't cover them all in this chapter, but we do highlight major CAM treatments that may help you with your pain management.

Getting the point about acupuncture

Acupuncture is a strange concept: Someone sticks needles into you to reduce your pain. The method most widely identified with acupuncture involves penetrating the skin with very thin, solid, metallic needles that are then moved by hand or electrical stimulation. The process is not particularly painful — it just feels like a small prick.

Acupuncture is based on the belief that health is determined by a flow of life energy, called *qi* (also spelled ki or chi and pronounced chee). Qi is believed to travel through your body along four invisible paths called *meridians.* The belief is that diet, stress, and many other things block these meridians. When the meridians become blocked, your energy flow becomes unstable, causing injury and disease. To regain balance, acupuncturists stimulate certain points, called *acupoints,* along meridians. (See Figure 15-1 for a view of meridians and their corresponding acupuncture points.)

Others who reject the meridian-blocking idea still support acupuncture because they believe it stimulates the production of *endorphins,* or pain-killing neurochemicals. But whether it's ancient Chinese beliefs or modern science that's right, the point is that acupuncture may help a person in pain, which may be you!

Dr. Kassan says, "Rheumatologists see a lot of patients with problems we can't do anything about, especially chronic pain. We become very frustrated. And this is where acupuncture makes its greatest impact: with patients who have failed conventional treatment."

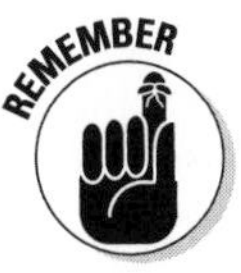

According to the National Institutes of Health, new research and a lot of anecdotal information have shown that acupuncture can be therapeutic for specific and very different conditions, including addiction, stroke rehabilitation, osteoarthritis of the knee, headache, menstrual cramps, tennis elbow, fibromyalgia, myofascial pain, osteoarthritis, low-back pain, carpal tunnel syndrome, and asthma.

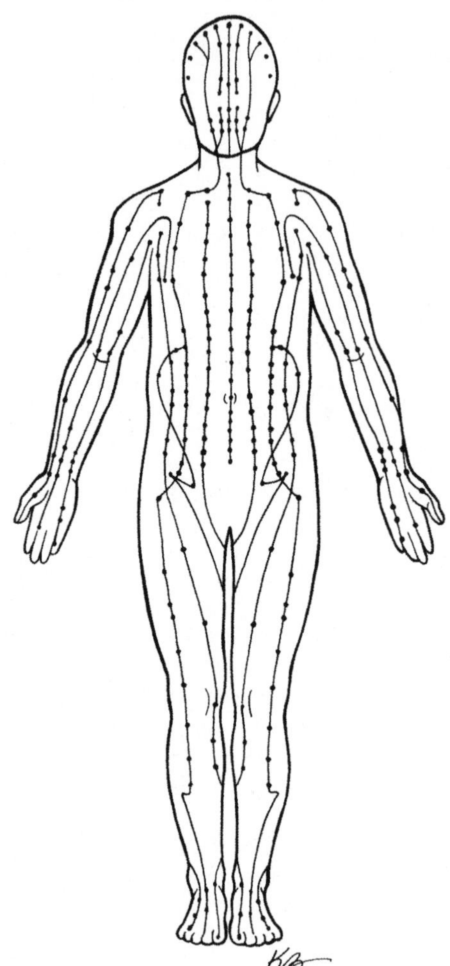

Figure 15-1: Acupuncture meridians.

Acupuncture is generally safe and won't harm you unless you use it to replace necessary medical treatment. However, be sure to select a reputable acupuncturist.

Many medical doctors are trained in acupuncture. About 40 states have established training standards for acupuncture certification, but they have varied requirements for obtaining a license to practice acupuncture. Two organizations provide searchable databases to help you find a practitioner certified in acupuncture: The National Certification Commission for Acupuncture and Oriental Medicine (`www.nccaom.org/find.htm`) and the American Academy of Medical Acupuncture (`www.medicalacupuncture.org`).

Don't rely on a diagnosis of disease by an acupuncture practitioner who doesn't have substantial conventional medical training.

Although acupuncture is usually safe, be sure to go to a practitioner who is diligent about sterilizing needles or who uses disposable ones. Possible dangers with reused needles are infection, nerve damage, and punctured organs.

Acupressure uses the same basic concepts as acupuncture, only without the needles. Putting pressure on the acupoints with your hands, feet, or knees is a form of massage known as acupressure or shiatsu. You can perform acupressure on yourself, or a loved one can learn the basics.

Calming down with biofeedback

Biofeedback uses your mind to control your body. It's a technique in which you use equipment to measure your brain activity, breathing, heart rate, blood pressure, skin temperature, and/or muscle tension (see Figure 15-2). By watching these measurements, you can find out how to change them by relaxing or holding pleasant images in your mind. Some psychologists and other therapists use biofeedback with reportedly good results.

During a biofeedback session, a trained practitioner monitors your heart rate, blood pressure, and skin temperature using electrical sensors. The sensors measure your body's response to stress and feed the information back to you on the monitor or through auditory cues.

Through biofeedback, you discover how to associate your pain with physical habits, such as muscles tensing or holding your breath. For example, you may figure out that your headaches come from tensed muscles.

You then discover how to relax specific muscles to prevent or stop your headaches. The goal is to produce these responses on your own without the help of technology.

The Biofeedback Certification Institute of America (BCIA) has a searchable database at `www.resourcenter.net` that you can use to find a qualified biofeedback therapist.

Although biofeedback is considered safe, talk to your doctor if you or a loved one has depression, severe psychosis, diabetes, or other endocrine disorders before using biofeedback.

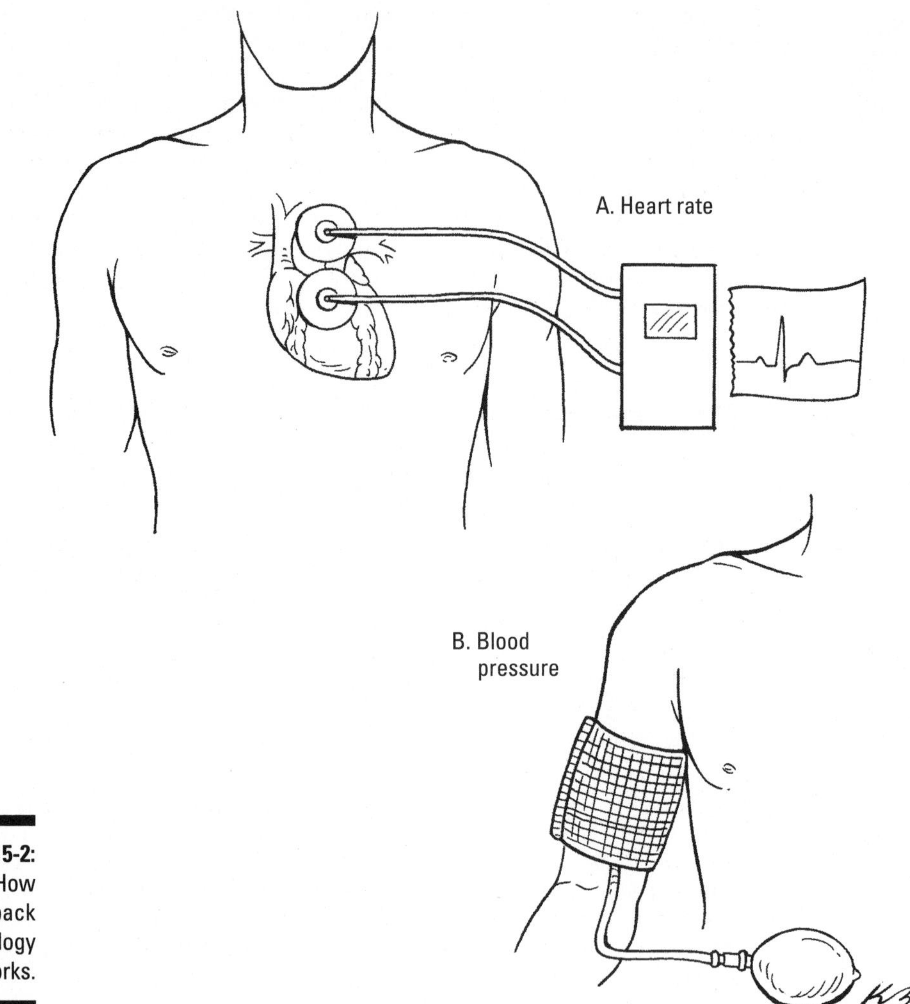

Figure 15-2: How biofeedback technology works.

Boning up on osteopathy

Osteopathy focuses on diseases that begin in the musculoskeletal system. The theory behind osteopathy is that all the body's systems work together, and instability in one system causes instability and pain in other parts of the body. Some osteopathic physicians practice osteopathic manipulation to reduce pain, restore function, and promote health and well-being. Osteopaths focus on joint, muscle, and nerve problems, such as back, neck, and head pain.

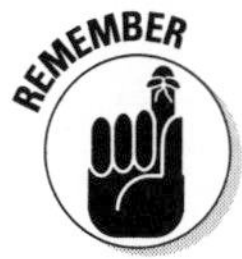

Osteopathy emphasizes a holistic approach to medicine and the use of a range of manual and physical therapies. The goal of the osteopathic physician is to boost the body's own recuperative powers by treating musculoskeletal or other types of dysfunction. A doctor of osteopathy (D.O.) inspects your posture, how you walk, and how you sit. The D.O. also checks to see whether your joints can move through their full range of motion and also looks at your body's symmetry.

Manipulating the spine, arms, and legs doesn't help every medical condition. However, because of their training, D.O.s can also treat conditions in conventional ways when appropriate.

A D.O. is also licensed to perform surgery and prescribe medication. Like an M.D., an osteopath completes four years of medical school, can practice in any specialty of medicine, and is licensed by the state. However, osteopaths receive an additional 300 to 500 hours in the study of hands-on manual medicine and the body's musculoskeletal system.

Osteopaths who want to specialize can become board certified by completing a two- to six-year residency within the specialty area and passing the board certification exams.

The American Academy of Osteopathy (`www.academyofosteopathy.org`) has a searchable database you can use to find a D.O. near you.

Getting cracking with chiropractic care

Chiropractic is a medical system that focuses on the relationship between your body's structures (primarily the spine) and how they function and how that relationship affects health. The goal of chiropractic is to normalize the relationship between your body's structure and function when it's out of whack.

Chiropractic professionals are doctors of chiropractic, or D.C.s. Chiropractors complete a four-year course in a chiropractic college, and must pass national and state examinations. Many people visit chiropractors for treatment of low back pain.

Chiropractic includes spinal manipulation, diet, exercise, X-rays, and other therapeutic techniques. Spinal manipulation is a method of adjusting the spinal cord using hand pressure, twists, and turns.

The premise behind chiropractic is that changes in the normal relationships between the bones of the spine (vertebral bodies) or joints can result in health problems in other areas of the body; consequently, manipulation of these areas may correct these changes and improve function.

Some practitioners also believe that abnormal spine or joint positioning may cause nerve damage or compression, muscle spasm, soft-tissue adhesions, or the release of toxic chemicals from damaged soft tissues. These conditions may be improved with manipulation. Scientific research backing up these theories is rarely reported in medical journals, although it does show up in chiropractic journals. Some people report relief from chiropractic techniques.

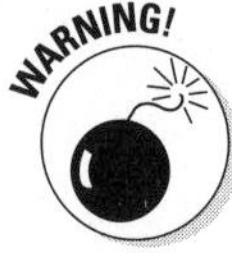

The safety of chiropractic is controversial. The most common side effects are stiffness, headache, and fatigue. Some evidence indicates that chiropractic can increase the chance of having a stroke. If you're at high risk for a stroke or have any of the following risk factors, stay away from manipulation of the neck: use of oral contraceptives, use of blood thinning medications, or high blood pressure.

In addition, if you or a loved one has any of the following conditions, be sure to use caution and talk to your doctor before using chiropractic, because it may cause bone fractures or nerve damage: a bone infection, cancer involving the bone, prior vertebral fractures, severe degenerative joint disease (osteoarthritis), osteoporosis, or ankylosing spondylitis.

Try to find a chiropractor whose practice is limited to conservative treatment of back pain and other musculoskeletal problems. Look for chiropractors who are members of the American Chiropractic Association (`www.amerchiro.org`), or the Canadian Academy of Manipulative Therapists (`www.manipulativetherapy.org`).

Getting hip to hypnosis

Hypnosis has been used since ancient times to relax the mind, reduce pain, and promote health. Hypnosis causes a relaxed state of mind in which the individual is open to reasonable suggestions. This aspect of the technique has made it the brunt of many comedy routines and TV dramas.

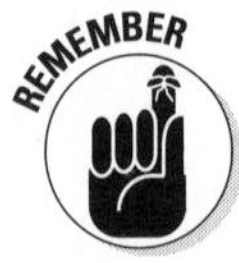

You can't be made to do something when under a hypnotic trance that you wouldn't do normally. However, you can use the suggestibility caused by hypnosis to your physical and mental benefit.

For example, you can work with a trained therapist to find out how to put yourself into a hypnotic state (see Chapter 21). You may also decide to use a therapist on an ongoing basis.

To treat chronic pain, the therapist gives you suggestions to help reduce your perception of pain and relax your tense muscles (which add to the pain), and so on.

Hypnotherapy has not been studied extensively for safety. The World Health Organization cautions that people with psychiatric illnesses, such as schizophrenia, manic depression (bipolar disorder), multiple personality disorder, or antisocial personality disorders, should not use hypnosis.

There's no national accreditation or licensing for hypnotherapists in the United States, but many different organizations provide certification for hypnosis therapists. One such organization is the National Board for Certified Clinical Hypnotherapists (`www.natboard.com`).

Chapter 16

Considering Surgery: The Last Resort?

In This Chapter

- Opting for surgery
- Choosing the right surgeon
- Identifying different types of surgery used for chronic pain
- Considering surgery when you're older
- Preparing for surgery

Your chronic pain may be so bad that you're totally fed up and desperate. You'd do just about anything to lessen the agony, including letting a surgeon cut into you while you're unconscious. Or maybe your doctor has told you that you *need* surgery. Alternatively, perhaps you simply want to know all your options for managing your pain, including surgical choices. Whatever led you to reading this chapter, you're probably approaching the idea of surgery with considerable trepidation. We don't know anyone who says, "Okay, I'll have surgery. No big deal." It's always a big deal.

But for many, surgery actually is a great option that can have stunning results. One of your authors (Elizabeth Vierck) has had two hip replacement surgeries, as well as surgery on both feet, all problems caused by arthritis. She says, "Fifty years ago, I'd be walking with two canes or in a wheelchair by now. Instead, I walk a few miles on most days, hike in the mountains, bicycle, and do water exercise four times a week. I'm not pain-free, but have a lot less pain than before the surgeries, and I'm active, best of all." A true testimonial for the surgery choice!

Benefits of surgery for those over age 65

Research conducted by the Agency for Healthcare Research and Quality has shown surgery can be a boost to older people in pain. Its study showed that, despite the risk of complications, the quality of life improves for older people after having knee replacement surgery. Older patients reported less pain and better physical function after surgery than younger patients.

Additional research confirmed the value of total knee replacement surgery in a study of patients whose average age was 65 years. After four years, nearly 90 percent of patients had a good to excellent outcome. After five years, 75 percent had no pain, 20 percent had mild pain, 3.7 percent had moderate pain, and only 1.3 percent had severe pain. These are good numbers!

Making the Decision

Most surgeries for pain are *elective*. In other words, the choice is really up to you. Surgery for chronic pain is usually not an emergency. Your life isn't in danger. You have time to find out as much as possible about the surgery and the surgeon and to review your options. You also have time to get a second opinion (or more, if need be). No rush decisions are required, which is good.

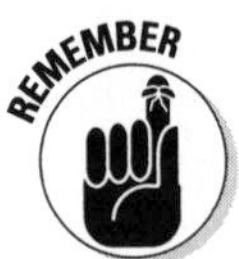

All surgery has risks and requires a recovery period ranging from days to months, depending on the type of procedure and your general health status. Outcomes can vary considerably, from thrillingly successful to not so great.

One of your authors (Dr. Kassan) cautions, "As a general rule, don't consider surgery until you've tried all other approaches, including medicines, physical therapy, and other techniques we discuss in this book. Even then, have surgery only when you feel that a not-so-great surgical outcome can't be worse than the pain you're in at present." He also warns, "There is an exception to this advice: If you have any neurological signs, such as numbness, weakness, or loss of bowel function, talk to your doctor about these symptoms right away."

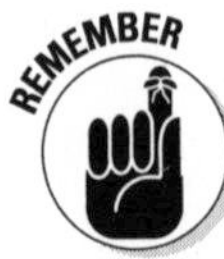

You and your primary care doctor should exhaust all other pain-relieving options before you even consider surgery or meet with a surgeon.

Your primary care physician is usually a good starting point to learn about surgery. For example, your doctor will know what type of surgery you may need and which surgeon you should interview for your operation, such as an orthopedic doctor, neurosurgeon, or general surgeon.

Although your doctor can refer you to a specific surgeon by name, also do some investigating on your own to make sure that person is a good fit. Before you meet the surgeon, think about issues you need to discuss:

- **Does my particular condition respond well to surgery?** For example, surgery for back pain is controversial. Many medical experts suggest that most back pain will eventually ease up or go away completely without surgery. And some spinal surgeries can lead to other problems, such as collapsing of the vertebrae above where the surgery was done or below the area that was operated on. You should discuss these types of issues with your primary care doctor, as well as the surgeon.
- **What results can I expect from surgery?** Ask such questions as, "Will my pain go away entirely?" or "If my pain will only be reduced, about how much pain will I still have?" or "Will my pain probably be reduced by 80 percent, 50 percent, 10 percent, or some other percentage?"
- **What lies ahead for me if I do *not* have surgery now?** Several things can happen. If you don't have surgery, your condition may worsen. Alternatively, depending on your medical problem, the condition may improve on its own. Or it may stay about the same. Find out which situation applies in your case.
- **Are there any emerging surgical techniques that may help even more or that would require less recovery time and may be worth waiting for a year or two down the road?**
- **Are there other nonsurgical treatments that I haven't tried yet to ease my pain?** Besides your doctor's response, this question also requires an honest answer from you. For example, have you carried out all the recommendations of your physical therapist? Do you take your medications as prescribed and on schedule? Do you control your weight? If not, now is a good time to start!

Checking Out a Surgeon's Resume

Two important attributes to look for in a surgeon are specialized training and a lot of experience. Be sure to find out about your surgeon's qualifications.

Obtain the following types of information about the surgeon's credentials and experience before you sign up to lie down on that operating table:

- **Is your surgeon certified by a surgical board approved by the American Board of Medical Specialties (such as the American Board of Orthopaedic Surgery, the American Board of Colon and Rectal Surgery, or another national surgical board)?** Board-certified surgeons have successfully completed training and passed exams for their specialty. If the surgeon or his group has a Web site, this information is usually included there.

- **Does the surgeon have the letters FACS after his name?** If so, the doctor is a Fellow of the American College of Surgeons. Fellows have passed a test of their surgical training and skills; they've also committed to high standards of ethical conduct. Doctors with FACS after their name are proud of this credential and often include the designation after their name in the Yellow Pages of the phone directory.
- **Is the surgeon board certified?** Most minimally invasive spine surgeries for pain control, such as disc decompression or spinal cord stimulation are performed by board-certified anesthesiologists or physiatrists with extra training in pain medicine. These physicians do not have the FACS designation (see preceding bullet), but have specialized training specifically in pain medicine, which may include a year of formal fellowship training.
- **Does the surgeon operate regularly?** You're looking for a surgeon who operates at least several times a week.
- **How many times has he performed the specific surgery you need in the past year?** Studies suggest that surgical outcomes are better when a surgeon has performed a surgery many times.

  So how many is many? We don't have a definite answer to this question. As a general rule, your surgeon should perform an operation like yours at least every few weeks, and much more often would be better.
- **Does the surgeon get good reviews from commercial services?** Check out sites such as bestdoctors.com (`www.bestdoctors.com`) and healthgrades.com (`www.healthgrades.com`).
- **Does the surgeon practice at a highly reputable, accredited hospital?** You want one that has a Gold Seal of Approval from the accreditation organization called The Joint Commission (`www.qualitycheck.org`) or those who make U.S. News and World Report's Best Hospitals list (`www.health.usnews.com`).

Knowing what to ask the surgeon

Interview at least two surgeons when you're considering surgery. Remember the surgeon isn't going to be your new best friend, so don't be put off by a brusque and busy manner. More importantly, does he have a lot of experience with the surgery you're considering? In other words, find a surgeon whose specialty is the specific procedure that you're going to be having. For example, if you're going to have your neck fused, pick a surgeon who performs neck fusions a hundred or more times per year.

Your author, Dr. Kassan, says that the best surgeons are usually the ones who are busiest. As a result, you may not get into see the surgeon of your choice right away.

If you have to wait to see a popular surgeon, ask to be put on the doctor's waiting list. Also, ask to be put on the cancellation list in case someone cancels her appointment. You may not get much notice, but you also may get your appointment much faster.

When you meet the surgeon, ask these questions, recommended by the National Institutes of Health:

- What type of surgery is recommended?
- Why do I need surgery?
- Can another treatment be tried instead of surgery?
- What if I don't have the surgery?
- How will the surgery affect my health and lifestyle?
- Are there any activities that I won't be able to do after surgery?
- How long will it take to recover?
- How much experience has the surgeon had doing this kind of surgery?
- Where will the surgery be done — in the hospital, the doctor's office, a special surgical center, or a day surgery unit of a hospital?
- What kind of anesthesia will be used? What are the side effects and risks of having anesthesia?
- Is there anything else I should know about this surgery?

You may want to create your own list of questions that relate to your specific case. Write down your concerns *before* you see the doctor. Ask the most important questions in case you run out of time — that way, at least the doctor has addressed those issues. Take notes on what the doctor says, in case you forget later. (You think you won't, but sometimes people do!)

Getting a second opinion

Many people worry that if they get a second opinion about surgery, they'll hurt their doctor's delicate feelings. Don't worry: Second opinions are standard medical practice, and getting them gives you several advantages. They're a good way to get expert advice from another doctor specializing in your particular medical problem. And second opinions can reassure you that your decision to have surgery is the right one. The opposite can also be true; the other doctor may just stop you from having unnecessary surgery. Medicare, many Medicaid programs, and many private health insurance companies help pay for a second opinion.

When getting another opinion, do the same upfront research that you did for the first surgeon and ask the second surgeon the same questions that you asked the first one (from the "Making the decision" and "Knowing what to ask the surgeon" sections, earlier in this chapter) so that you can compare answers.

How do second opinions work? If both doctors agree that your surgery is probably a go, you may choose to go to either doctor for the surgery. If the second surgeon doesn't come to the same conclusion as the first, you may want to see a third surgeon to break the tie. You should also get the opinion of your primary care doctor.

Before going for a second opinion, have your medical records sent to the second surgeon so that you won't have to repeat any tests. Also, if you've had recent X-rays and the evaluating doctor will probably need to see them, call the clinic (or wherever the X-rays are located) and tell the staff you want to check out your X-rays. Give them at least a few days notice.

Profiling Major Types of Pain-Relieving Surgery

Many conditions cause chronic pain, so many types of surgery are available. They range from procedures to implant electrical equipment to reduce your pain to surgery to replace entire joints. In the following sections, we cover major surgeries performed to relieve pain, but check with your doctor about specific surgeries available for your particular condition. New surgical procedures and technologies appear all the time; make sure that you're up on the latest and greatest options for your specific condition.

Spinal cord stimulation (SCS)

Spinal cord stimulation (SCS) is a nondestructive, surgical approach to reversible pain relief. This therapy is used to control such chronic pain conditions as neuropathic pain, post-herpetic neuralgia, complex regional pain syndrome, low back pain, pain that remains after back surgery (failed backs), and Raynaud's disease. (Check Part II for information about these conditions.) In fact, SCS is often the last resort for these conditions and provides welcome relief when all other approaches fail. The success rate for SCS is a stunning 50 to 70 percent, depending on the cause of pain.

In SCS, a surgeon installs a little generator and a *lead* (wire) under your skin. The generator sends electrical currents through the lead to your spinal cord. (You'll probably feel a tingling sensation.) These currents act like a jamming device. Installing the equipment is usually a simple outpatient procedure, and you'll have a small incision.

Two types of SCS systems are available — one type is placed totally inside your body, and the other type uses a remote control and sends radio frequency signals to communicate with a receiver in the body.

Implantable drug delivery systems

Implantable drug delivery systems send pain-relieving medications, such as morphine or other drugs, directly to receptors in the spinal cord. A major advantage is that smaller doses of medication are required to gain relief because you're receiving a steady dose.

The system is made up of a pump and *catheter* (a thin, flexible tube) surgically implanted under the skin. The pump is inserted just above or below the belt line. A catheter runs from the pump to the spinal cord where it delivers medication, usually an opioid. The pump releases medication at a set rate and eventually expands out and bathes pain receptors all along the spinal cord.

Some health problems are particularly amenable to drug delivery systems. If you or a loved one has any of the following conditions, implanted drug systems may help:

- Failed back surgery syndrome
- Complex regional pain syndrome (CRPS)
- Chronic abdominal pains
- Failed neck surgery syndrome

Morphine is usually used in implantable drug delivery systems. However, some people can't tolerate the side effects of morphine, but may be able to use other drugs such as Demerol, Dilaudid, methadone, Fentanyl, or sufentanil. (See Chapter 14 for more information on these drugs.) New drugs, such as Prialt, derived from the toxin of a Pacific cone snail, show promise but are currently extremely expensive.

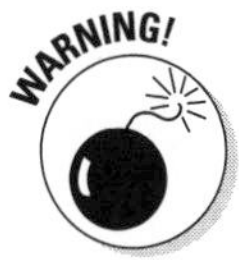

If you've used an implantable drug delivery system for awhile, you may develop tolerance to the drug delivered to your spine, or you may develop another condition that does not respond to opioids. If you have such a response, your doctor may try other medications such as local anesthetics.

Nerve blocks

Nerve blocks are injections of an anesthetic into or near a pain-conducting nerve. The procedure prevents pain signals from reaching the spinal cord or brain. A local anesthetic temporarily halts the transmission of pain signals in peripheral nerves.

Nerve blocks can be single injections or continuous infusions. They can relieve pain temporarily, for a few weeks, or several months.

According to the Cleveland Clinic, nerve blocks may help if you suffer from any of the following conditions:

- Neck pain
- Low back pain
- Sciatica resulting from herniated discs
- Lumbar canal stenosis
- Complex regional pain syndrome (reflex sympathetic dystrophy)
- Peripheral vascular disease
- Shingles pain
- Myofascial pain syndrome
- Cancer pain

Spinal fusion

Spinal fusion joins together two or more vertebrae with bone grafts, metals rods, or other hardware. If you have injured your vertebrae, have slipped discs, or curvatures of the spine, spinal fusion may be an option for you.

The surgery results in limited motion in the area of the fusion and may cause instability further up and down the spine. If you have spinal fusion surgery, you may be much more active than in the past, but if you don't stay in condition, you may still have pain.

Facet neurotomy

The purpose of a facet neurotomy is to destroy the root of a spinal nerve that is causing pain. The procedure is always considered a last resort because it can cause complete sensory loss to the destroyed nerve and can also lead to loss of motor function. However, it can also give major pain relief to some patients.

Minimally invasive disc procedures

Small to moderate-sized disc herniations and tears in the discs of the vertebrae can now be treated in ways that are far less invasive than previous surgeries. Many of these procedures are performed by pain medicine physicians and include the following:

- Devices such as mechanical instruments, laser tools, coblation tools (a type of radiofrequency energy), and high-pressure contained water jets can be used to repair discs. A radiofrequency probe, called an Intradiscal Electrothermal Therapy (IDET), can be used to repair tears in discs.
- Specialized tools can be inserted through a tube (endoscope) into discs. Then the tools are used through the scope to make pain-relieving repairs.

Surgery for cervical disc disease

If you have cervical (neck) disc disease, you may want to consider several surgical options. *Cervical disc disease* is caused by degeneration of the discs in the spine, narrowing of the spinal canal, arthritis, and, in rare cases, cancer or meningitis. Symptoms of the condition include pain in your neck or shoulder, tingling and numbness in your arms, and weakness in your arms or hands.

Several surgical procedures can relieve cervical pain. According to the American Association of Neurological Surgeons, they include

- **Anterior cervical discectomy (ACD):** ACD is widely performed to treat chronic neck pain. A disc (or discs) and bone spurs are removed from neck vertebrae. The surgery relieves pressure on one or more nerve roots or on the spinal cord.
- **Anterior cervical corpectomy:** This operation is performed together with anterior cervical discectomy. One or more parts of your vertebrae are removed, and then the space between the vertebrae is fused.
- **Posterior microdiscectomy:** This procedure is performed for a bulging disc on the side of the spinal cord. The surgeon carefully moves a nerve root to the side to free the offending disc.
- **Posterior cervical laminectomy:** In this procedure the surgeon uses a small incision in the middle of your neck to remove bone spurs or disc material.

Joint replacement

Some readers may remember an old '70s television show, "The Bionic Woman", in which many body parts of the injured Jaime Sommers were replaced, giving her incredible speed and mobility. Some people with joint replacement consider themselves bionic. Of course, joint replacement won't enable you to run so fast that people can't even see you, but it can often enable you to walk without pain once you recover, which sounds pretty good to people suffering from severe joint pain.

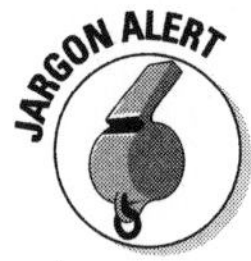

Joint replacement is the removal of a diseased joint and its replacement with an artificial one, called a *prosthesis.* The medical term for the procedure is *arthroplasty.* Over the last couple of decades, tremendous advances have been made in arthroplasty for knees and hips. The following are the most frequently performed joint replacements.

- **Hip replacement surgery** is one of the most successful orthopedic surgeries. It's evolving from a major surgery with a long recovery time to a less invasive procedure with a faster return to normal functioning. Regardless of the technique used, the process involves taking out diseased parts of the joint — the femur and acetebellum — and replacing them with artificial parts that allow smooth motion of the hip.

  If you have hip replacement surgery, you and your surgeon will decide whether your new hip will be fastened to your healthy bone using cement or something called *biologic fixation,* which involves giving your bone time to actually grow into the prosthesis. Your surgeon may also want to use a combination of methods. The advantage of cemented replacements is that you can go back to your normal activities soon after surgery.

- **Hip resurfacing** is a newer technique that enables the surgeon to remove less bone during a total hip replacement procedure. The femoral head, neck, and femur remain in your joint, allowing preservation of as much of the hip as possible. Resurfacing keeps a large portion of the hip joint intact for you to have total hip replacement surgery at a later date if needed.

- During **knee replacement surgery,** damaged bone and cartilage are taken from your thighbone, shinbone, and kneecap, and the areas are then reshaped. The surgeon inserts an artificial joint (*prosthesis*). As with hip replacement surgeries, knee replacements have benefited from new, minimally invasive surgical techniques. The procedure can be performed without large incisions, allowing for a quicker recovery than in the past. It also means you'll have less scar tissue.

Preparing for surgery if you have fibromyalgia

If you're having a major surgical procedure and you also have fibromyalgia or a similar chronic disease, talk with your surgeon and anesthesiologist about techniques to help you reduce a flare up of symptoms that often occurs after surgery. These techniques are adapted from materials developed by the Oregon Fibromyalgia Foundation (www.myalgia.com).

- If you'll have an endotracheal tube during surgery, ask for a soft neck collar to wear during surgery to minimize neck hyperextension.
- Ask that your arm with the intravenous line be kept near your body, not away from your body or over your head.
- Request a pre-operative opioid pain medication that you can take about 90 minutes prior to surgery. Pre-operative opioids can minimize the widespread body pain that you're already experiencing due to your fibro.
- Ask for a long-acting local anesthetic to be infiltrated into your incision — even though you'll be asleep during the procedure. This anesthetic minimizes pain impulses reaching your spinal cord and brain, which in turn drive central sensitization.
- You'll need more post-operative pain medication, and it'll usually need to be longer-acting medication. In most cases, opioids should be regularly administered or self-administered with a PCA pump (patient-controlled analgesia).

Most fibromyalgia patients require a longer post-operative convalescence, including physical therapy.

Recovering from Surgery

When you know in advance what to expect after surgery, you'll be less scared and more able to plan ahead for a successful recovery. Knowledge is power! Ask your surgeon how long you'll be in the hospital and find out what kind of supplies and equipment you'll need when you go home. Also ask your surgeon how much post-operative pain to expect and what kinds of activities you'll be able to do after surgery. For example, ask when you can take daily walks around the block again or when you can lift your 25-pound grandchild again safely.

Also, ask how long it will be before you can go back to work or start regular exercise. Find out whether you'll need any special equipment when you return to work. You don't want to do *anything* that will slow down your recovery! If you have other types of chronic pain in addition to the reason why you're having surgery, tell your surgeon and the health professionals helping you with rehabilitation. For example, not being able to perform physical therapy exercises after surgery may greatly impact your recovery.

Who can help on the Web

A number of great online resources are available for researching surgeries and surgeons. Start with the American College of Surgeons (www.facs.org/index.html; click on "Public Information" and then click on "Search for Members of the American College of Surgeons") to find surgeons who are members.

Also check with the American College of Medical Specialties (www.abms.org/login.asp) to find out whether the surgeon you're considering is certified in his specialty:

The following Web sites also provide interactive services where you can find board-certified surgeons in your area.

- American Academy of Orthopedic Surgeons, www.aaos.org
- American Association of Neurological Surgeons, www.aans.org
- American Pediatric Surgical Association, www.eapsa.org
- Society of American Gastrointestinal Endoscopic Surgeons, www.sages.org
- Society of Reproductive Surgeons, www.reprodsurgery.org

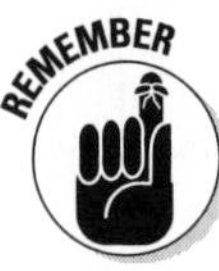

When you have surgery, remember that it's normal to have pain afterward. It even has a name: *post-surgical pain.* It will be awhile before you know how much pain relief you're going to have as a result of the surgery because the post-surgical pain will dominate for awhile. Many people also have pain due to inflammation and/or muscle spasms after surgery. You'll also have pain at the site of the incision and in the area where the operation was performed. Your body has had a major assault, and these reactions to surgery are all normal. As your body heals, this discomfort should decrease. If it doesn't, be sure to discuss your situation with your surgeon and primary care doctor.

Part IV
Managing Your Pain with Lifestyle

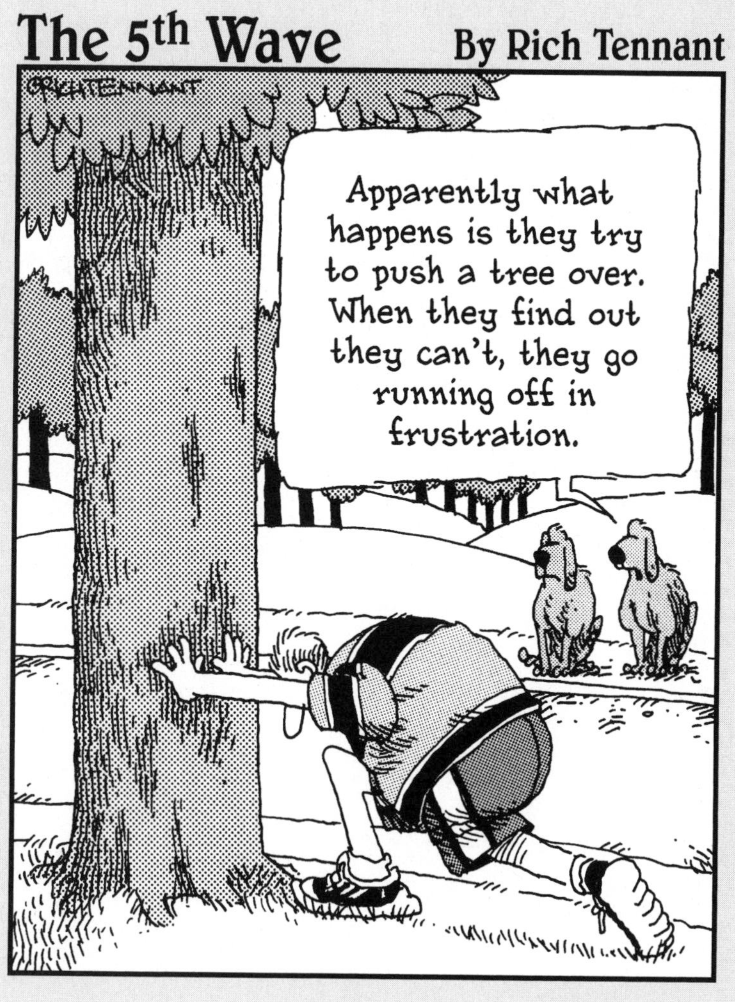
The 5th Wave
By Rich Tennant
Apparently what happens is they try to push a tree over. When they find out they can't, they go running off in frustration.

In this part . . .

In this part, you discover how to manage your pain with your lifestyle. We show you how to track and manage that pain and discuss how good nutrition, deconditioning, and sleep all affect your level of chronic pain.

We also take a look at how pain can be heightened or reduced by how you think and how your body reacts to that thinking and how to alleviate stress in your life.

Chapter 17

Tracking and Avoiding Pain Triggers

In This Chapter

- Identifying tools to track your pain
- Understanding how gadgets can help you
- Discovering good body mechanics
- Tracking how pain affects your life

Have you ever been sitting in your doctor's office when she asks you how intense your pain has been, and you suddenly blank out? Maybe you say, "Uh, maybe a 7 when it started. Oh, maybe a 3 now. Uh, well, okay, maybe it's more of a 5," you stammer. You're confusing your doctor and embarrassing yourself, but you can't help it. This so-called doctor-visit amnesia is a common phenomenon. It happens to most of us, so don't feel bad. (Just plan ahead, so you can hopefully avoid it!)

Many people grit their teeth, bear the pain, and avoid keeping track of the details. They don't remember or have any sort of record of what they were doing on the day the pain was its worst, nor do they know what was going on when the pain started in the first place. But, as the saying goes, the devil is in the details.

Tracking the minutiae of your individual chronic pain can help you and your doctor tame that wild demon. For example, if you honestly rate your maximum pain on a scale of 1 to 10 for a week at the end of every day, you may find that it is ever-so gradually going down. It may be subtle, but it means that your treatment is working.

This chapter provides you key suggestions for evaluating the intensity of your pain and also tracking and managing that pain. If you share this information with your loved ones, caregivers, doctors, and other health professionals, they'll better understand the impact your chronic pain has on you and be more adept at helping you manage it.

Tracking Your Pain

Medical research has shown that if you measure the level of your pain, and you also record the location of your pain, how long it lasts, and other characteristics, such as how it's affecting your quality of life, you'll have the most reliable gauge of your pain. And this information can really help you and your doctor.

The following sections provide you with a wealth of materials you can use to track your pain and improve its management.

Describing your pain

Are you at a loss for what words to use to describe your pain at its worst? One reason for your pain amnesia may be that people can't remember exactly how pain felt when they feel better again. It's over, and they know that it hurt, but they just can't recollect how it felt. (This is nature's way of keeping you sane!) When you're in severe pain, look at the following list and see which words best describe your pain so that you can report this information to your doctor later:

Aching	Burning	Buzzing	Crampy	Crushing
Cutting	Deep	Dull	Electric	Itching
Knot-like	Gnawing	Lightning-like	On the surface	Piercing
Pinching	Pins and needles	Prickling	Pounding	Pulling
Pulsing	Sharp or stabbing	Shooting	Stretching	Tender
Tight	Zapping			

Recording your pain

A pain log can help you identify your particular pain triggers. (*Pain triggers* are things in your life — such as too much exercise or too little sleep — that set off a pain cycle.) When you know what your own personal pain triggers are, you can deal with them more proactively.

Keeping a pain record can also help you and your doctor assess your pain and evaluate how well your medications and other treatments are working. And it can help you keep track of your pain management goals and whether you're reaching them. (We discuss goal setting in the "Taking Control"

Detect someone else's pain with nonverbal cues

If you're helping another person develop his pain diary or you want to explain his pain to a health professional, you may find it difficult to get a true picture of how he feels. It's often hard to tell what's going on, even when you know someone is in pain. Sure, he hurts, but how bad is it?

In fact, many people won't tell you, particularly if they're part of an older generation or naturally stoical. However, people in pain also display nonverbal clues to how they're feeling. You can use these clues developed by the National Institutes of Health to tell whether someone else is in pain:

- **Vocal complaints:** Moans, groans, grunts, cries, gasps, or sighs
- **Facial grimaces and winces:** Furrowed brow, narrowed eyes, tightened lips, dropped jaw, clenched teeth, distorted expression
- **Bracing:** Clutching or holding on to things during movement
- **Restlessness:** Constant or intermittent shifting of position, rocking, intermittent or constant hand motions, inability to keep still
- **Protecting:** Clutching or holding the affected area
- **Self soothing:** Rubbing and massaging the affected area of the body

section, later in this chapter.) If you suffer from chronic pain, you should be recording it at regular intervals to track your improvement and how well your treatments are working, as well as times when you worsen.

Many methods for keeping a record of your pain are available, and we describe several in the following sections. This way, you have no excuse because you should be able to work with at least one method here.

For example, if you don't like to keep handwritten notes, try using a picture log. Figure 17-1 shows one we really like, developed by the American Chronic Pain Association. Make copies of the form and then circle the number under the pictures that most apply to you.

Also consider combining methods — for example, using both this picture method and the quality of life scales in Figure 17-3.

Keeping a diary

A diary can help you track your pain. A student notebook or a pad of paper and a folder both work well.

Keep in mind that the more details that you include in your notebook, the better for you and your doctor.

Be sure to answer these questions in your pain diary:

- Exactly where does it hurt? Is your pain limited to one spot, or does it move around to other parts of your body?

Live Better with Pain Log

Date ______________

Name ______________

Pain Level

No Pain — Worst Pain

1 2 3 4 5 6 7 8 9 10

Stress

No stress — Very Stressed

1 2 3 4 5 6 7 8 9 10

Exercise

Exercise daily — No exercise

1 2 3 4 5 6 7 8 9 10

Activity

Normally active — No activity

1 2 3 4 5 6 7 8 9 10

Sleep

Fully rested — Poor-quality sleep

1 2 3 4 5 6 7 8 9 10

Courtesy of American Chronic Pain Association.

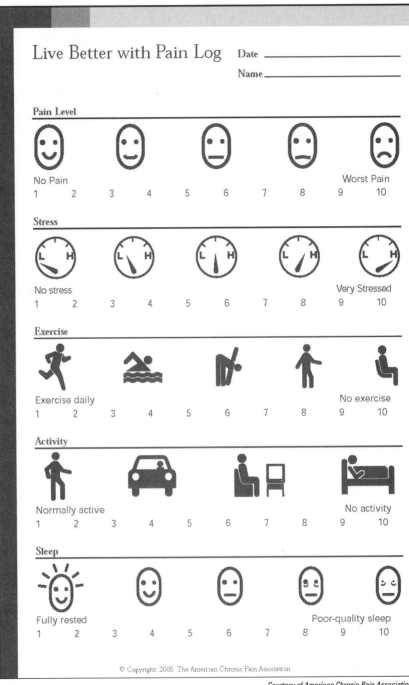

Figure 17-1: Live Better with Pain log.

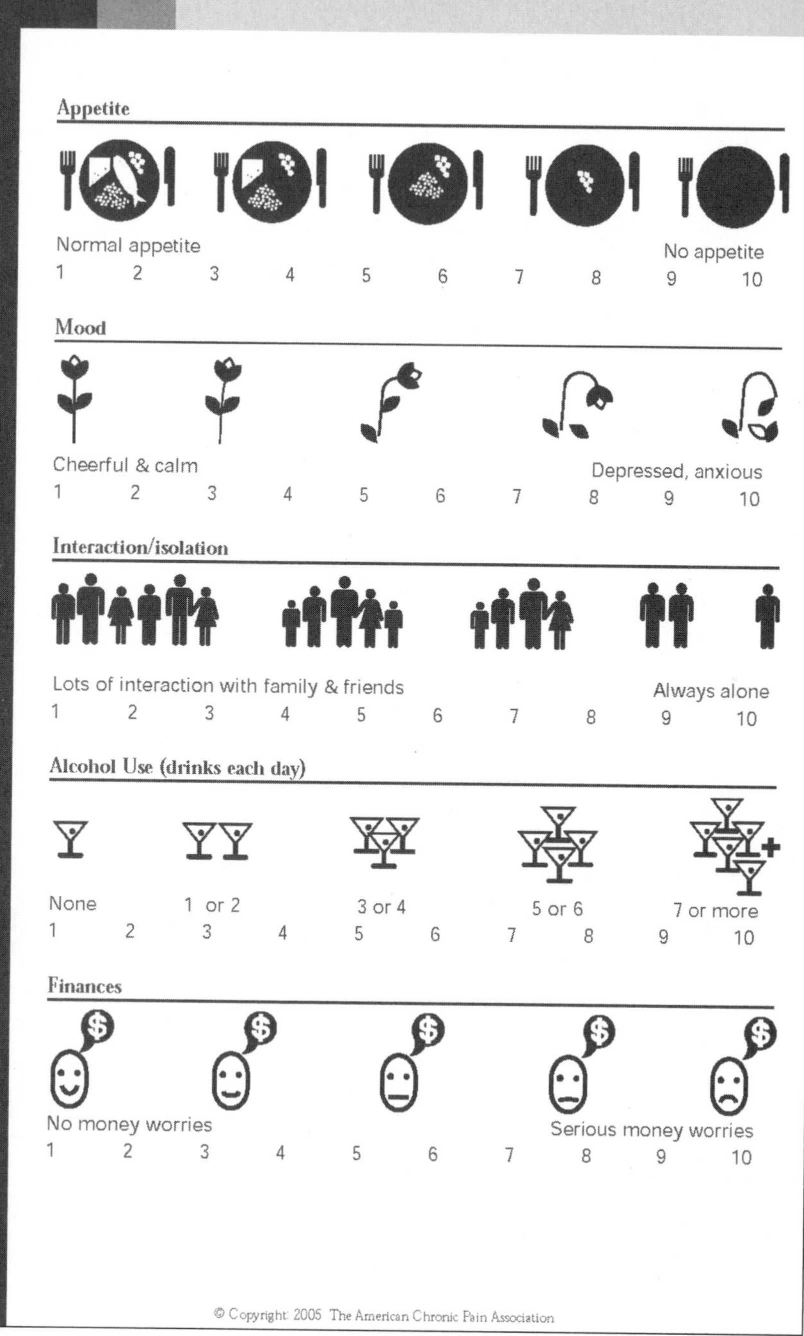
Appetite
Normal appetite
No appetite
1 2 3 4 5 6 7 8 9 10
Mood
Cheerful & calm
Depressed, anxious
1 2 3 4 5 6 7 8 9 10
Interaction/isolation
Lots of interaction with family & friends
Always alone
1 2 3 4 5 6 7 8 9 10
Alcohol Use (drinks each day)
None
1 or 2
3 or 4
5 or 6
7 or more
1 2 3 4 5 6 7 8 9 10
Finances
No money worries
Serious money worries
1 2 3 4 5 6 7 8 9 10
© Copyright 2005 The American Chronic Pain Association

Finding your environmental pain triggers

Some people's pain worsens when they eat certain foods or they're under stress. Others find weather changes greatly exacerbate their pain. Heavy lifting can trigger pain in some people. Some contorted positions (for whatever reason that you're contorted!) can zap your body with pain. Once you've identified your environmental triggers, you can start working on limiting their effects on your life!

Following are some basic suggestions for limiting some common pain triggers:

- Avoid lifting more than 15 to 20 pounds whenever possible. Extra weight can trigger pain in many people.
- Falls can be pain generators, and some people suffer for years from a seemingly minor slip and fall. Keep your house and driveway debris-free and watch where you're walking (hopefully not into a pothole!) when away from home. If you have small children or grandchildren, watch out for the tiny items they spread around that are too easy to trip over.
- When the weather is bad, you can't somehow transform a cold, snowy day into a sunny day at a tropical beach. But you can dress warmly, be careful, and decrease the probability of ratcheting up your pain quotient.
- Sometimes foods trigger pain. Track what you eat to find out whether spicy foods, caffeinated drinks, milk, or other types of food put you in Painland, a place where you don't want to be. If so, avoid those foods.
- If you're under a lot of stress, find some de-stressing activities. Do something fun or just take a nap — whatever works for you.

- What does the pain feel like? Is it a stabbing, throbbing, or aching pain, or would you describe it in another way?
- How strong is the pain? Use a 1 to 10 scale, with 0 for no pain and 10 for the worst that you can possibly imagine. You may want to use the scale at the top of Figure 17-1. In addition, the next section, "Using pain scales to determine pain intensity," provides the address for a Web site where you can download and print scales for free.

  Do not amplify your pain on the pain scales. For example, a 10 usually means that the pain sufferer has been in the emergency room getting IV narcotics. People who say their pain is a 20 are frequently viewed as not being truthful and are prone to exaggeration, which may negatively impact pain care. Consider recording a range of daily pain instead of simply picking a number.
- How frequent are your pain episodes? (For example, are they several times a day or week or some other frequency?) Do these pain episodes occur only when you get up in the morning, or whenever you've been resting for awhile? Or is the pain constant and unremitting?
- How long does each pain episode last? Do you have it all the time, on and off, the same all day long, or is it worse at a particular time?

- Do you have more than one type of pain? For example, you may have some constant aches, as well as a shooting pain in your shoulder that comes and goes.
- What are your pain triggers, if you know? What activities or times of day seem to set off the pain, make it worse, or make it better? For example, did you carry a heavy suitcase through the airport yesterday, and now you're paying for it with major pain? Did you stop taking a pain medication? Have you been avoiding exercise or over-exercising? (Yes, some people do exercise too much and for too long!)
- What pain medications are you taking, and how often do you take them?
- Is the medication giving you pain relief?
- If you get relief from the medication, how long does it last?
- Do you have any other symptoms associated with pain, such as sweating, loss of appetite, or insomnia?

Using pain scales to determine pain intensity

Pain scales are frequently used by health-care professionals who work with people in pain when they need to know how bad it hurts. You may decide to use a pain scale by itself or along with a diary to describe your pain intensity. (See the preceding section for more on a pain diary.) The National Institutes of Health provides free and downloadable pain scales on the following Web site: `http://painconsortium.nih.gov`. Click the Other Resources link and then click Pain Intensity Scales.

The pain scales include the number scale, the visual scale, the categorical scale, and the pain faces scale. People usually prefer one scale over the other:

- On the number rating scale, you explain how much pain you're having by choosing a number from 0 (no pain) to 10 (the worst possible pain).
- The visual scale is a straight line. The far left equals no pain, and the far right end equals horrible (the worst) pain. You mark on the line where your pain is.
- The category scale has four categories: none, mild, moderate, and severe. You circle the category that best describes their pain.
- The faces scale uses six faces with different expressions of pain on each face. You choose the face that best describes how you are feeling. This rating scale is easy to use by people from age 3 and up.

Using body diagrams to show where it hurts

A body diagram to describe *where* your pain is and whether it moves around can help your doctor greatly. Copy the body diagram in Figure 17-2. For each part of your body where you have pain, draw an outline that includes the pain area on the body diagram. Use different colored pencils or pens to describe pain that's inside or outside your body. For example, you can use green if the pain is inside your head and blue if it's on the top of your head.

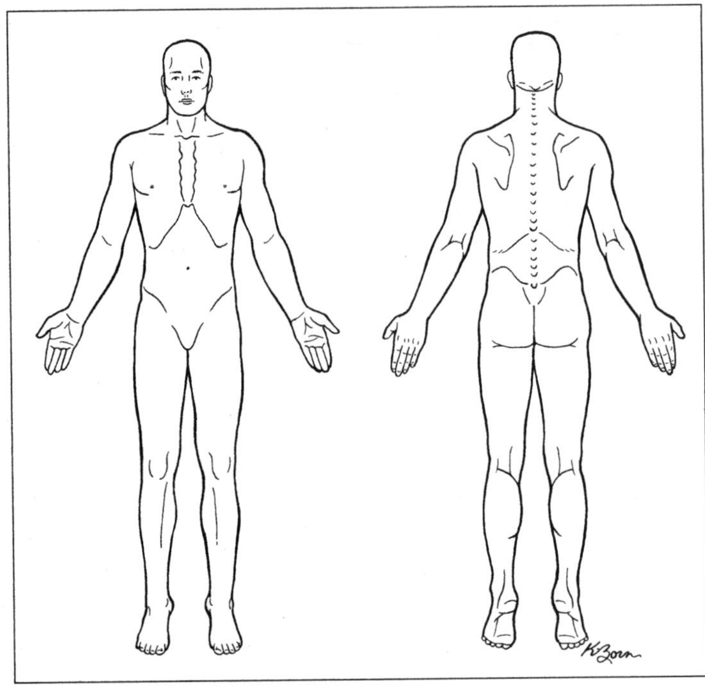

Figure 17-2: Body diagram.

Measuring your quality of life

Chronic pain affects all areas of your life. The staff at the American Chronic Pain Association say it's important to look at not just your physical level of pain, but also how much your pain limits your ability to live a full life. The organization's Quality of Life Scale, shown in Figure 17-3, takes into account your ability to work, enjoy your family, and participate in social activities. The ACPA suggests that you download the scale, print it, and show it to your doctor and other members of your medical team.

Taking your pain records to your doctor

After you create a pain diary and other pain tracking records of your choice (described earlier in the "Tracking Your Pain" section), you can describe to your doctor just what your pain is like and how it changes with different treatments. But how do you relay this information to your doctor during your 15-minute (or less) visit? Creating a summary of all your lists can help you accurately portray your pain to her. Your summary of all the careful records you've been keeping should make the following points:

- When did the pain start? For example, did it begin suddenly or come on gradually?

- Did a specific event seem to set off the pain?
- What does the pain feel like? If you're having trouble describing it, use the list of pain descriptors provided in the "Describing your pain" section, earlier in this chapter.

Quality of Life Scale
A Measure of Function
For People With Pain

0 Non-functioning	Stay in bed all day Feel hopeless and helpless about life
1	Stay in bed at least half the day Have no contact with outside world
2	Get out of bed but don't get dressed Stay at home all day
3	Get dressed in the morning Minimal activities at home Contact with friends via phone, email
4	Do simple chores around the house Minimal activities outside of home two days a week
5	Struggle but fulfill daily home responsibilities No outside activity Not able to work/volunteer
6	Work/volunteer limited hours Take part in limited social activities on weekends
7	Work/volunteer for a few hours daily. Can be active at least five hours a day. Can make plans to do simple activities on weekends
8	Work/volunteer for at least six hours daily. Have energy to make plans for one evening. Active on weekends
9	Work/volunteer for at least six hours daily. Have energy to make plans for one evening. Active on weekends
10 Normal Quality of Life	Go to work/volunteer each day Normal daily activities each day Have a social life outside of work Take an active part in family life

Courtesy American Chronic Pain Association

Figure 17-3: Quality of Life Scale.

- How intense is the pain on most days? This point is where the pain scale in Figure 17-1 that you choose comes in handy.
- Where is the pain on your body? Refer to the body chart shown in Figure 17-2, earlier in this chapter.
- What seems to trigger the pain or make it worse?
- What, if anything, makes the pain better?
- Does your pain affect your ability to carry out daily activities?
- Does your pain affect your mood and sense of well-being?
- Do you feel depressed or anxious?

Your doctor will probably ask you about past and present medical problems or injuries that may have a role in causing or worsening the pain. (For a complete list of the things you should discuss with your doctor, see Chapter 13.) And, of course, your doctor will give you a physical examination.

Developing a Pain Management Plan

Work with your professional anti-pain team to create your pain management plan and then be sure to write it down. (For more information on anti-pain teams, see Chapter 13.) Post your plan somewhere you'll easily see it, such as on your refrigerator or on your nightstand. You also may want to make a copy of your plan and keep it in your pain diary or folder.

Here's a list of the type of items to include in your plan:

- **Goals:** List your goals and update the list regularly. (See the "Getting smart about goals" section, later in this chapter.)
- **Medications:** List the medications you take, the dosage for each drug, and when you take them. You may want to make copies of the medication log in Figure 17-4 and insert your own medication information. (See Chapter 14 for information about the medications frequently used to manage pain.)
- **Pain triggers:** List your pain triggers and your strategy for avoiding them.
- **Exercise and stretching:** List the type of exercises you're doing and plan to do. (See Chapter 19 for information about exercise appropriate for you if you have chronic pain.)
- **Rest:** Plan to make rest and adequate sleep part of your daily routine. (See Chapter 20 for information on getting adequate sleep and rest.)
- **Other healthy habits:** List other healthy habits you'll practice, such as maintaining a healthy diet. (We list many throughout this book.)

- **Questions:** List any questions you have for your anti-pain team. (See Chapter 13 for information about forming your anti-pain team.)
- **Doctor's names and contact information:** Keep this information handy.

Name of Medication	Date Started	Dosage	How much and when	Effects Experienced (reduced pain, sleeplessness, etc.)	Side Effects (nausea etc.)	Name of Prescribing Doctor	Name of Pharmacy

Figure 17-4: Medication log.

- **Rehabilitation plan:** List any special exercises or techniques you're using to lessen your pain and build up strength and stamina.
- **Contact information for your physical and/or occupational therapist and pharmacist:** Include names, addresses, and phone numbers.
- **Contact information for other members of your health-care team such as your fitness instructor or dietician:** Include names, addresses, and phone numbers.

Taking Control

Once you develop a pain management plan with your doctor and other members of your anti-pain team, be sure to use it. A plan that you don't use isn't any good, even if you've got the best doctors in the world!

An important part of making the plan work is to focus on your health:

- Take care of yourself by eating a balanced diet, exercising regularly, and following your pain management plan.
- Be positive and stop negative thinking (see Chapter 21).
- Laugh and smile a lot. (Learn some jokes, read a funny book, or take the kids to an amusement park; see Chapter 22 for more ideas).
- Surround yourself with positive people.
- Enjoy activities with family and friends.

Getting smart about goals

After you're keeping track of your pain, you're ready to set some goals to use in your pain management plan. Select your greatest area(s) of concern and then use the following techniques to set goals to deal with those issues.

Set realistic and achievable pain management goals. If your goals are out of reach (such as a total cure or being pain-free), it's almost impossible to achieve them, so you'll feel discouraged. Conversely, if your pain management goals are too low (too pessimistic), then you'll be selling yourself short. Avoid both errors!

A surefire way to make smart goals is to use the following SMART system, which means your goals are specific, measurable, attainable, realistic, and timely.

- **Specific:** You have a much greater chance of accomplishing a specific goal than a general goal. One way to set a specific goal is to ask the six W questions:

- **Who:** Who is involved?
- **What:** What do I want to accomplish?
- **Where:** Where do I want to accomplish it?
- **When:** When should the goal be reached?
- **Which:** Which requirements and constraints must I pay attention to?
- **Why:** Why I am doing this? (List the specific reasons, purpose, or benefits of accomplishing the goal.)

For example, a general goal is, "Feel less pain." A specific goal is, "Join the pool and go to aqua exercise three days a week, to increase flexibility."

- **Measurable:** Choose a goal with measurable progress so that you can actually see and feel the change occur. When you measure your progress, you stay on track, reach your target dates, and experience the exhilaration of achievement that spurs you on to continued effort required to reach your goals.

  An example is, "My goal is to walk three blocks without stopping by June 1." When June 1 arrives and you find yourself walking down the fourth block without stopping, you've surpassed your goal! Good for you!

- **Attainable:** Set goals that make you stretch a little, but that that you also can realistically reach. If your goal is to lose 10 pounds in a week, that's unrealistic. But losing a pound a week is something you can achieve and also feel great about.
- **Realistic:** Realistic means do-able. Make a plan that makes the goal realistic. For example, a goal of totally giving up "empty calories" is a formula for failure if you love sweets and treats and eat them regularly. It may be more realistic to set a goal of eating an apple in the afternoon in place of your usual oatmeal cookie. You can then work toward reducing empty calories gradually, a much more reasonable goal.
- **Timely:** Set a timeframe to achieve your goal, such as a week from today, in three months, or by your daughter's graduation. Putting a target on your goal gives you something to work toward and to celebrate when you achieve it. Without a time limit, you have no urgency to start taking action now. Time should be measurable, attainable, and realistic.

Using a contract to monitor progress

Using pain records is a great way to track your progress toward your goals. Many pain programs and counselors also recommend making a contract with yourself to set and work toward your goals. They find that making a personal commitment makes it more likely that you'll follow through on your goals. For example, your contract might look something like this:

I agree for the next three months to:

- Take my medications every day.
- Walk for 20 minutes.
- Stretch for five minutes before and after walking.
- Get at least seven hours of sleep every night.

Sidestepping Pain Triggers

When you're aware of your personal pain triggers, you can deal with them more proactively. You may already know that chewing bubble gum gives you headaches, jogging makes your knees swell, or eating spicy food is a no-no for your irritable bowel syndrome.

You may also discover your triggers by tracking your pain. Keeping a diary, using pain scales, or using a similar technique — all described earlier in this chapter — work because they make you pay attention to your body and your environment. And when you pay attention to your body and the world around you, you'll have an easier time identifying what makes your pain worse or better.

Make a checklist of your pain triggers and then develop your strategies for avoiding them. For example, if you've identified using a backpack is a trigger for your neck pain, make it your goal to stop using one and instead purchase a tote bag on wheels. (A better choice: Stop carrying around so much stuff!)

Using handy gadgets

Literally hundreds of assistive products can help people adjust to chronic pain of all types. We like to call these products handy gadgets. They're also known as *assistive devices, assistive technology,* or *adaptive devices.*

These gadgets help people with chronic pain accomplish the activities they've always done but must now do differently. One of their biggest advantages is that they can help people avoid pain triggers. These handy gadgets include the following:

- **Aids for daily living:** Gadgets to help with activities of daily living, such as bathing, carrying items, getting dressed, and managing personal hygiene. For example, if you love to garden, consider pruning shears especially designed for individuals with arthritis, carpal tunnel syndrome, or similar problems. If you have trouble moving from a seated position, some products can help considerably, such as lift chairs that enable people to sit comfortably and safely and get up easily.

- **Computers:** Gadgets, software, and accessories that enable people with limitations to use desktop and laptop computers and other kinds of information technology. For example, software and hardware that enables sight-challenged people to read text in large fonts or that converts text to speech may be just what you need.
- **Controls:** Gadgets that enable people with limitations to start, stop, or adjust electric or electronic devices. For example, a one-handed camera gives you the ability to operate the zoom lens. Some products enable people with chronic pain and limitations to drive or ride in cars, vans, trucks, and buses.
- **Housekeeping:** Gadgets that assist in cooking, cleaning, and other household activities. They include everything from adapted appliances to smart homes, which use computers to control appliances and other parts of the house remotely or to respond automatically to the people living in it. Without flicking a switch, smart homes do everything from filling bath tubs half full with water of a predetermined temperature to lifting cupboards up and down so that they will be at the most appropriate position for different people.
- **Recreation:** Many gadgets and products help people with chronic pain with their leisure and athletic activities. For example, a knitting needle holder that enables you to knit with one hand, a glove that can help you grasp the handles of pool cues, and The HandBike, a hand-propelled bicycle for people with problems in their lower bodies or with spinal cord injuries, are all products that may work well for you.

You can identify many gadgets through ABLEDATA, a government program that provides an Internet database on assistive devises and rehabilitation equipment available from domestic and international sources. ABLEDATA (`www.abledata.com`) doesn't sell products listed on the database, but it provides information on how to contact manufacturers or distributors of the products.

Maintaining the right body mechanics

When you have chronic pain, learning the right body mechanics enables you to move in a way that avoids further injury and triggering of more pain. Body mechanics are related to *biomechanics,* which, among other things, is the study of how your body reacts to its own weight and the environment's gravity.

Why do you need good body mechanics? People with chronic pain often sit, stand, and walk in very awkward and even rigid positions to avoid irritating the painful parts of the body. The result can be new pain in a new area of the body, which is the result of awkward positioning. Learning how to keep your body in the right position can help protect your skeleton, organs, and soft tissues and allows you to use your body in a safe way.

Different professionals, including physical and occupational therapists, can teach you good body mechanics. (See Chapter 13 for information about physical and occupational therapists and the many services they provide.) In addition, you may want to consider a practitioner in one of the following methods. They are trained in body mechanics:

- The **Feldenkrais method** is a system that gives people a greater understanding of their bodies. The method uses movement and awareness, and is thought of as a complementary and alternative technique, but we include it here because of its value for learning good body mechanics.

  The Feldenkrais Method is used by people who want to reduce their pain or limitations while walking and moving around. Many people feel that the method improves movement-related pain in their backs, knees, hips, or shoulders. It also can lead to better recovery for people who have had strokes. To find out more about Feldenkrais go to `www.feldenkrais.com`. To find a class near you, click Practitioners/Classes and Events and then Find an ATM class. (ATM stands for Awareness Through Movement.)

- The **Alexander Technique** is an educational system with the intention of teaching practitioners to recognize and overcome bad habits in their posture and movement. As with the Feldenkrais Method, the Alexander Technique is thought of as a type of complementary and alternative technique. Students of the technique are taught to stand, walk, and sit in ways that are not stressful on the body. To find out more about the Alexander Technique, go to `www.alexandertech.com`. To find practitioners near you, click the Find a Teacher link.

Chapter 18
Nutrition and Weight Control

In This Chapter

- Discovering how a healthy diet decreases pain
- Understanding the principles of healthy eating
- Shunning trigger foods
- Maintaining a healthy weight

I keep trying to lose weight, but it keeps finding me!"

"I'm on a seafood diet. I see food, and I eat it."

"Inside some of us is a thin person struggling to get out, but she can usually be sedated with a few pieces of chocolate cake."

Probably more jokes are told about the struggle to lose weight than any other topic, including blondes! That's because losing weight is such a universal phenomenon and so ridiculously difficult for most people that almost everyone can relate to it. Even the string beans of the world get the jokes because they know numerous people who've tried countless diets to no avail. Yet weight control and good nutrition are both possible. In fact, they're inextricably linked. In addition, weight control and good nutrition also directly affect your level of chronic pain. Too many pounds equal a higher level of pain, and some foods can actually trigger pain.

Healthy nutrition is a very important topic for anyone who has chronic pain. Because, as Carol Ann Rinzler says in *Nutrition For Dummies* (Wiley), "Food is life. All living things, including you, need food and water to live. Beyond that, you need good food, meaning food with the proper nutrients to live well." And when you have chronic pain, living well is a priority.

This chapter focuses on following healthy diet guidelines and keeping your weight under control, which, in turn, can help tame the wild lion of your chronic pain into an annoying kitty.

Paying Attention to Nourishing Your Body

Are you malnourished? Your answer may be, "Are you kidding? My T-shirts are XL!" We hear you! Yet it's very common to be both overweight *and* malnourished. Not the starving-in-a-poor country kind of malnourished, but malnourished nonetheless.

You may be malnourished if you have any of the following food issues:

- **A diet deficient in nutrients because it's unbalanced:** For example, do you shun fruits and vegetables, thinking they're reserved for children or aging hippies or because you just don't like them? Do you consume a lot of sweets and soda? We know one 20-something-year-old who goes to college full time and works two jobs. Her diet consists of colas (love that sugar and caffeine!) and candy bars. If scenarios such as these apply to you, you may be malnourished.
- **A diet deficient in nutrients because you have an eating disorder:** Eating disorders are severe disturbances in the way an individual eats, such as a woman who's eating so little that she's literally starving herself. Or conversely, binging on food (and maybe purging, too) is another form of an eating disorder. All eating disorders can cause serious malnourishment and health problems.
- **A diet deficient in nutrients because of a medical problem:** Some medical problems dramatically affect nutrition. For example, people with kidney problems must restrict the amount of protein they eat, causing shrinking of muscle tissue, a buildup of fluids (*edema*), anemia, and other medical problems. Another example: People with a severe allergy to gluten can develop a deficiency in vitamin B6, which is essential to good health. For example, vitamin B6 is needed for more than 100 enzymes involved in protein metabolism. It's also essential for red blood cell metabolism.
- **A diet deficient in nutrients because of medications you take:** Some medicines block the absorption of nutrients. For example, if you have an ulcer or acid reflux and have been taking acid-reducing drugs for a long time, they can cause vitamin B12 deficiency. Your body needs vitamin B12 to help maintain healthy nerves and red blood cells.

  In addition, some drugs are known to *lower* vitamin C levels, such as estrogen and also aspirin, if taken frequently.

If any of these issues apply to you, then you may be malnourished because your body is lacking one or more key nutrients. Here are some signs of malnutrition:

- Loss of appetite
- Weight loss or a very thin body structure
- Lack of energy
- Dull hair, skin, and eyes
- Swollen abdomen
- Water retention

If you have any of these symptoms, discuss them with your doctor who may draw some blood from you to test for deficiencies caused by lack of adequate nutrition.

Healthy Eating

The key principle of a healthy diet is to eat a well-balanced variety of wholesome foods so that you'll take in all the nutrients required for good health and disease prevention. Probably the best nutritional advice comes from Dr. Walter Willett and his colleagues at the Harvard School of Public Health (HSPH).

Dr. Willett's premise is that your diet should consist mostly of health-promoting foods and drinks, which you eat frequently. Foods that aren't health-promoting should be eaten far less often and in small amounts. "Duh," you say! "That's pretty obvious!" Well, Dr. Willett made this simple concept even simpler by recommending health-promoting foods that you can (and should) eat a lot of and the foods you should limit.

Dr. Willett organizes his nutrition guidelines into levels similar to the government's food pyramid. For our purposes, we give you the amounts in each level in a checklist that you can copy and use for meal planning.

Each level that Dr. Willett specifies has its own special significance:

- **Level 1:** Exercise daily and control your weight. (See Chapter 19 for information on exercise.)
- **Level 2:** Whole-grain foods are healthy carbohydrates your body needs for energy. Eat them at most meals. Whole grains contain the essential parts of the grain's seed or the equivalent. Examples of generally accepted whole-grain foods and flours are amaranth, barley (lightly pearled), brown and colored rice, buckwheat, bulgur, corn and whole cornmeal, millet, oatmeal and whole oats, popcorn, quinoa, whole rye, whole or cracked wheat, wheat berries, and wild rice.

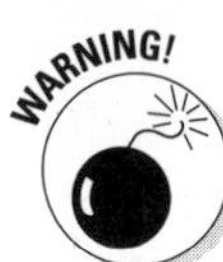

Stay away from anything made with "white" flour. All the good nutrition has been refined right out of the grain!

Level 2 also includes plant oils. Because most people get one-third or more of their calories from fats, they're in the first level of Willet's guidelines. However, the fats you eat should be health promoters. Stay away from trans fats, animal fats, and palm, palm kernel, and coconut oils. Replace them with olive or canola oil. Flaxseed and nut oils are also great for your heart and for fighting inflammation. Fried foods are on the forbidden list, along with margarines, unless they contain an ingredient called *sitostanol,* a plant sterol that lowers cholesterol absorption. Benecol, Take Control, or other margarine-like spreads include this ingredient.

- **Level 3:** Produce (vegetables and fruits) make up the third level. Men should eat nine servings of fruits and vegetables a day, and women should eat seven servings. Eating lots of fruits and vegetables can help prevent many chronic diseases. They're also great for your digestive system. Because they're low in calories and high in fiber, fruits and vegetables are great foods for weight control, particularly if you cut back on high-calorie foods.

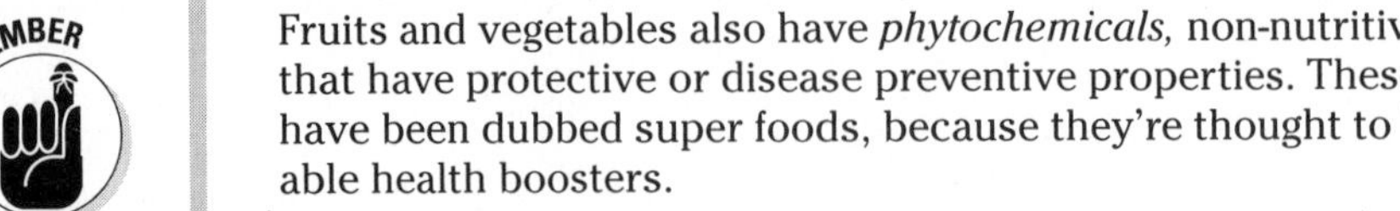

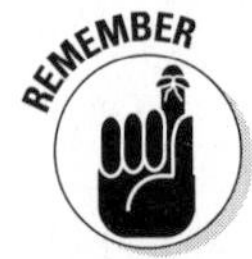

Fruits and vegetables also have *phytochemicals,* non-nutritive chemicals that have protective or disease preventive properties. These chemicals have been dubbed super foods, because they're thought to be remarkable health boosters.

By sampling one food of every color a couple of times a day, you're more likely to eat the recommended five to nine servings of vegetables and fruits every day. For example, at lunch you could have a salad with 1 cup of green spinach, and the following sprinkled on top: 1 tablespoon chopped white onion, 1/2 cup of red tomatoes, 1/2 cup of yellow pineapple chunks, orange slices equivalent to half an orange, and 1/2 cup of blueberries.

- **Level 4:** Nuts and legumes are the fourth level. They should be enjoyed one to three times daily. Nuts and legumes are excellent sources of protein, fiber, vitamins, and minerals.

Nuts are often overlooked as the elegant source of protein that they are. Yes, nuts are high in fat, but the fat is heart-healthy and may help lower low-density lipoproteins. In fact, nuts are recommended as part of the DASH (Dietary Approaches to Stop Hypertension) diet, a dietary plan supported by the National Heart, Lung, and Blood Institute and clinically proven to significantly reduce blood pressure. Legumes are healthy, too, and include many vegetables, such as string beans, lentils, dried beans, and peas. The DASH diet recommends four to five servings per week of nuts, seeds, and legumes.

Would you like some nuts with that?

The FDA recommends eating up to 1.5 ounces of nuts daily. Here are some tips:

- A handful of nuts equals about 1-ounce.
- On average, a 1.5-ounce serving is equivalent to about 1/3 cup of nuts.
- In terms of protein 1/3 cup of nuts or 2 tablespoons of peanut butter equals about 1 ounce of meat.

Legumes are low in fat, high in protein, and absorb the flavor of spices and herbs. Beans and other legumes have many nutrients important to prevent heart disease, cancer, and obesity. They're also high in complex carbohydrates, fiber, vitamins, and minerals.

When lentils are eaten with rice, they become a complete protein, which means that they contain all the amino acids that you need in your diet. Many classes of dry beans are available in the United States, including black beans, black-eyed peas, chickpeas, cranberry, and Great Northern, kidney, lima, navy (pea), and pinto beans.

- **Level 5:** Fish, poultry, and eggs are important sources of lean protein, and you should eat them up to two times a day. Lean animal proteins are healthful proteins. The best choices are fish, shellfish, skinless lean chicken or turkey, low-fat or fat-free dairy (such as skim milk and low-fat cheese), egg whites (no yolks), and egg substitute.
- **Level 6:** You need dairy or calcium supplements one to two times a day. Dairy products are great sources of protein but can contain a lot of saturated fat. In fact, three glasses of whole milk have as much saturated fat as 13 strips of cooked bacon! No-fat or low-fat dairy products are great. You can also get your calcium from other sources, such as broccoli and soybeans.
- **Level 7:** Remember the old joke? If it tastes good, spit it out! Most of us love the way fat, starch, and sweets taste. But, stay away from these foods as much as possible. Eat them only occasionally for special treats. Here's why:
  - Red meat, and butter: Foods in these two categories contain lots of saturated fat, which is very bad for your cardiovascular system and is also high in calories.
  - White rice, white bread, potatoes, white pasta, soda, and sweets: These foods are also forbidden because they are empty calories. In other words, they're high in calories, but have absolutely no nutritional value. Notice that even potatoes are restricted, so potatoes and butter are really no-no-nos!

Getting the truth about nutrition

A lot of confusing information about nutrition appears on the Web, in the media, and in bookstores. The Nutrition Source cuts through all that, providing clear tips for healthy eating and dispelling nutrition myths along the way. Go to its Web site at `www.hsph.harvard.edu/nutritionsource/index.html` to find out what you should eat and why.

Cutting Back on Calories to Avoid Obesity

Due to the lack of activity that often accompanies chronic pain, you can easily gain weight and even become obese. Putting on unnecessary pounds can become a serious problem even if it was never an issue in the past. In other words, even if you were a Skinny Minnie or a Slim Jim before chronic pain struck, you're not immune to becoming super-sized when you have chronic pain.

Being super-sized is a big health risk. Obesity can cause early death, strokes, diabetes, heart disease, and blood clots that can break off and travel to the lungs, in addition to causing a large number of other life-threatening conditions.

If you have chronic pain and are inactive, you should not keep eating the same amount of calories as you did before pain became a permanent intruder in your life.

And here's more bad news: Weight gain can happen sooner than you may think. Therefore, cut down on overall calories and adjust your eating habits whenever you reduce your activity level.

Maintaining a Healthy Weight

To live as well as possible with chronic pain, your weight should be under control. That means you're not too fat or too thin.

The formula for weight control is calories in = calories out. If the amount of calories you take in equals the amount that you spend through daily activity and exercise, your weight will remain the same. If the amount of calories is more than your activity and exercise expenditure, you'll put on weight. If the amount of calories is less than you spend, then you'll lose weight.

So, weight loss is basically a process of eating less and exercising more. A pound of body weight is equal to 3,500 calories. If you eat 500 fewer calories less per day than the amount you need, you'll lose 1 pound per week. The same rule applies to exercise. If you exercise the equivalent of another 500 calories per day — such as exercising on an elliptical machine for 30 minutes — and also eat 500 fewer calories a day, you'll lose two pounds. (Exercising can also be great for chronic pain!)

One way to judge whether you're overweight, underweight, or in a normal range is by using a number calculated from a person's weight and height called the *Body Mass Index* (BMI). To determine your own BMI, check out the table at the Centers for Disease Control at `www.cdc.gov/nccdphp/dnpa/bmi/index.htm`.

Avoiding Trigger Foods

If you have food allergies or intolerances that trigger your chronic pain, taking those foods out of your diet can bring relief. If you're allergic or intolerant to a food (and maybe you don't know it because you've had a reaction that wasn't severe), eating this food can increase your chronic pain level.

If you have a *food allergy,* your immune system reacts to a protein that it thinks is poison. In the most extreme cases, your body reacts with swelling, hives, asthma, or other symptoms of an allergy.

Ninety percent of all food-allergic reactions are caused by one of eight foods:

- Lactose in milk
- Eggs
- Peanuts
- Tree nuts, such as walnuts and cashews
- Fish
- Crustacean shellfish
- Soybeans
- Gluten (found in wheat and some other grains)

The Food and Drug Administration (FDA) now requires food labels to clearly state if products contain any proteins from these foods.

A *food intolerance* is a problem with the body's metabolizing certain foods. Milk lactose and wheat gluten are common triggers. If you're sensitive to these foods, your symptoms can include gas, bloating, abdominal pain, and headaches.

Some people don't realize that they have a food intolerance. Try eliminating milk or wheat from your diet for at least one week and see whether you feel better. If you do, you may have a food intolerance.

Nodding Yes to Nibbling

Now is your chance to eat all day long! Nibbling throughout the day has many health benefits, such as reducing the symptoms of diabetes, lowering cholesterol, and reducing the chance of heart disease. Nibbling can also help you control your weight as long as you keep the portions under control.

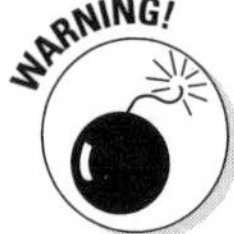

Here's the catch. You have to give up those large three square meals a day.

Here's why: In 1989, researchers led by Dr. David J. A. Jenkins, a professor at the University of Toronto, conducted a study in nibbling. In the study, seven men ate food equaling 2,500 calories a day. For two weeks, they ate the way most Americans do — three meals a day. Then for another two weeks, they ate the same amount of calories in 17 snacks throughout the day.

The results were reported in *The New England Journal of Medicine*. The nibblers' diet had the benefit of reducing cholesterol levels and low-density lipoprotein (the bad one). Nibbling also caused the release of smaller amounts of insulin and evened out its secretion, preventing the yo-yo effects of surges of insulin after large meals.

Try to eat many small meals throughout the day rather than three large ones. Just remember, though, that when you nibble, you need to stay away from those saturated fats and empty calories. Focus on grains, fruits and veggies, and lean protein.

Chapter 19

Getting Physical: Flexibility, Strength, Endurance, and Balance

In This Chapter

- Reversing deconditioning
- Discovering how to exercise even though you have chronic pain
- Looking at key exercises for people with chronic pain

Is this scenario familiar to you? So many areas of your body are sore that you find yourself trying to protect the painful parts and avoid moving in ways that make you hurt more. You're moving like a stick person, *and* you're limping to lessen the pain. Also, when you're sitting down, you slouch over to guard your hurting joints and muscles. You say to yourself (often), "Forget exercise. It just hurts too much!"

Here's another scene that you may recognize. You're exhausted from your chronic pain (which may be caused by any condition included in this book). And your fatigue is accompanied by the blahs. In other words, you're totally worn out and a little depressed. "I can barely move," you say. "How could I possibly go to the health club?" (Or go for a walk, or do the exercises that the physical therapist gave you.)

Situations like these cause a cascade effect throughout your body that results in a physical state known as *deconditioning*. For example, if you limp on your left leg, it throws off your right leg, which is now carrying most of the burden). And, if you're overweight, the excess pounds intensify the stress on the other leg. Or, if you're a couch potato and avoid all types of exercise, you quickly get out of shape, which makes your chronic pain worse and exacerbates the fatigue and depression.

This chapter covers how to prevent deconditioning through exercising and also offers you the best exercises for people with chronic pain.

Why exercise?

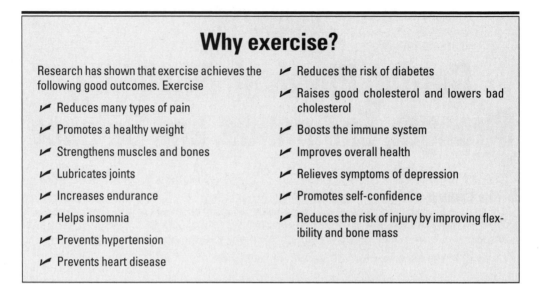

Research has shown that exercise achieves the following good outcomes. Exercise

- Reduces many types of pain
- Promotes a healthy weight
- Strengthens muscles and bones
- Lubricates joints
- Increases endurance
- Helps insomnia
- Prevents hypertension
- Prevents heart disease
- Reduces the risk of diabetes
- Raises good cholesterol and lowers bad cholesterol
- Boosts the immune system
- Improves overall health
- Relieves symptoms of depression
- Promotes self-confidence
- Reduces the risk of injury by improving flexibility and bone mass

Turning Around Deconditioning through Physical Therapy

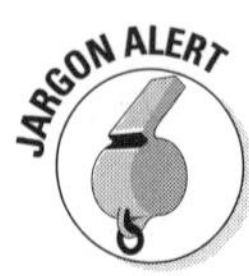

When your movement is very limited for an extended period (weeks, months, or longer!), you develop a physical state that the health community calls *deconditioning.* The way you move, the way you protect the sore parts of your body, the way you hold your body, and the amount of exercise you get all affect the overall condition of your body.

If you're deconditioned, it's important to work on reversing this state. Deconditioning makes it much more likely that you'll have health problems, such as coronary artery disease and some types of cancer. In fact, research has shown that physical inactivity doubles the chance of getting coronary artery disease. Conversely, regular exercise helps protect you from colon and some cancers of the breast, endometrium, and ovaries.

One of the best things you can do when you have chronic pain and you're starting an exercise program is to work with a qualified physical therapist. (For a description of what physical therapists do and how to find a qualified professional, see Chapter 13.) The goals of physical therapy (PT) are to get your body functioning again, relieve your pain, and teach you how to keep up the recovery on your own.

A physical therapist can help you turn around your deconditioning and make you stronger and more flexible than ever. You'll also have more endurance. In addition, PT can also boost your self-confidence. Having more strength, flexibility, endurance, and better balance will make you proud of your abilities. You've done yourself a very big favor and accomplished something really major.

When you start working with a physical therapist, he'll also play an important role in helping you set your exercise goals. He'll evaluate your condition and design an exercise program appropriate for your pain level, abilities, and condition.

Exercising Right for Your Pain Condition

Many people despise exercise of all types and find every excuse not to do it. Describing working out in her magazine, *O*, Oprah Winfrey, purportedly the richest woman in the world, said: "There's no easy way out. If there were, I would have bought it. And believe me, it would be one of my favorite things!" So, you may be rich or poor, a star or an average Joe or Jane, but you still have to get moving or live with the unhappy consequences of a deconditioned body.

The No. 1 rule for exercise and chronic pain is to do as much as you can as often as you can. As you probably know all too well, exercise can cause *a little* pain, particularly when you're first starting out after a long period of inactivity.

The reason why you sometimes feel pain when you start exercising is that it causes small injuries to the soft tissues of your body. As the injuries heal, your tissues get stronger, helping you become conditioned! So, if you feel *a little* pain during or after exercise, don't let it stop you. Keep going. In general, more exercise means less pain unless you've overdone it, which is another matter. Be sure to build up your exercise program gradually to prevent doing too much and too soon.

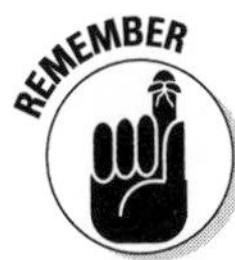

An important rule concerning chronic pain and exercise is to try to experience all four of the major types of exercise on a regular basis:

- Endurance
- Strength
- Flexibility
- Balance

Performing all four types helps you rebuild your body and become fully conditioned. Sure, it's okay to do just a little bit in each of the four types when you're first getting started, but do be sure you cover all four categories.

The following sections offer key details about the four important categories of exercise.

Exercising for endurance

If you have trouble climbing stairs or walking more than a few blocks, your body probably needs to build up endurance. Endurance exercise, which is another name for aerobic exercise, builds stamina. Endurance exercise increases your heart rate and breathing. It's also great for your cardiovascular system and lungs. Endurance exercise is the key to becoming conditioned.

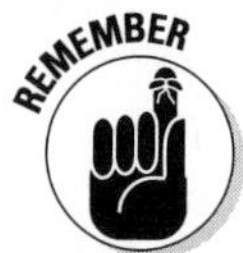

When beginning endurance exercise, start slowly and build up gradually. A good rule is to work up gradually to 30 minutes of endurance exercise a minimum of four times a week.

Endurance exercise includes such activities as bicycling, walking, running, swimming, rowing, skating, and working out on equipment, such as elliptical trainers or stair-step machines.

Building up strength

Strength exercises accomplish what they claim in their name: They make you stronger. This type of exercise also helps you control your weight because, happily, it speeds up your metabolism. Strength exercises also give you the vigor for a more active life, and they help you complete tasks such as carrying groceries or performing your endurance exercises more easily!

To get the benefits of strength training, exercise all your major muscle groups at least twice a week. But — and this is very important! — don't exercise the same muscle group two days in a row. Doing strength exercises too often can end up harming rather than helping you.

Here are a few strength-training exercises to consider:

- **Weights:** Perhaps the most well-known method of strength training is using weights, which are sold in most sports and department stores and are available in health clubs. You can also use soup cans or water bottles filled with equal amounts of fluid. It's important to get instruction from your physical therapist or a qualified trainer on the proper way to lift weights.
- **Resistance bands:** *Resistance bands* are giant rubber bands that you pull against (resist) to strengthen certain muscle groups. Resistance bands are more convenient than most weight-lifting gear, and they're also inexpensive and easily carried in a purse, pocket, or small bag. Resistance

bands come in different levels, from easy-to-stretch to progressively more difficult. Ask your physical therapist or a qualified trainer how to use resistance bands.

- **Pilates:** The goal of the Pilates program is to build strength in the core of your body. Pilates teaches body awareness, good posture, and easy, graceful movement. The program emphasizes proper breathing, correct spinal and pelvic alignment, and complete concentration on smooth, flowing movement. Pilates classes use machines called *reformers* or floor mats. Many instructional video programs are available, but if you're a beginner at Pilates, it's important to start by getting instruction from a well-trained professional. A great resource is *Pilates For Dummies* (Wiley) by Michelle Dozois.

Gaining flexibility

A program of stretching can do wonders to reverse stiffness and soreness. Stretching and moving your joints and supporting tissues through their full range of motion promote flexibility, which, in turn, helps to hold back deconditioning and its result: increased pain.

You need to stretch properly, so be sure to get your instruction from a well-trained professional. The techniques in the "Exercises for Conditioning" section, later in this chapter, include some important movements that you can do at home.

If you do these exercises regularly, you can prevent overly tight muscles. Do your stretching exercises after performing your endurance and strength training, and when your muscles are warm.

Getting balanced

Loss of balance is common for people with chronic pain conditions, leading to falls and difficulty walking. Here's the good news: Strength and balance exercises overlap, so one exercise can work for both problems. (For more on strength exercises, see the section "Building up strength," earlier in this chapter.) Balance exercises build up your leg muscles. Any of the lower-body exercises for strength in the next section are good for balance.

Exercises for Conditioning

The following exercises can help you prevent deconditioning. If you're a beginner or you haven't exercised for awhile, you can expect to have sore muscles for the first week or two of your exercise program.

If the soreness doesn't go away or you're hurting so much that you're not exercising, be sure to talk this issue over with your physical therapist and/or doctor. Most importantly, if any of these exercises cause moderate to severe pain, then stop right away and wait to do the exercise again only after you talk to your physical therapist or doctor.

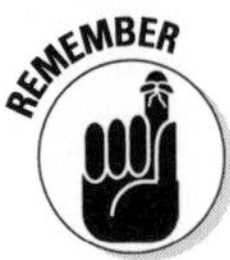

Keep in mind that breathing correctly is important during all exercise. Exhale during the initial movement and inhale slowly when returning to the original position. Never hold your breath during any exercise. Be smooth and deliberate in all your movements. Don't bounce while stretching or performing any exercise.

Biceps curl

The biceps curl, shown in Figure 19-1, strengthens your upper-arm muscles.

Here's how you do a biceps curl:

1. **Sit in an armless chair or on a bench with your feet flat on the floor, spaced apart so that they are even with your shoulders.**
2. **Hold hand weights, soup cans of equal weight, or a resistance band in each hand with your palms facing your hips.**

   Your arms should be straight down at your side.
3. **Take 3 seconds to lift your left hand weight toward your shoulder by bending your elbow; as you lift, turn your left hand so that your palm is facing your shoulder, holding the position for 1 second.**

   Do not use your upper arm!
4. **Take 3 seconds to lower your hand to the starting position.**
5. **Pause and then repeat Steps 3 and 4 with your right arm.**
6. **Alternate until you have repeated the exercise 8 to 15 times on each side.**
7. **Rest and then do another set of 8 to 15 alternating repetitions.**

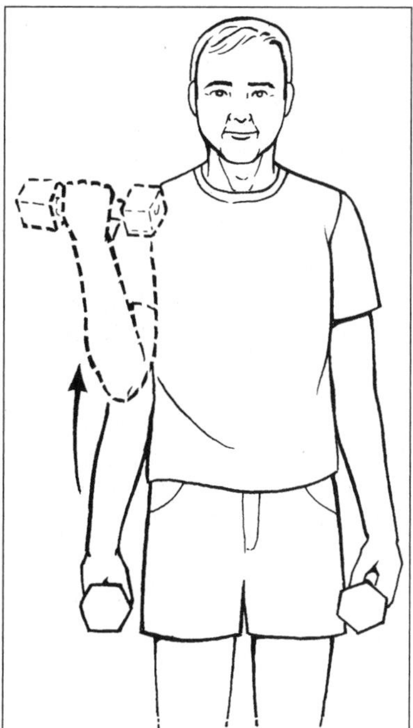

Figure 19-1: The biceps curl.

Here are some tips to follow when doing a biceps curls:

- You can do this exercise while standing.
- Keep your elbows glued to your sides all the way through the exercise.
- Avoid rocking back and forth.
- Don't bend your wrist. Keep it straight with your forearm.
- Don't let the weight pull your arm down when lowering it. Let it down slowly resisting its weight.
- Do not lift the weights higher than your neck.

Chair stands

The chair stand exercise, shown in Figure 19-2, strengthens the muscles in your stomach and thighs. Here's how it works:

1. **Sit toward the middle or front of a chair and lean back so that you're in a half-reclining position, with your back and shoulders straight, knees bent, and feet flat on the floor.**

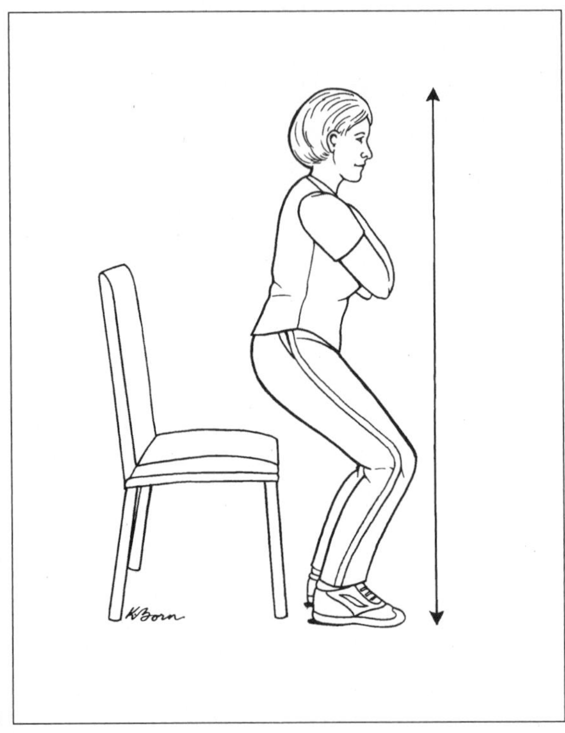

Figure 19-2: The chair stand exercise.

2. **Cross your arms and put your hands on your shoulders.**
3. **Keeping your head, neck, and back straight, bring your upper body forward and then stand up slowly.**
4. **Sit back down slowly and return to your original position.**
5. **Repeat four to six times; build up gradually to 8 to 12 repetitions.**

   Your goal is to do this exercise without using your hands as you become stronger.
6. **Repeat 8 to 15 times.**
7. **Rest; then repeat 8 to 15 times more.**

You should feel your abdominal muscles working as you do this exercise.

Here are some tips to follow when doing chair stands.

- Be sure not to lean forward with your shoulders as you rise.
- Don't sit down too quickly.
- Don't lean your weight too far forward or onto your toes when standing up.

Arm raise

Arm raises, shown in Figure 19-3, strengthen your shoulder muscles. Here's how you do the arm raise exercise:

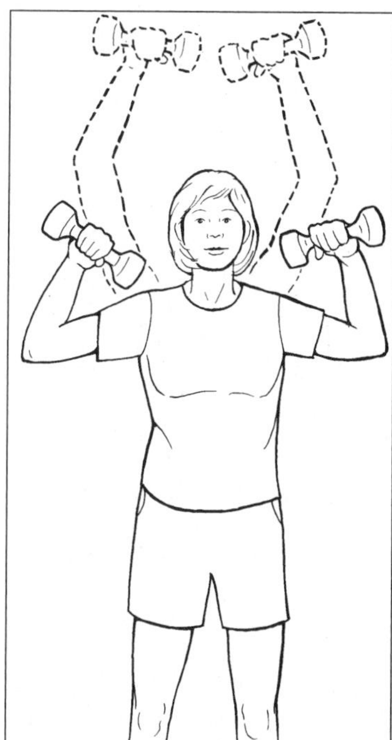

Figure 19-3: Arm raise

1. **Sit on a chair and place your feet flat on the floor, spaced apart so that they're even with your shoulders.**
2. **Hold a 1- to 2-pound weight or a soup can with one hand and raise your right arm until the elbow is straightened; hold for 5 seconds.**

3. **Lower your arm slowly.**
4. **Repeat ten times with each arm.**

Two other important arm exercises are similar to this one, but you move your arms in front of you or to the side.

- **Arms in front:** Sit in a chair. Hold the weights straight down at your sides, with your palms facing inward. Take 3 seconds to lift your arms in front of you, keeping them straight and rotating them so that your palms are facing upward. Stop when your arms are parallel to the ground. Hold the position for 1 second. Take 3 seconds to lower your arms so that they're straight down by your sides again. Pause. Repeat 8 to 15 times. Rest; do another set of 8 to 15 repetitions.
- **Arms to the side:** Sit in a chair. Hold the weights straight down at your sides, with your palms facing inward. Take 3 seconds to lift your arms straight out, sideways, until they're parallel to the ground. Hold the position for 1 second. Take 3 seconds to lower your arms so that they're straight down by your sides again. Pause. Repeat 8 to 15 times. Rest; do another set of 8 to 15 repetitions.

Plantar flexion

The plantar flexion exercise, shown in Figure 19-4, strengthens the ankle and calf muscles. You can use this exercise for developing balance following the instructions in the "Getting balanced" section, earlier in this chapter.

Here's an example of how to do it:

1. **Stand straight, feet flat on the floor, holding on to the edge of a table or chair for balance; take 3 seconds to stand as high up on tiptoe as you can; hold for 1 second, and then take 3 seconds to slowly lower yourself back down.**

   As you become stronger, do this exercise first on your right leg only, then on your left leg only, for a total of 8 to 15 times on each leg.

2 **Repeat this exercise 8 to 15 times; rest a minute and then do another set of 8 to 15 repetitions.**

3. **Rest a minute and then do another set of 8 to 15 alternating repetitions.**

You can also use ankle weights if you feel strong enough.

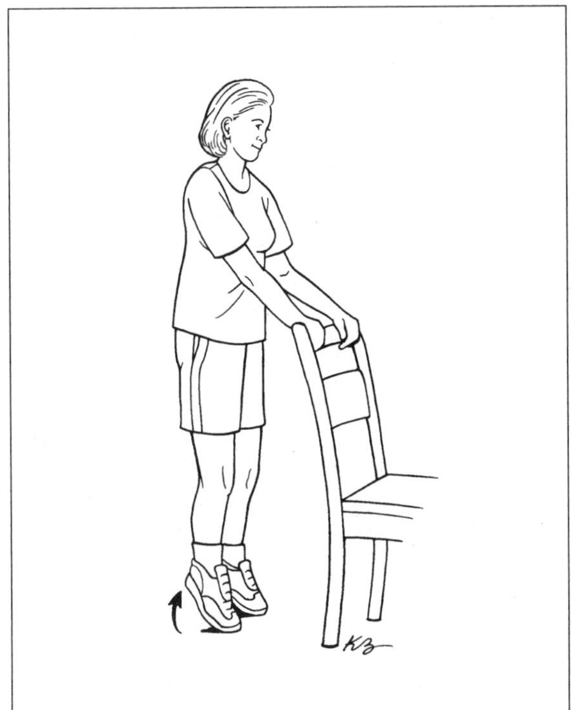

Figure 19-4: Plantar flexion.

Knee flexion

The knee flexion exercise, shown in Figure 19-5, strengthens muscles in the back of your thigh. You can use this exercise for developing balance following the instructions in the "Getting balanced" section, earlier in this chapter.

Here's how it works:

1. **Stand straight.**

   If you need to, you can hold on to a sturdy table or chair for balance.

2. **Slowly bend one knee as far as possible so that your foot lifts up behind you; hold position for 1 second.**
3. **Slowly lower your foot all the way back down to the floor.**
4. **Repeat with your other leg for a total of 8 to 15 times on each leg.**
5. **Rest a minute and then do another set of 8 to 15 alternating repetitions.**

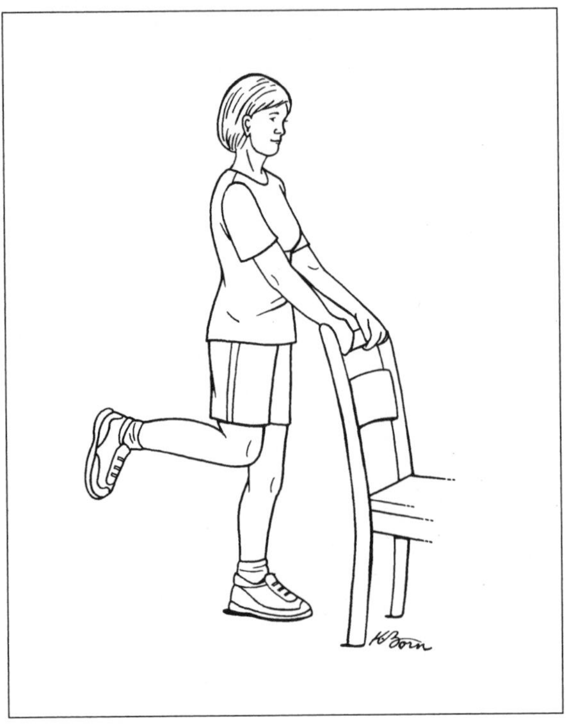

Figure 19-5: Knee flexion.

You can also use ankle weights for this exercise.

Hip flexion

The hip flexion, shown in Figure 19-6, strengthens your hip and thigh muscles. Here's how it works:

1. **Stand straight.**

   If you need to, you can hold on to a sturdy table or chair for balance.

2. **Slowly bend one knee toward chest, without bending waist or hips, and hold this position for 1 second.**
3. **Slowly lower your leg all the way to the floor.**
4. **Repeat with your other leg for a total of 8 to 15 times on each leg.**
5. **Rest a minute and then do another set of 8 to 15 alternating repetitions.**

You can use this exercise for developing balance following the instructions in the "Getting balanced" section, earlier in this chapter. You can also use ankle weights for this exercise.

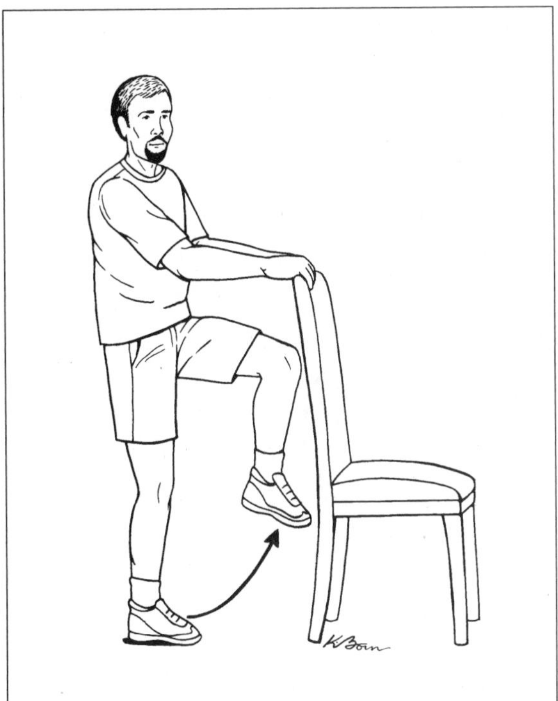

Figure 19-6: Hip flexion.

Hip extension

The hip extension, shown in Figure 19-7, strengthens the buttock and lower-back muscles. Here's how to do it:

1. **Hold on to a table that's 12 to 18 inches away from you.**
2. **Slowly lift one leg straight backward and hold for 1 second.**
3. **Slowly lower your leg.**
4. **Repeat with the other leg for a total of 8 to 15 times on each leg.**
5. **Rest a minute and then do another set of 8 to 15 alternating repetitions.**

You can use this exercise for developing balance following the instructions in the "Getting balanced" section, earlier in this chapter. You can also use ankle weights for this exercise.

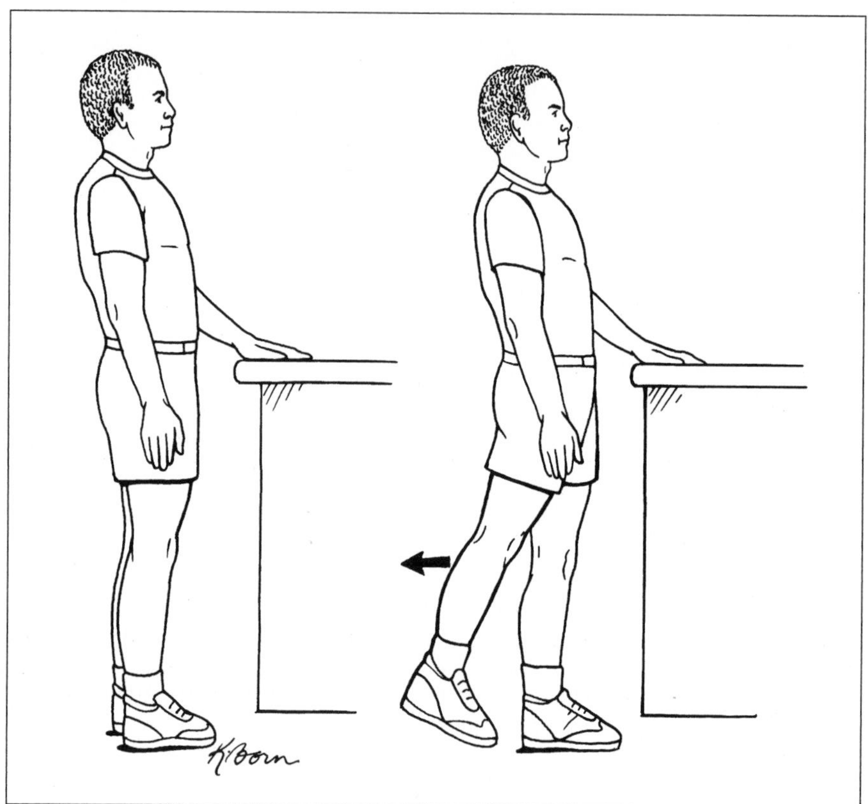

Figure 19-7: Hip extension.

Hamstring stretch

This exercise, shown in Figure 19-8, stretches your hamstrings, which are the mid-rear thigh muscles.

You can do this exercise many different ways. Here's one way!

1. **Lie with your back and head flat against the floor.**
2. **Bend your knees and place both feet on the floor.**
3. **Straighten your right leg and point your toes.**

   Your left knee should be on the floor, slightly flexed.
4. **Slowly raise your right leg toward the ceiling, keeping your leg straight. Extend your leg until you feel a stretch in your right hamstring; hold stretch for a count of 8.**

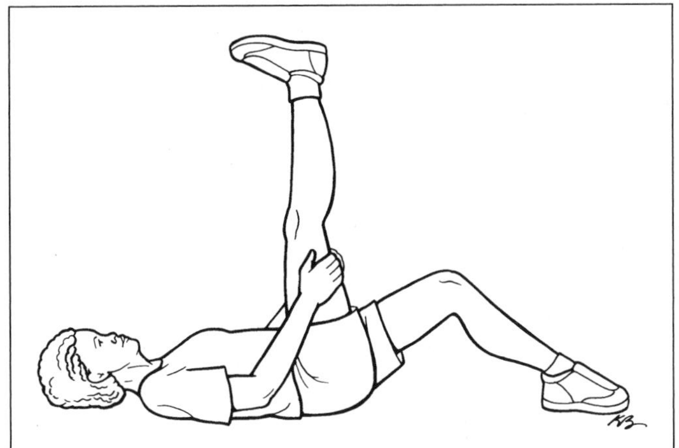

Figure 19-8: Hamstring stretch.

5. **Repeat on your left leg.**
6. **Repeat three times on each side.**

Here are some tips to follow when doing the hamstring stretch exercise.

- Do not do this exercise if you have pain radiating down your leg, or you have a bulging disc or herniated disc.
- Keep your head and back against the floor.
- Don't lift your leg too quickly when preparing to stretch your hamstring.

Thigh and calf stretch

The thigh and calf stretches, shown in Figure 19-9, stretch your thigh and calf muscles. Here's how to do them:

The thigh stretch:

1. **Hold on to something for balance; standing on one leg, grasp the foot of the other leg.**

   Keep your knee pointing down.

2. **Pull up your leg with light pressure; hold your foot in this position, behind you for 30 seconds and then relax.**

   You should feel the stretch in the front of your thigh.

3. **Repeat this stretch three times for each side.**

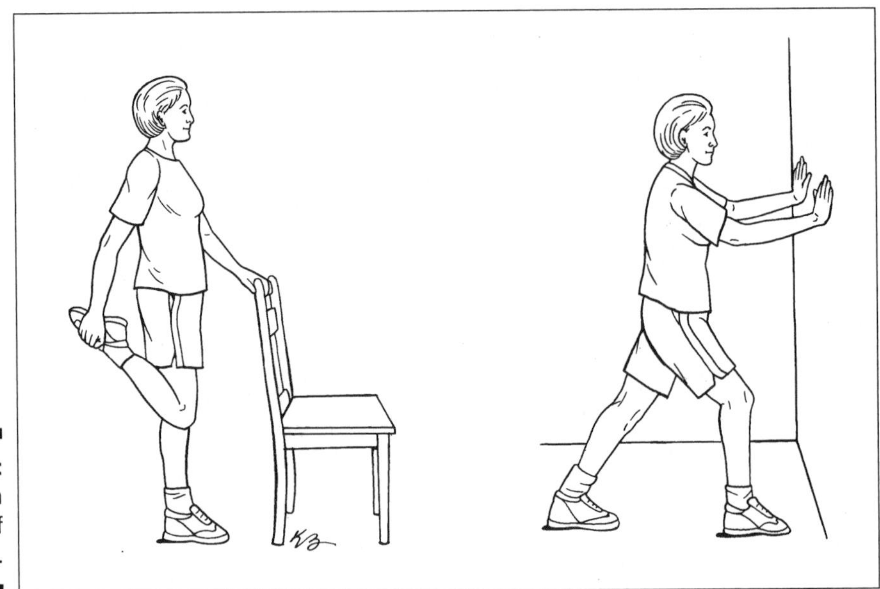

Figure 19-9: Thigh and calf stretches.

Here are some tips to follow when doing the thigh stretch:

- Be careful not to arch your back.
- You do not need to pull your leg up all the way to your buttocks.

The calf stretch:

1. **Rest your hands on a wall at about shoulder height and place one foot forward in a lunging position.**
2. **Stand upright, making sure that both toes are facing forward and your heel is on the ground.**
3. **While keeping your back leg straight, lean toward the wall.**

   You should feel the stretch in the calf of your back leg.

Here are a couple of tips to follow when doing the calf stretch:

- Don't stick your bottom out.
- For a deeper stretch, try bending your back knee so that you're sitting down with your weight over the back leg.

Neck exercises

Neck exercises can help relieve pain and stiffness in your neck. They strengthen your neck muscles and keep them flexible. They can also help reduce the frequency and severity of your headaches. You can do these exercises every half hour throughout the day to prevent neck strain.

To do neck exercises, gently tense your neck muscles for a few seconds in each position. If you do them every day, the neck movements will increase your muscle strength.

Here's what you do:

- **Tilt from front to back:** Tilt your head slowly back, far enough so you can look up, and hold for 5 seconds. Return slowly to front position. Repeat five to ten times.
- **Rotate head from side to side:** Slowly turn your head as far as you can and hold for 5 seconds . Return your head to the center. Move your head in the opposite direction. Repeat five to ten times.
- **Tilt from side to side:** Keep your head straight as you slowly tilt it over to the side and hold for 5 seconds, as shown in Figure 19-10. (Don't go so far that you touch your ear with your shoulder.) Return your head to center position. Move your head to your opposite shoulder and repeat five to ten times.

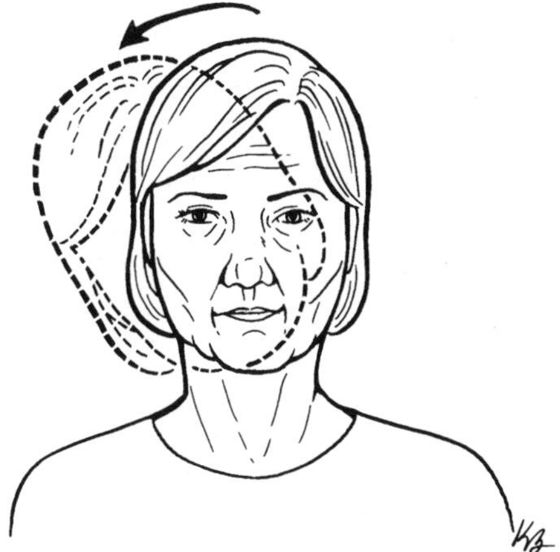

Figure 19-10: Head tilt.

Achieving balance!

Would you like to ace the balance class? You should have someone stand next to you when you do this! Do your strength exercises for the lower body and hold on to your support with only one hand. Eventually hold on with only four fingertips, then three, and so on. Then try not holding on at all. Finally, when you're ready, don't hold on at all, and also keep your eyes closed.

Other ways to build up your balance are to stand on one leg or use a wobble board. Of course, do not try these exercises without the guidance of a physical therapist or other exercise professional. (As well as gaining the approval of your medical doctor.)

Another great way to develop balance is to try Tai Chi, which is a martial art in China and a popular movement in the West. Classes in Tai Chi are widely available in the United States and offer increased balance and flexibility when aerobic exercise isn't possible or desirable.

Chapter 20

Tackling Fatigue

In This Chapter

- Pondering the importance of sleep in your daily life
- Considering specific sleep problems
- Mapping your sleep patterns
- Creating strategies to ratchet up your hours of sleep time

If you have chronic pain (and maybe chronic stress as well), getting enough sleep may be a major challenge for you. You may toss and turn while trying to get to sleep, and then once you're "there," sudden jabs of pain jolt you awake. Or you may have other sleep problems, such as sleep apnea or restless legs syndrome. Whatever the causes, a sleep deficit can impair your thinking and memory and make you groggy, affecting your alertness, causing your energy levels to plummet, and also making you downright grumpy. In addition, loss of sleep and the weariness it causes can even make you accident-prone, resulting in injuries, accidents, and crashes.

Finally, sleep loss can make you more sensitive to pain, according to the National Sleep Foundation. One study found that sleep deprivation caused by continuous sleep disturbances throughout the night increased spontaneous pain and impaired the body's ability to cope with painful stimuli.

This chapter discusses major sleep problems that can cause or aggravate pain and what you can do about them.

Losing Sleep Is a Bad Thing

Sleep is a daily period of rest, during which you're inactive and experience different levels of consciousness. If you're getting adequate sleep, you spend about one-third of each 24-hour day (give or take an hour) in this rest state.

The science of sleep is still in its infancy, and researchers have a limited understanding of the biological function of sleep. However, it is known that a lot goes on inside your body while you sleep. For example, during different stages of sleep, the body temperature changes, breathing and heart rhythm slow and then return to normal, and blood flow to the brain increases. In addition, hormone levels change. In addition, growth hormone increases during the first two hours of sleep. (So, when you were a kid and your mother told you that you had to go to sleep so you'd grow, she wasn't kidding!)

Sleep happens in stages: rapid eye movement (REM) sleep and nonrapid REM (NREM) sleep. Adults spend about 20 percent of their sleep time in REM and 80 percent in NREM sleep. Elderly people spend less than 15 percent of their sleep time in REM sleep.

Most dreams occur during REM sleep. During REM sleep, your eyes move back and forth rapidly. However, your muscle activity is very quiet during this sleep stage.

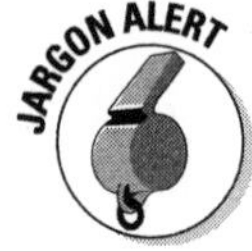

Microsleeps are quick, involuntary episodes of sleep when you're otherwise awake, and they can be another sign of sleep deprivation. They last from 2 seconds to 2 minutes, and you may not even be aware that you're having them. Symptoms include blank stares, nodding your head, and closing your eyes for much longer than it takes for a normal blink. Microsleeps are dangerous. While experiencing them, you can't take in what is going on around you, such as Stop signs when you're driving.

How much sleep is enough?

How much sleep you need depends on your individual physical needs, and no magic number applies to all people. However, most adults need 7 to 8 hours of sleep each night, according to the National Sleep Foundation. Children need more sleep than adults; for example, babies need 16 to 18 hours a day of sleep, and preschool children sleep 10 to12 hours a day. School-aged children and teens need at least 9 hours of sleep a night. (They're still growing, after all.)

The elderly need about the same amount of sleep as younger adults — between 7 and 8 hours each night. As people age, they tend to go to sleep earlier and get up earlier than in previous decades, and they may nap more during the day.

If you feel drowsy during the day, even during boring activities, you haven't had enough sleep, according to the National Sleep Foundation. In addition, if you normally fall asleep within 5 minutes of lying down, you're probably sleep-deprived.

Fatigue and chronic pain

Fatigue, a common problem for people with chronic pain, is dangerous when combined with driving. Falling asleep at the wheel causes at least 100,000 crashes and 1,500 deaths each year, according to the National Highway Traffic Safety Administration. Close to half of American adult drivers drive while drowsy, and nearly two out of ten admit to falling asleep at the wheel, according to a 2002 poll conducted by the National Sleep Foundation. If you have trouble keeping your eyes focused, if you can't stop yawning, or if you can't remember driving the last few miles, you're probably too drowsy to drive safely.

A lack of sleep is bad for your health because you may lose important time in one of the two major stages of sleep. In addition, one of sleep's major functions is to aid mental functioning. (The parts of the brain that control learning and memory are still active during sleep.) Studies show that people who are taught mentally challenging tasks perform significantly better after a good night's sleep.

Lack of adequate sleep can also:

- Make it tough to mentally focus
- Slow your reaction time
- Make you irritable
- Increase the chances that you'll be overweight or obese (Yes! Not sleeping enough can make you fat!)
- Put you at risk for depression and diabetes
- Increase your risk for high blood pressure and heart disease
- Magnify alcohol's effects on your body

Chronic Pain and Sleep Problems

Chronic pain and the sleep problems it causes can make you hurt even more. For example, if you're exhausted from coping with your migraines, and on top of that you toss and turn all night, the result can be even worse migraines. (And you thought they couldn't get any worse! Wrong!)

The major forms of sleep problems, described in the following sections, are sleep apnea, insomnia, sleepwalking, restless legs syndrome, narcolepsy, snoring, teeth grinding, and *hypersomnia* (sleeping too much).

Resources for getting enough rest

From information centers to sleep labs, the following organizations are great resources for managing sleep problems:

American Academy of Sleep Medicine (AASM), 1 Westbrook Corporate Center, Suite 920, Westchester, IL 60154; phone 708-492-0930, fax 708-492-0943; Web site `www.aasmnet.org/AboutAASM.aspx`. AASM is the professional society of the medical subspecialty of sleep medicine. AASM membership consists of more than 7,000 physicians, researchers and other health-care professionals. AASM specializes in studying, diagnosing, and treating disorders of sleep and daytime alertness, such as insomnia, narcolepsy, and obstructive sleep apnea. AASM sponsors a site called `http://sleepcenter.org` that provides lists of medical sleep centers by state.

American Insomnia Association (AIA), 1 Westbrook Corporate Center, Suite 920, Westchester, IL 60154; phone 708-492-0930; Web site `www.americaninsomniaassociation.org`. AIA is a patient-based organization that assists and provides resources to individuals who suffer from insomnia. The AIA encourages the formation of local support groups.

American Sleep Apnea Association, 1424 K St. NW, Suite 302, Washington, DC 20005; phone 202-293-3650; Web site `www.sleepapnea.org`. The ASAA is a nonprofit organization dedicated to reducing injury, disability, and death from sleep apnea and to enhancing the well-being of those affected by this common disorder. ASAA's Sleep Apnea Support Forum sponsors live chat groups on various issues, such as sleep apnea in children.

National Sleep Foundation (NSF), 1522 K St. NW, Suite 500, Washington, DC 20005-1253; phone 202-347-3471; Web site `www.sleepfoundation.org`. NSF sponsors public education and awareness initiatives, such as *National Sleep Awareness Week* and *Drive Alert . . . Arrive Alive.*

Restless Legs Syndrome Foundation, 1610 14th St. NW, Suite 300, Rochester, MN 55901; phone 877-463-6757 (toll-free), 507-287-6465; Web site `www.rls.org`. The Restless Legs Syndrome Foundation is a nonprofit organization that provides the latest information about the condition. The Web site provides an online community.

Sleep apnea

Apnea is Greek for "without breath." People with sleep apnea snore loudly, and they actually stop breathing for brief periods during sleep. Breathless episodes can last for a minute or longer and can occur hundreds of times during sleep. During apnea spells, your brain wakes you up so that you'll restart breathing. It's sort of like jump-starting your brain, but the result is nonrestful sleep. Sleep apnea causes fatigue and drowsiness during waking hours and can cause chronic morning headaches, as well as cluster, tension, and migraine headaches.

Sleep apnea affects more than 12 million Americans, according to the National Institutes of Health. The condition is more common in men, men and women who are overweight, and those age 40 or older.

The standard treatment for sleep apnea is use of a *continuous positive airway pressure (CPAP) machine.* A CPAP machine is about the size of a shoebox. A flexible tube connects the machine to a mask or other device you wear during sleep. CPAP machines work by pushing air through your airway passage at a pressure that doesn't cause snoring.

If you have sleep apnea, or think you may have it, add an ear, nose, and throat doctor *(otolaryngologist)* to your health-care team. She can also help you choose the right CPAP machine for you.

Insomnia

Insomnia is a lack of sleep or fitfull sleep when the chance for restful sleep is present — such as when you're wide awake at 2 a.m. watching the shopping channel on TV or reading historical novels because you just can't get to sleep.

Insomnia can be temporary or chronic. Most people have had insomnia at least several times in their lives, usually during stressful periods. Symptoms include difficulty falling asleep or waking up during the night and not being able to go back to sleep. As with sleep apnea, insomnia can cause chronic morning headaches, as well as cluster, tension, and migraine headaches. For treatment of insomnia, see the "Getting Some Shuteye the Natural Way" and "Knocking Yourself Out with Medications" sections, later in this chapter.

Sleepwalking

During *sleepwalking* (somnambulism), people perform actions as if awake, but they're actually asleep. Sleepwalking usually occurs during deep non-REM sleep. About 1 in 6 people sleepwalk, and the condition is more common in children and teenagers than adults. Some medications, such as Ambien (used to treat sleep disturbances), are associated with sleepwalking.

Sleepwalkers don't remember their actions. So, if you're a sleepwalker, you may wander around your neighborhood or clean out your basement while asleep, and you'd never know it unless someone woke you up during your sojourn. Sleepwalking most often afflicts stressed or anxious people and those with a family history of the condition.

If there's a possibility of injuring yourself during sleepwalking, taking antidepressants, such as trazodone (Desyrel), or an anti-anxiety drug, like clonazepam (Klonopin), which is sometimes used to treat seizures, may be a necessity.

Snoring and snoring partners

Snoring is noisy breathing during sleep. It's the result of a blockage to the free flow of air during breathing, which causes structures at the back of your mouth to strike each other and vibrate. Forty-five percent of adults snore at least occasionally, and 25 percent are habitual snorers, according to the American Academy of Otolaryngology. Men are most at risk for snoring. Being overweight or obese is another major snoring risk factor.

You and/or your sleep partner may snore away every night or occasionally. Snoring often causes disturbed and restless sleep, resulting in fatigue the next day.

Snoring has many possible causes, including the following:

- Relaxation of throat muscles, due to aging
- Inflammation of the nose and/or throat due to colds, allergies, and related problems
- Alcohol or medications that loosen the muscles of the throat
- Anatomical problems, such as nasal polyps or a deviated septum in the nose
- Blockage by cysts, tumors, or excess fatty tissue in the throat (the latter is due to being overweight)

Don't sleep on your back, which causes the soft tissues in the back of your throat to block your airway. Many people are successful with the "tennis ball technique" in which you attach a tennis ball to the back of your night clothes. You won't be able to lie on your back, forcing you to turn on your side. Eventually, you'll naturally sleep on your side, and you can dump the ball.

Don't underestimate the negative impact of snoring on a relationship. A snoring partner can wake you up often or keep you from getting any sleep. The result is drowsiness and irritation — and sometimes, it's separate bedrooms or even a separating couple.

Fortunately, you're not doomed to lifelong snoring. Instead, consider the following suggestions to reduce your risk for snoring.

- Lose weight if you're overweight, which will reduce fatty tissue in your airway.
- Consider a specially designed pillow for snorers, available in retail or online stores. One option is the Sona Pillow available at `www.sonapillow.com` and some retail stores.

- Elevate the head of your bed four inches, which causes your tongue and jaw to move forward and out of snoring position. Try placing rolled up towels under the head of the mattress to raise it.
- Avoid alcohol at night. Alcohol worsens snoring.
- Avoid sedatives before bed. Sedatives relax throat muscles.
- Avoid high-fat dairy products or soy milk before sleeping. They can cause mucus buildup in your throat, blocking air passages and causing snoring.
- Try nasal decongestants, but stay away from antihistamines. *Decongestants,* which increase mucus flow, can help clear your air passages. However, *antihistamines,* which dry up the mucus, relax the throat muscles, leading to snoring. (Some people take Benadryl or Tylenol PM, which contain antihistamines. These drugs help you fall asleep, but increase your risk for snoring!)
- A number of devices can help keep your airway open. Ask your dentist or otolaryngologist about them.

Surgery can open blocked airways by removing structures such as tonsils or fatty tissue blocking them. A new outpatient surgery called *palatal implantation* involves putting small plastic implants into the soft palate. Scar tissue forms around the implants, hardening the soft palate in the back of the throat so that it does not vibrate.

Restless Legs Syndrome

If you have Restless Legs Syndrome (RLS), you have an uncontrollable desire to move your legs constantly. You may also have strange feelings in your legs such as a creeping or crawling, cramping, burning, tingling, soreness, or pain. RLS is particularly uncomfortable when you're trying to fall asleep. It can cause sleeplessness and daytime fatigue. RLS affects about 10 percent of adults.

If your legs twitch and jerk spasmodically, you may have a sleep condition called *periodic limb movements* (PLMS). If you have this problem, your leg movements may be severe enough to awaken you.

According to the National Center on Sleep Disorders Research, Restless Legs Syndrome is underdiagnosed yet treatable. The key treatment for RLS is taking a dopaminergic drug, such as L-Dopa, which increases the levels of a neurotransmitter called dopamine in the central nervous system. Other treatments include opioids, mild tranquilizers, anticonvulsants, and iron supplements.

Narcolepsy

Narcolepsy is extreme daytime drowsiness and sudden attacks of REM sleep while still awake. Insomnia, dreaming while awake, and a condition called *sleep paralysis* (the inability to perform voluntary movements either while falling asleep or when waking up) are also symptoms.

Narcolepsy affects both sexes equally and develops with increasing age. The condition may be caused by a deficiency in *hypocretin,* a substance that helps to regulate sleep cycles.

Some medications improve the constant lapsing into sleep that people with narcolepsy suffer from. Some examples of meds that may help this condition are

- Stimulants, such as Methylphenidate (Ritalin), and amphetamines, such as Adderall, the main drugs prescribed for narcolepsy. They act on the central nervous system to help people stay alert and awake during the day. Stimulants are effective, but may have strong side effects, such as nervousness and heart palpitations.
- Antidepressants, such as protriptyline (Vivactil) and fluoxetine (Prozac) help narcolepsy by suppressing REM sleep.
- Sodium oxybate (Xyrem), a central nervous system depressant, can control symptoms that some people with narcolepsy have, such as episodes of *cataplexy,* a condition characterized by weak or paralyzed muscles. But sodium oxybate has unpleasant side effects, such as nausea and urinary incontinence.

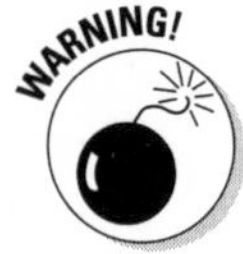

If you have narcolepsy, don't drive, skydive, or take any other actions that may be dangerous if you suddenly fell asleep. You may want to wear a medical alert charm to notify others if you have a narcolepsy spell. (MedicAlert charms are available through `www.medicalert.org`.)

Teeth grinding

Some people unknowingly grind their teeth at night, a habit known as *bruxism.* This relatively common condition is like the nervous habit of tapping your foot or twisting a lock of hair, but you're asleep while you're doing it. Eight percent of adults grind their teeth at night, and more than a third of parents report symptoms of bruxism in their children.

Among other things, bruxism can cause chronic facial, mouth, and/or jaw pain and damage to the teeth and gums. It can greatly reduce the quality of your sleep and also cause headaches. Sleep apnea and bruxism often go hand and hand, and in those cases, treating your sleep apnea can reduce episodes of bruxism. Whether or not you have sleep apnea, the standard treatment for bruxism is an oral device designed by a dentist to protect your teeth.

Hypersomnia

Do you feel compelled to nap a lot during the day? In fact, do you sometimes feel so compelled to nap that you have to leave important activities, such as work or a conversation with your best friend, to take a nap? You may have *hypersomnia,* which are recurrent episodes of excessive daytime sleepiness or oversleeping at night that don't result in feeling rested.

According to the National Sleep Foundation, up to 40 percent of people have some symptoms of hypersomnia from time to time.

Why are you getting too much shuteye? The cause may be one or more of the following:

- Sleep deprivation
- Excessive use of tranquilizers
- Being overweight
- Drug or alcohol abuse
- A head injury, tumor, or neurological disease, such as multiple sclerosis
- A genetic predisposition to hypersomnia
- Prescription medications, including opioid narcotics, sedatives, antidepressants, muscle relaxants especially Soma, and anticonvulsants

The medical treatment of hypersomnia includes prescribed stimulants, antidepressants, or two newer medications: Provigil, a drug that keeps you awake (used for performance enhancement by military pilots and soldiers), and Xyrem, used for treating people with narcolepsy who have episodes of *cataplexy,* a condition characterized by weak or paralyzed muscles. CPAP machines can also be helpful. (See the earlier section on sleep apnea for more on these devices.)

Charting Your Sleep Patterns

In order to detect what type of sleep problems you have, keep a sleep diary for a couple of weeks. Each morning, jot down such things as the quality of your sleep, how long you slept, and how often you woke up. Also, note whether you snored (ask your partner or use a tape recorder) and how loudly, whether you were tired during the day, how many naps you took, and so on.

Be sure to note anything unusual, such as feeling drowsy during an activity you usually enjoy (such as playing tennis) or falling asleep in class. Also note all medications and all alcohol or other mind-altering substances you take. (Be honest! This list is only for *your* eyes!) Track these events for a couple of weeks if you can. Then check your diary to see what your sleep patterns are. Summarize your diary for your doctor and anyone else helping you with your sleep problems.

Getting Some Shuteye the Natural Way

Whether your problem is chronic pain by itself, a sleep disorder such as insomnia or sleep apnea (see sections on these topics earlier in this chapter), or a combination, proven practices can aid your search for restful sleep, if not solve the problem. Make these practices part of your daily regimen until they become regular habits like brushing your teeth and washing behind your ears.

- Go to sleep and get up at the same time each day, even on weekends.
- Don't nap! It can keep you awake at night.
- Develop a regular bedtime schedule. Every night, about half an hour to an hour before you go to bed, do the same ritual so that your body knows it's time to sleep. For example, walk your dog, set the coffee to start perking at 6 a.m., brush your teeth, and then read (nothing scary or violent!) for ten minutes before turning off the light.
- Avoid exercising within three hours of your bedtime.
- Don't eat large meals close to bedtime.
- Remember the old coffee lover's joke that "Sleep is a symptom of caffeine deprivation." Don't consume products that contain caffeine after dinner. Caffeine is found in coffee, tea, cola, and chocolate.
- Be moderate in drinking alcohol.
- Use your bed only for sleeping, sex, and reading no longer than 15 minutes before you go to sleep. No TV! No page-turner novels!

Knocking Yourself Out with Medications

Sometimes you may need a little help from prescribed medications to get to sleep. The following list covers the major types of drugs used to help people sleep.

- **Benzodiazepines** are part of a class of drugs called hypnotics. These drugs include Klonopin, Valium, Restoril, Prosom, Xanax, and Ativan. In addition to being sleep aids, benzodiazepines are also used to stop teeth grinding. These habit-forming drugs should be used only under doctor supervision. Benzodiazepines can cause withdrawal and rebound insomnia.
- **Nonbenzodiazepine** hypnotics include Ambien, Sonata, and Lunesta. These habit-forming drugs should be used only under doctor supervision. Nonbenzodiazepine hypnotics can cause withdrawal and rebound insomnia.
- **A melatonin receptor stimulator,** Ramelteon (Rozerem), was approved in July 2005 and is in a class all by itself. Ramelteon does not produce dependence or rebound insomnia.

Chapter 21

Treating Pain and Stress Using the Power of Thought

In This Chapter

- Overcoming stress-inducing thoughts
- Challenging your negative thoughts
- Adopting new ways of thinking

Did your mother ever say to you (or maybe you say it to your own children), "Don't believe every little rumor that you happen to hear." In the same spirit, consider this tip: Don't believe all the negative or panicky thoughts you may have about your chronic pain. In fact, you may find that your internal grumbles about your pain are actually making it a whole lot worse.

People with chronic pain often have distorted, extreme, or negative thoughts about their condition. For example, when Jim gets a migraine aura, his thoughts are often "I'm going to become deathly ill!" or, "I know that the pain is going to eat me up alive." But migraines don't kill, and they don't devour people either. In addition, such thoughts aren't helpful when you have chronic pain, and they can actually kick the pain up a few notches, the opposite of what you need.

Numerous studies have shown that paying attention to your thoughts about pain can really help you. Identifying thoughts that reflect internal inaccurate or negative beliefs and replacing them with new positive ones can help you experience your pain more realistically — and usually less painfully. In this chapter, you find steps to help you treat your pain using the power of thought.

Understanding the Pain/Stress Link

Pain causes stress, which in turn causes more pain and more stress and so on, in a downward negative spiral.

How you interpret or appraise your pain directly influences how your pain feels. For example, doctors know that any two patients with identical damage shown on their x-rays do *not* experience pain the same way. Each person has their own experiences, beliefs, and physical condition that influence how they feel pain. Once you discover your underlying thinking that affects *your* pain, you'll gain better control over it.

The writer Natalie Goldberg aptly says in her book *Wild Mind,* "Stress believes that everything is an emergency." The thoughts that you have under the stress of pain are often exaggerated because your body and your mind both think they're in the middle of a red alert, so sound the pain klaxons! But with chronic pain, red alert is the opposite of what you want.

Recognize that stress is heightened or reduced by how you think and then how your body reacts to how you think. For example, if every time you awaken with stomach pain you think, "This is going to be *another* bad day," then your negative expectation will *cause* the bad day to happen, just like you anticipated. On the other hand, try thinking, "I'm going to try some things to make me feel better," such as taking your medicine or soaking in a hot bath.

When you think positive thoughts, the result is often that you do feel better. You're not as stressed, and your pain lessens.

Decreasing Stress Using Your Thoughts

Use this tactic. Observe, identify, and write down your automatic thoughts about your pain. Carry a pen and paper with you so that you can jot them down as you go about your daily activities.

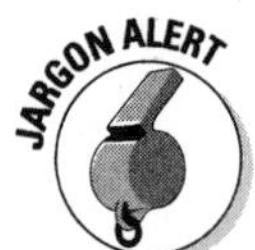

Automatic thoughts are habitual thoughts that spring to mind, and you often accept them unquestioningly. But many people in chronic pain have negative automatic thoughts that need a serious spring cleaning! Use the advice in this chapter to revamp your automatic thoughts.

Following are some examples of automatic thoughts:

- **Catastrophic thinking:** "I know this stomach flare-up means I have cancer, not just irritable bowel syndrome." Or, "I'll never be able to travel again because of my stomach problems."
- **All-or-nothing thinking:** "I can't do sports anymore, so there's no point in exercising at all." Or "I can't stand for long periods of time any more, so that means that I can't do any work at all."
- **Fortune telling** (predicting the future with a negative outcome): "By next year, I'll be in a wheelchair." Or "This new medicine will never work."

- **Labeling:** "All doctors hate people with fibromyalgia." Or "I move slowly because I'm old. All old people move slowly."
- **Mind reading:** "If I tell my fellow churchgoers that I get migraines, they won't let me join the choir." Or "My friends have given up on me because I'm disabled."

These thoughts and others like them add to your pain, just like in football when three or four players pile on the guy with the ball. Don't pile on to your pain!

Notice what happens to your body when automatic thoughts occur. Do your muscles tense up? Does your posture become more stooped? Do you clench your teeth or wring your hands? Or pace around? These stress responses may occur when you have these negative thoughts, and they amplify your pain. Once identified, they're easier to change.

Challenging Negative Thoughts

Don't automatically accept your negative automatic thoughts. Instead, ask yourself whether they're really valid. Are they realistic? Are they based on fact?

For each negative thought, ask yourself these questions.

- Are my thoughts exaggerated?
- Could my thoughts be distorted?
- Are my thoughts overly negative?
- Are there any positive aspects to my thoughts? For example, if I have a headache today, is it just a minor one?

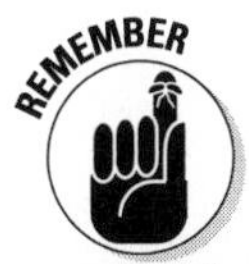

While you're challenging your thoughts, don't chastise yourself if any of them seem out-of-whack. Blaming yourself just adds to the stress and pain.

For all the negative automatic thoughts and their challenges you identify, create new beliefs to replace them with that could change your thinking. For example, Fred, age 83, has a bad knee and thinks of himself as old and decrepit. But Fred could think of himself as a healthy older person (which he is) who happens to have one bad knee. (The other one is still just fine.)

Creating New Automatic Thoughts

Replace your old negative thoughts with new ones. Here's an example of more positive thinking. "When I'm in pain, I can still do a lot. I can work on my craft project. I can also call my friend in my chronic pain group." Another example: "When I'm in pain, I can do more than sit in front of the TV. Instead, I can do a crossword puzzle or read the newspaper, and use my brain." Practice using these new thoughts in place of the old ones.

Many good techniques are effective at reducing stress, such as distraction, framing, and expressive writing, all which can effectively counter your negative thoughts. Read about these techniques in Chapter 22.

Adopting new thoughts as habits

Keep it up, and your new thinking patterns will become habitual. Changing your thoughts can be hard but doable! And it's well-worth every effort you make, because these new thoughts will often translate into considerably less pain.

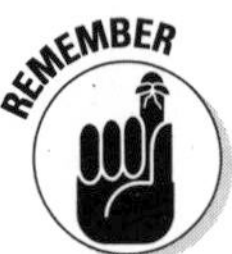

Your new thoughts should be based on reality. For example, if you were just diagnosed with cancer, saying to yourself, "I'm getting better and better every day in every way," isn't appropriate. Your mind will respond with something like, "I'm *not* getting better, I'm getting worse!"

Instead, use thinking that is more along the lines, of "I'm going to do everything I can to become as healthy as possible." This thought is positive and realistic.

Challenge Your Thoughts worksheet

To work on challenging your negative thoughts, copy the worksheet in Table 21-1 and keep notes for a couple of days (or longer). This process can help you develop new patterns of thinking.

First write down the event that has set off the negative thought, then the thought itself, and, last but not least, a positive statement that you're going to use instead.

Use the example in Table 21-2 as a guide.

Table 21-1 Challenge Your Thoughts Worksheet

Event	*Negative Thought*	*New Thought*

Using thought-control resources

These resources can help you think more clearly and more positively:

The Albert Ellis Institute (AEI), `www.albertellisinstitute.org`: AEI's network of therapists practice an action-oriented therapy that teaches individuals to examine their thoughts, beliefs, and actions and replace self-defeating thoughts with more life-enhancing alternatives.

Cognitive Behavioural Therapy For Dummies (Wiley) by Rob Willson and Rhena Branch: This helpful book shows you how to identify and change unhealthy modes of thinking.

Table 21-2 Challenge Your Thoughts Example

Event	*Negative Thought*	*New Thought*
Cleaning up around the house	It hurts too much. I can't do anything. I'm a mess.	Well, I'll just break up the chores into small steps, and I'll reward myself by sitting down for five minutes every time I complete a small chore. I can make it fun!

Chapter 22

Relaxing, Praying, and Creating

In This Chapter

- Understanding the major types of stress
- Easing your stress levels
- Self-hypnotizing stress away
- Rubbing out stress with self-massage

When you have chronic pain, you're also very stressed out, and too much stress is bad for your body. Stress causes clenched muscles, an upset stomach, and — at its peak — a heart beating so fast you can feel the thump, thump, thumping in your chest. Even when things are at an even keel, if you are overly stressed, you still feel awful. And when a situation heats up, then watch out! You're in stress overdrive.

In this chapter, we share many ways that you can minimize stress — and therefore the pain — in your life.

Exploring Stress

Stress is the feeling that the demands in your life are greater and stronger than your physical and personal abilities and resources to cope with them. It's the condition you experience when you feel that you've lost control of your health or your circumstances. When you're stressed out for whatever reason, your body releases the same hormones into your bloodstream that would be pumped out if you were being chased by a big black bear. Stress sets off your body's fight-or-flight response, as if you had to either fight that furry beast or run as fast as you can away from it.

Stress hormones speed up your heart and breathing. In addition, as your body prepares for battle, your muscles tighten. Your liver secretes glucose so that your body will have needed fuel to either struggle in place or run like crazy. Your body also produces sweat to cool itself down. These examples are only a few body processes in full play when you're having a major stress attack.

Sizing up stress

If you're stressed out, you're not alone! One-third of Americans live with extreme stress, and nearly half of Americans (48 percent) believe that their stress has increased over the past five years, according to a 2007 poll conducted for the American Psychological Association (APA).

Chronic pain also causes stress, and your pain can elicit physical and psychological stress symptoms. For example, the APA poll showed that many people experience both physical symptoms (77 percent) and psychological symptoms (73 percent) that are directly related to stress in the last month.

Physical symptoms that the poll respondents reported were fatigue (51 percent); headache (44 percent); upset stomach (34 percent); muscle tension (30 percent); change in appetite (23 percent); teeth grinding (17 percent); change in sex drive (15 percent); and feeling dizzy (13 percent).

Psychological symptoms reported included irritability or anger (50 percent); nervousness (45 percent); a lack of energy (45 percent); and sadness, or feeling as though you could cry (35 percent). In addition, almost half (48 percent) of Americans report lying awake at night due to their excessive stress levels.

Many people cope with stress in unhealthy ways. For example, four in ten Americans (43 percent) say they overeat or eat unhealthy foods to manage their stress, while about one-third (36 percent) skipped a meal in the last month because of stress. Those who drink (39 percent) or smoke cigarettes (19 percent) were also more likely to engage in these unhealthy behaviors during periods of high stress.

Some people cope with their stress in more positive ways; for example, significant numbers of Americans report listening to music (54 percent); reading (52 percent); exercising or walking (50 percent); spending time with family and friends (40 percent); and praying (34 percent). These behaviors are the kind you should emulate!

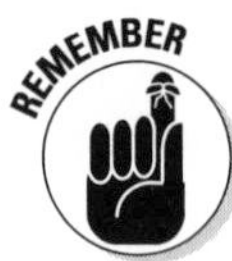

Stress doesn't occur solely in response to immediate dangers, such as rampaging bears. Just as a person can have chronic pain, she can have chronic stress. Long-term challenges, such as coping with chronic pain, can produce a low-level, long-term stress that simply wears you out and wears you down. That's why you need to work on easing your stress levels.

The American Psychological Association (APA) has identified three major types of stress: acute stress, episodic acute stress, and chronic stress. Your chronic pain can cause one or all three of these forms of stress, which are described in the following sections.

Acute stress

When you experience a traumatic event, acute stress is your instantaneous response. You may have been injured or witnessed a violent event. You may have been fired or betrayed. Whatever the incident, your initial response was fear and a feeling of vulnerability. Fortunately, acute stress is brief and usually doesn't do extensive physical and emotional damage *unless* it turns into the longer-lasting response of episodic acute stress or chronic stress.

Interestingly, acute stress, such as a near-miss automobile accident, actually temporarily relieves chronic pain ostensibly due to the release of endorphins.

Episodic acute stress

This type of stress usually occurs for Type A personalities. Type As are said to be excessively competitive, aggressive, impatient, and have a harrying sense of time urgency.

Constant worrying can also cause this type of stress. Worrywarts, for example, see disaster around every corner. If you're constantly worrying about your chronic pain or other major stressors in your life, then you need to chill out!

The symptoms of acute and episodic acute stress are the same. However, if you have the symptoms during episodic stress, they usually last longer than symptoms triggered by acute stress alone.

These symptoms include

- Persistent tension headaches
- Migraines
- Hypertension (high blood pressure)
- Chest pain
- Heart disease

Chronic stress

Chronic stress is the grinding strain that wears you down, day after day, year after year. Chronic stress results when you feel trapped by a miserable situation. It's the stress of poverty, of working in a despised job, of living in a war zone. And far too often, it's the stress of chronic pain.

According to the APA, a terrible aspect of chronic stress is that you can actually get used to it. It starts to feel like your situation is hopeless, and it's just the way things are. You don't realize that things could actually change for the better. The APA literature on chronic stress says, "People are immediately aware of acute stress because it is new; they ignore chronic stress because it is old, familiar, and sometimes, almost comfortable."

Coping with Stress and Pain

Wouldn't it be great if you could just inhabit a stress-free zone and eliminate all your troubles from your life? Say good-bye to the jitters and the stomach aches. And especially say goodbye to the relentlessness of it all!

But when you have chronic pain, you have to deal every day with the stress it creates. The best approach is to curb the stress as much as you can and when you can. Fortunately, numerous techniques can help you alleviate stress. From meditation to yoga, the techniques described in the following sections can help reduce both your stress and pain.

Using guided imagery

Guided imagery can help you use your imagination to calm the stress that reality brings to your life every day. This technique involves creating positive images, sounds, smells, tastes, and feelings with your mind. An instructor — in person or on audiotape — guides you through the process of forming your own imagery. One commonly used technique is to imagine a safe, comfortable place, such as a beach on a pleasant clear day or a peaceful chapel in the autumn woods.

Guided imagery is frequently used in hospital settings due to the success of a study conducted at the Cleveland Clinic in the mid-1990s. Clinic researchers found that employing guided imagery reduced their patients' anxiety and pain, as well as their use of narcotic medication both before and after surgery. The technique has become so popular that Kaiser Permanente, a major health maintenance organization, provides patients and the public with free downloads of guided imagery to use during medical procedures and for overall wellness (`http://members.kaiserpermanente.org/redirects/listen`). Guided imagery tapes are also widely available through bookstores and the web.

Meditating through the hurting

Meditation is a group of techniques rooted in spiritual traditions. Many people use meditation for stress and pain reduction and to promote wellness. When meditating, you use one of a range of techniques, such as repeating a word over and over again (a *mantra*) or paying attention to your breathing. These approaches help focus your attention and quiet down your stress-related thoughts. No one really knows how it works, but for many people, meditation leads to physical relaxation, pain reduction, and psychological balance.

All techniques used for meditation have four elements in common:

- A quiet location with as few distractions as possible
- A comfortable posture
- A focus of attention, such as an object in the room
- A feeling of letting go so that any distractions come and go gently, and your focus does not remain on them

Here's a sample meditation exercise to try at home:

1. **Find a peaceful place where you'll be free of interruptions.**
2. **Choose a focus word, a phrase, or an image you find relaxing.**

   Examples of words are "grace" and ooohmmm." (Some practitioners believe that the mantra should be syllables or words that have no meaning to you. That is why many people use "ooohmmm" or "aaaaummm.")

   Example of phrases you can use are "May I be well," or "May I have patience and gratitude." Examples of images to concentrate on include statues of a spiritual figure or a photograph of the sun.
3. **Sit quietly in a comfortable position.**

   The easiest posture is a comfortable sitting position, with your spine straight and erect. If you lie down, you'll probably fall asleep, and you can't meditate when you're unconscious!
4. **Close your eyes and relax your muscles, starting at your head, working down your body to your feet.**
5. **Breathe slowly and naturally, focusing on your breathing or a word, phrase, or image; continue for 10 to 20 minutes.**

   If your mind wanders, that's OK. Gently return your focus to your breathing and to the word, phrase or image you've previously selected.
6. **After the time is up, sit quietly for a few minutes with your eyes closed; then open your eyes and sit in silence for a few more minutes.**

Relaxing your breathing

Stress causes rapid, shallow breathing. If you slow down and deepen your breathing, you can reduce the effects of stress. Here's one frequently used approach to achieve this goal:

1. **Inhale.**

   With your mouth closed and your shoulders relaxed, inhale as slowly and deeply as you can, to the count of six. At the same time, push your stomach out. Allow the air to fill your diaphragm.

2. **Hold.**

   Keep the air in your lungs as you slowly count to four.

3. **Exhale.**

   Release the air through your mouth as you slowly count to six.

4. **Repeat the inhale-hold-exhale cycle three to five times.**

Driving to distraction

Multitasking is good, but many people take it too far and ratchet up their stress to bad levels that increase their chronic pain.

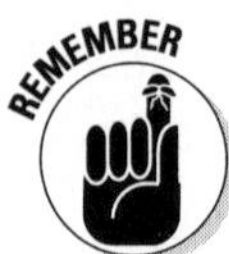

You can concentrate on only so many things at one time: organizing your To-Do List for the next day, preparing dinner, finding your son's soccer gear, all the while talking to your mother on the phone. Multitasking too much is a setup for burning the rice! When your brain is crowded with too many tasks, attention to some things will inevitably drop off. You can turn around this principle and use it in a positive way to manage pain.

Sidetrack your mind away from your hurting by focusing on things that compete for attention in your brain. The approach is called *distraction.* The idea is to find activities that you can be totally absorbed in. Try the activity at least an hour every day and see how you feel.

For example, Elizabeth Vierck (one of your authors) had a difficult hip replacement surgery and subsequently spent a week transfixed by her husband's fish tank, watching the clown fish swim in circles. It was fun. It was soothing. And it helped ease the pain. Other people have tried activities like learning to count to 400 in Chinese or teaching a child a hobby, such as sewing or whittling.

Here are a few other ideas that may help you distract yourself from your pain:

- Read or listen to a book or listen to music.
- Do Sudoko puzzles, crosswords, or jigsaw puzzles.
- On your computer, go to `http://zefrank.com` to play games, draw flowers, or practice meditation by watching a flower move slowly across your screen.
- Take up creative pursuits, such as needlework, painting with acrylics, or learning carpentry.
- If you're physically fit enough, take up a new activity, such as golf or bocce ball.

- If you don't have a pet, consider adopting a puppy or kitten. (Or an adult dog or cat, which are usually already trained and less stressful!) They demand attention, are by nature distracting, and are also entertaining and funny.

Using self-hypnosis

The goal of self-hypnosis is to draw your attention away from your pain and help you relax. You can also use it to change negative thoughts. In fact, if you try this stress-reduction technique, make sure that you use only positive words and images throughout your self-hypnosis experience.

You may want to consult a certified hypnotherapist to teach you specific techniques for using self-hypnosis for pain reduction. The National Board for Certified Clinical Hypnotherapists has an online directory available at `www.natboard.com`. In addition, many self-hypnosis instructional programs are available for purchase on audio through bookstores or online.

Keep in mind that hypnosis typically involves four stages: induction, deepening, suggestion, and termination.

- In the *induction stage,* you achieve a deep state of relaxation.
- The second stage, *deepening,* involves increasing your hypnotic state.
- The third stage is *suggestion.* Tell yourself soothing phrases that will help your pain, such as "The muscles of my back are totally relaxed."
- *Termination,* where you end the hypnosis, is the last stage of the process.

The following steps walk you through a self-hypnosis script to try. You'll want to have about a half hour available.

1. **Find a quiet, comfortable spot where you can avoid distractions.**
2. **Choose a suggestion that will help your pain. Whisper it silently to yourself.**

   For example, try something like, "My muscles are relaxing, and I am calm" or "I feel warmth soothing my joints."
3. **Take a deep breath, hold the breath for a count of three, and then exhale with a sigh; repeat three times.**

   Let go all your tension when you breathe out.
4. **Take another deep breath through your nose, hold for a count of five, and let it go through pursed lips; repeat three times.**

   Really let go on the exhale, releasing all your body tension. You should begin to relax.

5. **Repeat to yourself the suggestion you chose in Step 1 and imagine yourself in that state.**

   For example, if you say to yourself, "My body is relaxing," imagine yourself as relaxed, with your arms and legs limp.

6. **Focus on the spots on your body where you have pain.**

7. **Deepen your hypnotic state.**

   You can try several techniques:

   - Repeat to yourself, "I am going deeper and deeper into a hypnotic state."
   - Use imagery: Tell yourself that your eyelids are getting heavier and heavier. Imagine this wonderful feeling.

   Repeat the suggestion to yourself several times.

8. **Tell yourself that you're coming out of your trance and give yourself a positive message.**

   For example, "I will count from one to five. When I reach five, my eyelids will open, and I will be wide awake and relaxed, and I will be in less pain.

Healing with your own hands: Self-massage

Of course, you'd probably prefer to have a professional give you a massage than do it yourself. Who wouldn't? But, if you're like most people, you don't always have the time or money to see a massage therapist. Self-massage is a great option at these times. (If your insurance covers massage, consider yourself lucky! But you still may want to do self-massage in between your appointments with a therapist. It will help keep those sore muscles relaxed!)

The idea behind self-massage is to rub and stroke the areas on your body that a massage therapist would stroke, concentrating on the most painful areas. You probably do some self-massage without even thinking about it — rubbing your head when you have a headache, stroking your shoulders after hunching over a keyboard all day, or massaging your sore feet after a long hike.

Following are some self-massage ideas to help you get started. You also may want to get a massage therapist to instruct you in these moves. See Chapter 13 for information on how to find a licensed therapist.

- **Back massage:** Find a tennis ball and sit in a straight back chair. Place the tennis ball on any sore spots on your back. Lean into the chair. Lean your back into the ball. Take ten deep breaths. Repeat at least once more.
- **Head massage:** Spread your hands out on your scalp. Massage in a clockwise motion, beginning at your hairline and moving backward to the nape of your neck. Take deep breaths and massage as you breathe. Change direction.
- **Foot massage:** Wash your feet and put a light coat of lotion or oil on them. Sit on a comfortable chair and rest one foot on the thigh of the other leg. Thread the fingers of one hand through the toes of your foot, spreading out your toes. Place the palm of your hand against the bottom of your foot. Rotate the joints of your forefoot back and forth for one minute with the palm of your hand. Repeat with the other foot.

  Next, hold your ankle with one hand and gently rotate your foot with the other hand. Start with small circles and make then increasingly larger. Switch directions. Repeat with the other foot.
- **Neck massage:** Clasp your fingers behind your neck, pressing the heels of your palms into your neck on either side of your spinal column. Move the heels of your hands up and down slowly.

  Then place the fingers of your right hand on the muscle along the left side of your neck just below the base of your skull (the trapezius muscle). Press into that muscle, tilt your head to the left, and rub downward toward your shoulder. Repeat three times and then switch sides.
- **Shoulder squeeze:** Cross your arms over your chest and grab a shoulder with either hand. Squeeze each shoulder and release three times. Move your hands down your arms, squeeze, and release.

Praying and using other spiritual techniques

Prayer can be a powerful pain reducer for those who practice it. A *USA Today* poll found that 59 percent of its respondents reported that they used prayer to control pain. Of the people who use prayer for pain, 90 percent said it works well, and 51 percent said it works "very well." Many people find that repeating a word or prayer many times is soothing. Choose a prayer that will work best for you based on your religious beliefs.

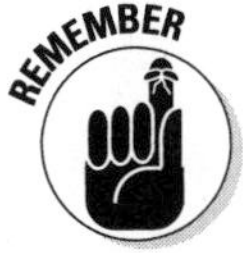

Some people who worry a lot say that it helps to give over their problems to God or a higher power to solve. By letting go of your problems, you can work toward relaxing.

Ironically, many people find that when they pray, solutions to their problems suddenly occur to them. Before praying, the intense worry was blocking the answers that they sought.

Journaling for wellness and pain management

Many people find that writing their thoughts in a journal relieves their stress and helps them manage their pain better. The concept behind journaling for stress relief and pain management is to write specifically about your thoughts, feelings, and frustrations on your pain, health, and related issues. Journaling also includes writing about positive things. For example, maybe your pain condition has brought you closer to your family or you've started a new hobby to replace old ones you can no longer perform. Write down the positives as well so that you can celebrate the good!

Think of your journal as a nonjudgmental best friend or therapist, to whom you can pour your heart out. Also, keep in mind that your journal should be different from your pain diary. (For information about keeping a pain diary, see Chapter 17.) Think of your pain diary as a spreadsheet where you keep details about your pain and overall health, while your journal is an open and honest conversation with yourself.

Journaling can be done with pen and paper or on a computer. If you're a perfectionist, let it go! Don't worry about using correct grammar or spelling or perfect penmanship. Journaling is for your eyes only.

Laughing through your stress and pain

"There's nothing like a good laugh." How many times have you said that to yourself (or your best friend) after a particularly good joke? The great editor Norman Cousins famously discovered the therapeutic effects of laughter when he developed heart disease and arthritis. He described his laughter-as-therapy approach in the 1979 book *Anatomy of an Illness.*

While the pain-ridden Cousins was in the hospital, he watched Marx Brothers films. "I made the joyous discovery that ten minutes of genuine belly laughter had an anesthetic effect and would give me at least two hours of pain-free sleep," he reported. Cousins said that "Laughter is inner jogging."

Tips to bring humor into your life

Laugh more and feel better! Watch comedy on DVD, TV, and even on your computer. Most TV comedy shows include highlights of popular episodes on their Web pages. For example, the site for the late-night host, Jay Leno, shows the clip "Impressing Ed Asner" from one of his episodes in which a spry 90-year-old woman does a dance routine that ends with her doing impressive splits. Watch this piece, and not only will you laugh in pure delight at the enthusiasm of the performer, you'll also cheer in awe. (And, you will forget your pain, if only for a minute.)

Here are a few more ideas:

- **Go to comedy clubs.** Most large cities have comedy clubs featuring standup comics. Many acts are top-notch; most great comedians, such as Jerry Seinfeld and Tim Allen, got their starts in comedy clubs.
- **Read or listen to funny books.** Many good comedy writers can tickle your funny bone: Steve Martin, Woody Allen, Whoopi Goldberg, and Ellen DeGeneres, to name just a few. You can also listen to them on CD while in your car. A great resource for purchasing CDs designed for laughs is Laugh.com at `http://laughstore.stores.yahoo.net`.
- **Check out funny things wherever you go and whatever you do.** If the comic section in your local paper doesn't interest you, try the Web. Some funny sites are `www.funny2.com`; `www.ahajokes.com`; `www.comedycentral.com/jokes/index.jhtml`; and `www.knock-knock-joke.com`.
- **Be funny.** Make yourself and other people laugh. If it doesn't come naturally, take a class from the Laugh Tour (`www.worldlaughtertour.com`; 1-800-NOW-LAFF). They travel around the country teaching people to laugh. Or read the classic and still great *How To Be Funny* by Steve Allen, (Prometheus) the founder of late-night TV.

Since Cousins' time (he died in 1990), the power of laughter as an anecdote for pain and stress has caught on around the world. The Laughter Tour (`www.worldlaughtertour.com`) is very popular in rehab centers and long-term care facilities. The Laughter Arts and Science Foundation (`www.laughterfoundation.org`) supports and creates programs that capitalize on laughter to promote harmony in the world. The Association for Applied and Therapeutic Humor (`www.aath.org`) is a network of laughter authorities and enthusiasts. And the International Society for Humor Studies (`www.hnu.edu/ishs`) is a scholarly and professional organization dedicated to the advancement of humor research.

Interest in laughter is based in part on its positive effects on health and pain reduction. For example, using laughter-provoking movies to gauge the effect of emotions on cardiovascular health, researchers at the University of Maryland School of Medicine in Baltimore showed that laughter is linked to the healthy functioning of blood vessels. Laughter appears to cause the tissue that forms the inner lining of blood vessels, the *endothelium,* to dilate or expand in order to increase blood flow — a very good thing!

When the same group of study volunteers was shown a movie that produced mental stress, their blood vessel linings constricted, reducing blood flow — a very bad thing.

Other research has shown that laughter

- Lowers blood pressure
- Increases vascular blood flow and oxygenation of the blood, which assists healing
- Exercises your diaphragm, abdominal, respiratory, and other muscles
- Reduces levels of stress hormones in your body, which surge when you feel stress, anger, or hostility. These hormones cause all sorts of harm in your body: They can suppress your immune system, obstruct your arteries, and raise blood pressure.
- Increases natural killer cells (such as T and B cells) that destroy tumors and viruses

Humming through your stress and pain

Using music to soothe pain isn't a new phenomenon. The medical community recognized its success during the first and second world wars, when nurses used music with wounded soldiers in veterans' hospitals.

More recently, U.S. researchers tested the effects of music on 60 patients who had endured years of chronic pain. Those who listened to music reported decreases of up to 21 percent in their pain levels and up to 25 percent in depression levels, compared to those who did not listen to music. They had suffered from osteoarthritis, disc problems, and rheumatoid arthritis for an average of more than six years.

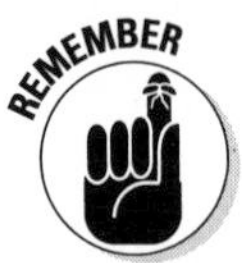

Music is an individual taste. What soothes one person may jangle the nerves of another. But if listening to the music of your choice gives you relief from pain and stress, then we say, "Listen up!"

Playing with crayons and clay: Art therapy

Art as a healing tool is mainstream in medicine. In a 2004 survey, the Joint Commission on Accreditation of Healthcare Organizations found that about 2,000 hospitals nationwide offer some kind of art programming or therapy (including music).

Recent research has underscored the benefits that practicing art can have for pain reduction and other symptoms. A study of cancer patients published in the *Journal of Pain and Symptom Management* found that participating in art programs reduces uncomfortable symptoms in cancer patients. The researchers found reductions in eight of nine symptoms: pain, tiredness, depression, anxiety, drowsiness, lack of appetite, well-being, and shortness of breath. Nausea was the only symptom that didn't change as a result of participating in the program.

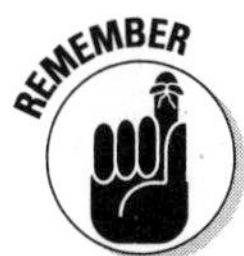

You don't have to be a gifted artist to practice art for pain reduction. In fact, the purpose is to paint as you did as a child — to be distracted by the process of creating something from within yourself. Use any medium you want, including crayons, clay, or colored pencils.

To try your hand at art to reduce pain, you may want to start by locating an art therapist in your local area. Contact the American Art Therapy Association, Inc., 5999 Stevenson Ave., Alexandria, VA 22304; phone 888-290-0878; e-mail `info@arttherapy.org`.

Part V

Understanding Pain Throughout the Life Cycle

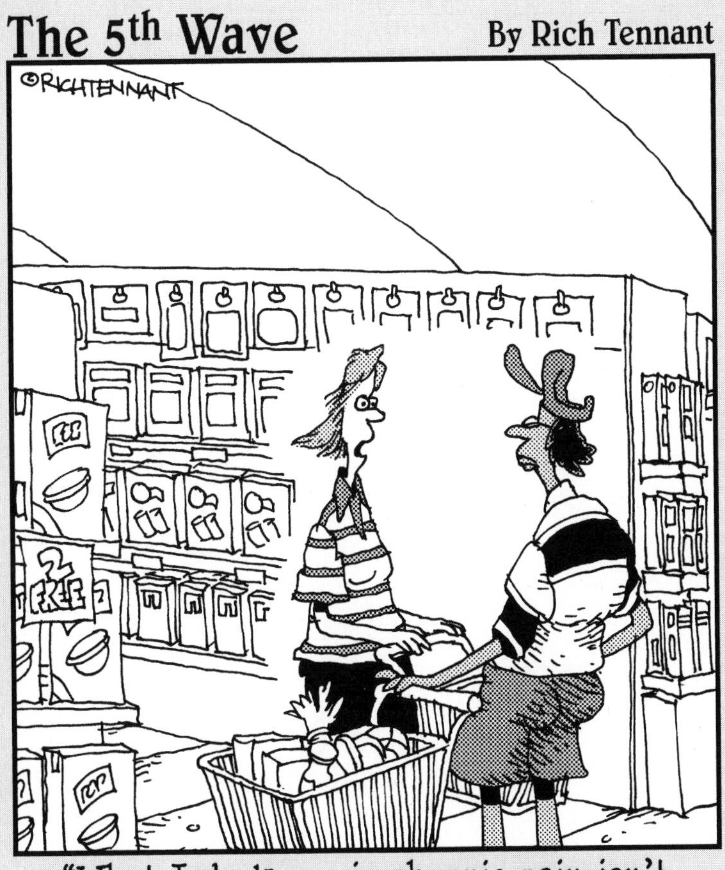

"What I do know is chronic pain isn't contagious. Unless your child has it."

In this part . . .

In this part, we give you practical advice on detecting and managing chronic pain during three stages of the lifecycle: childhood, the later years, and during the end of life. Pain during each of these stages requires different treatments and solutions than during adulthood. For example, the types and dosages of drugs that you can give a child with chronic pain differ greatly from those an adult can take. And the same is true people over age 65.

So, if you have a child with chronic pain, if you or a loved one is over age 65, or if you (or a loved one) have a terminal illness, this part is for you.

Chapter 23

Pain in Children

In This Chapter

- Understanding children's experience of pain
- Identifying chronic illness in your child
- Considering children's pain meds

If you have a child in chronic pain, you're all too familiar with the heartbreak and challenges of seeing a kid who's hurting. And you're not alone — many other parents know exactly how you feel. The American Pain Society estimates that 15 to 20 percent of children are affected by chronic pain. Many experts say that this number actually is an underestimate because a lot of pain in kids goes undiagnosed.

Many conditions, including cystic fibrosis, chronic headaches, and cancer, cause chronic pain in children. But kids experience the pain these conditions cause much differently than adults. For example, until about age 3, children don't think abstractly about pain and have no experience to draw on to realize that the pain of a needle prick will go away fast. To the child, it hurts right now! And it hurts a lot! And, that's really, really scary!

This chapter gives you tips to detect the severity of your child's pain and covers the medicines commonly used to treat pain in children.

Understanding How Children Experience Pain

Until the last few decades, pain was often ignored in infants. It's incredible to think about now, but physicians believed that infants didn't feel pain as intensely as older children or adults do (or they believed that babies didn't feel pain at all). The medical profession assumed that an infant's nervous system was just not mature enough to transmit pain the way that an older child's or an adult's does. But the truth is that infants can feel pain. However, they don't know how to tell you about pain and don't show it the same way that adults do.

Resources

The following resources may be useful when your child suffers from chronic pain:

The American Academy of Family Physicians (AAFP), P.O. Box 11210, Shawnee Mission, KS 66207; phone 800-274-2237, 913-906-6000; Web site `http://familydoctor.org`. AAFP's Parents and Kids section on its Web site provides information about health conditions that affect children. Its Find a Family Doctor page provides an interactive directory of family physicians by state.

KidsHealth, Web site `www.kidshealth.org`. KidsHealth provides health information about and for children from before birth through adolescence. KidsHealth has separate areas for kids, teens, and parents.

American Academy of Pediatrics, 141 Northwest Point Blvd., Elk Grove Village, IL 60007; phone 847-434-4000; Web site `www.aap.org/parents.html`. The Parenting Corner of the AAP offers many helpful hints on a broad array of topics. In addition, you can search its database to locate a pediatrician.

Children also don't have any life experience to draw on to compare one type of pain to another. In addition, a child's pain may be ignored because she may not be able to tell an adult about it — she doesn't have the words to describe "pain in the sinuses" — or she may try to hide her pain because she's afraid of the events that may be set in motion if she does talk about it.

For example, maybe the last time she complained about something that hurt, her dad took her to the doctor's office, and a very tall stranger drew blood from her arm — and the idea of going to the doctor's office and going through that ordeal again is a lot scarier than the headache she's having at the moment.

Whether a child feels pain in relationship to a chronic illness and how she expresses it depends on the individual child and the disease process. For example, some children with juvenile rheumatoid arthritis have pain, and some other (luckier) kids don't. Some children will also keep playing in spite of their pain, while others withdraw or scream bloody murder — and they all have the same level of pain.

Measuring Pain in Children

With so many ways that a child can respond to pain, how do you tell what's really happening with your kid? Fortunately, health professionals have developed methods for measuring pain in children:

- **Self-reported (subjective) pain,** which is assessed by asking questions and using scales. (Experts say that children 6 to 7 years and older are as accurate as adults at assessing pain using self-reporting methods.)

- **Physiologic measures of pain,** noted by signs such as elevated blood pressure and sweating.
- **Behavioral signs of pain,** observed by contorted facial expressions and crying.

Measuring self-reported pain

To make it easier for your child to describe her pain and help you determine how much pain your child is experiencing, try one of the following techniques. To use these measures, your child must be talking and able to answer questions — it won't work on baby!

- Ask your child to draw or describe the color of her pain. Give your child a box of crayons and some paper and ask her to draw her pain. Children's pain drawings are usually very detailed and emotionally powerful, and they often use red or black to draw areas where they feel the most pain.
- Use the chips game to determine pain. *Note:* For this method, your child must be able to understand that adding one thing to another thing results in creating something bigger. Use four identical chips — poker chips or checker pieces are fine. Tell your child that you want to talk to her about the pain she's having right now. Then line the chips across (not up and down) in a row on a kitchen table, tray, or other flat surface.

  Starting at the far left, describe the chips to your child. Say something like, "This chip is a little hurt." (If your child doesn't understand the concept of "hurt" very well, use words she does understand, such as "This chip is a *little* owie.") Point to the next chip and say "This chip is *more* hurt." Point to the next one and say "This one is *a lot* of hurt." Then point to the last one and say, "This chip is the *most* hurt you can have!" Then ask your child, "Show me how many chips you feel like right now?"

  Make sure that you understand what your child is expressing by saying something like, "Oh, that means you have a little hurt" if she picks only the first chip. If she then says, "No, hurts a *lot*," then re-explain the concept one more time. (Don't try a third time if it still doesn't work. Use one of the other measures.)
- Use the faces scale to determine pain. Particularly after about age 5, some children describe their pain accurately using the faces scales, such as the one shown in Chapter 17. If you use this scale, try using these descriptions for the five faces:
  - **First face:** Doesn't hurt at all.
  - **Second face:** Hurts a little.
  - **Third face:** Hurts more.
  - **Fourth face:** Hurts a lot.
  - **Fifth face:** Hurts the most.

Reading physiologic measures of pain

An increased heart rate, sweating, an elevated pulse or blood pressure, or rapid breathing can all indicate that a child is in pain and feeling stress. However, these signs must be used along with the self-reporting and behavioral measures because these physical responses can be caused by other factors, such as anxiety or hunger. And, just as in adults, infants in pain sometimes don't show any abnormalities in heart rate or blood pressure.

Reading behavior to detect pain

Children show pain by crying and pulling away from the cause, such as a needle or catheter that hurts. They also may hold their breath; clench their fists; show pain, anxiety, or fear on their faces; and hold or stroke the area where it hurts. Children in pain may also be less active and sleep more or less than normally. They may refuse to eat.

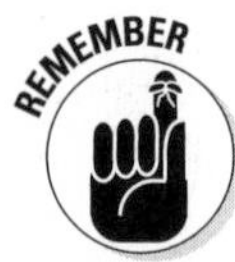

The most reliable way to tell pain in an infant is by facial expression. The following expressions show an infant is in pain: quivering chin, eyes squeezed shut, mouth wide open, and grimacing. An inability to be comforted and crying with a tone that is higher and louder than usual also may indicate pain. Cries from pain also tend to be sharp, not melodious.

Detecting Chronic Illness in Your Child

A myriad of medical conditions can cause chronic pain conditions in children. If you think that your child is in pain and notice any of the following signs, report them to your pediatrician or family doctor, because they may be symptoms of a chronic or serious illness.

- Breathing problems such as coughing or wheezing
- Marked changes in weight, behavior, sleep patterns, eating, or drinking
- Vomiting or diarrhea that doesn't improve
- Crankiness and crying
- Rashes that don't improve

Assessing Pain Medications for Children

Most drugs used to treat pain haven't been studied in children, and the FDA doesn't give guidelines for giving painkillers to children. So, doctors must extrapolate from studies performed with adults.

In part, because of the lack of guidelines, many health professionals are afraid of overdosing a child, so, they sometimes don't give them *enough* medicine to handle the pain.

Acetaminophen, ibuprofen, and opioids are used most often for pain control in children. However, ibuprofen and other nonsteroidal anti-inflammatory drugs (NSAIDs), such as Motrin, are not recommended for infants younger than 6 months old. (Their livers can't metabolize it.) Pain medicines for children are available as lollipops, syrups, or nasal drops, which can make administration easier.

Don't give your child Motrin and Tylenol at the same time or within the time on the dosage schedule given to you in this chapter, by the drug's manufacturer, or by your pediatrician. In other words, if the bottle for your child's Motrin says, "give every six hours," don't give him either drug during that six-hour period. Giving your child Tylenol and Motrin close to each other in time can cause her to have kidney failure.

Acetaminophen and ibuprofen are the most frequently used OTC pain relievers in children. They're effective for both acute and chronic pain. The two OTC drugs are similar in their ability to relieve moderate to severe pain, but ibuprofen is better at reducing fever. The dosage to give your child is based on weight.

Acetaminophen

Administering the correct dosage of acetaminophen is extremely important to avoid accidentally overdosing your child. For example, giving your child too many OTC drugs that include acetaminophen (Tylenol and Datril) can damage his liver. Not only is the drug sold under the brand name of Tylenol (and other names), but it's also available in many cough and cold products. Be sure to read the labels on all OTC drugs your child will be taking *before* administering them and also total the amount of acetaminophen in them. Don't exceed the recommended dosage even though the acetaminophen comes from different sources. Also, don't give your child acetaminophen for more than the days recommended by your pediatrician.

If your child is prescribed a drug that includes acetaminophen, ask the pharmacist how much acetaminophen is included in the drug and whether it's okay to also give the child OTC painkillers.

An overdose of acetaminophen can cause liver damage. The signs of liver damage include abnormally yellow skin and eyes (jaundice), dark urine, light-colored stools, nausea, vomiting, and loss of appetite. The signs are similar to the symptoms of the flu, so they easily can go unnoticed.

Table 23-1 shows the recommended dosages for acetaminophen according to the age of the child.

Table 23-1 Acetaminophen Dosage Chart

Age	*Weight*	*Drops (0.8 ml)*	*Syrup (5 ml)*	*Chewable Tablets (80 mg)*
0–3 mos.	6–11 lbs.	0.4 ml	n/a	n/a
4–11 mos.	12–17 lbs.	0.8 ml	1/2 tsp	1 tab
1–2 years	18–23 lbs.	1.2 ml	3/4 tsp	1 1/2 tabs
2–3 years	24–35 lbs.	1.6 ml	1 tsp	2 tabs
4–5 years	36–47 lbs.	2.4 ml	1 1/2 tsp	3 tabs

Dosages may be repeated every four hours, but they should not be given more than 5 times in 24 hours. (*Note:* Milliliter is abbreviated as ml; 5 ml equals 1 teaspoon [tsp].)

Don't use household teaspoons, which can vary in size. Instead use the medicine spoon or syringe provided by the pharmacy (usually for free).

Ibuprofen

Ibuprofen works better than acetaminophen in treating high fevers (103° F or higher). However, ibuprofen should be given only to children older than 6 months (see Table 23-2). Never give ibuprofen to a child who is dehydrated or vomiting because it can cause renal failure. Dosages may be repeated every 6 to 8 hours, but should not be given more than 4 times in 24 hours.

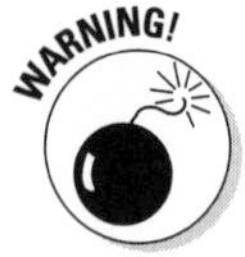

If your child has kidney disease, asthma, an ulcer, or another chronic illness, ask your pediatrician whether ibuprofen is safe. Don't give your child ibuprofen or acetaminophen if he's taking any other pain reliever or fever reducer, unless your pediatrician says it's okay to do so.

Table 23-2 Ibuprofen Dosage Chart

Age	*Weight*	*Drops (1.5 ml)*	*Syrup (5 ml)*	*Chewable Tablets (50 mg)*
6–11 mos.	12–17 lbs.	1.5 ml	n/a	n/a
1–2 years	18–23 lbs.	2.25 ml	n/a	n/a

Age	Weight	Drops (1.5 ml)	Syrup (5 ml)	Chewable Tablets (50 mg)
2–3 years	24–35 lbs.	3 ml	1 tsp	n/a
4–5 years	36–47 lbs.	n/a	1 1/2 tsp	3 tabs

Other pain-reducing options

The two opioids used most often in children are morphine (MS Contin) and Fentanyl (Duragesic). However, many doctors are reluctant to prescribe these drugs because of the lack of research on side effects in children. Opioids are available in pills for swallowing, tablets to put under the tongue, rectal suppositories, nasal sprays, intravenous shots, and subcutaneous injections.

In addition, children who are 4- to 6-years-old in extremely severe pain can, with supervision from an adult, use patient-controlled analgesia (PCA). This implanted device can be triggered when pain occurs and doesn't allow more than a specific level of medication to be released. Older children can often use PCAs without supervision. (See Chapter 14 for information on PCAs.)

Prescription drugs

Unfortunately, no research shows the effectiveness of giving children prescription drugs, such as antidepressants and anti-epileptics, which are often used to treat chronic pain in adults. (See Chapter 14 for information for adults regarding taking these types of drugs for chronic pain.) However, many doctors do prescribe the following drugs for pain control in children:

- Anti-anxiety medications, such as lorazepam (Ativan) and diazepam (Valium), to enhance the effects of opioids
- Tricyclic antidepressants, such as amitriptyline (Elavil), to treat chronic pain and headaches
- Corticosteroids to eliminate inflammation and bone pain
- Anticonvulsants, such as phenytoin (Dilantin) and gabapentin (Neurontin), to treat neuropathies. (See Chapter 11 for information on neuropathies.)
- Neuroleptics, which are antipsychotic drugs with sedative and pain-killing effects, to help relieve cancer pain and other severe pain
- Anesthetics, such as the topical painkiller EMLA cream, which is available for children over 1 month old and is given ahead of time, to reduce pain caused by medical procedures

Chapter 24

Pain and Aging

In This Chapter

- Admitting to chronic pain
- Realizing how medicines act in the bodies of older people
- Understanding the medical risks of ignoring pain in seniors
- Detecting pain in people with cognitive problems

Have you heard of *ageism?* It's prejudice against older people, and it's partially reflected in society's worship of youth, as well as its anxiety and horror over wrinkles and graying hair. Strangely, most people wish for a long life, and yet they don't seem to want to think about becoming old. (How you achieve long life without actually aging is a mystery.)

Most people (including some doctors!) have preconceptions of older age. One of them is that getting old means you're *supposed* to live with aches and pains. Well, it's true you're more likely to have arthritis and other pain-inducing disorders as you age. However, chronic pain isn't inevitable, and it's caused by an actual disease or disorder, not by whatever age you are. If you're older, you don't have to let your aches and pains bench you altogether, nor should your doctor assume that you should accept all pain as normal. Fight back! You *can* take action against chronic pain. This chapter offers suggestions for older people in pain, as well as for the people who love them.

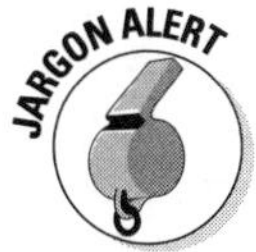

What is meant by older Americans, senior patients, or seniors? These are all terms that generally apply to people age 65 and older, a common definition of the elderly in the United States.

Older People Have Real Pain

Many doctors say that a lot of senior patients deny that they have pain. Even people who are bent over, stiff, and in obvious discomfort may deny that they're in pain. When asked if they hurt, they say, "I'm fine" or "At my age, who can complain?" But if doctors probe a little further, many older patients say that they "always" feel stiff and sore.

Sometimes older people have adapted society's ageist beliefs and *expect* aching and discomfort to appear or accelerate as their birthdays stack up. So they don't report it to their doctors. Their thinking is, "Of course, I'm in pain. I'm old!" Other older individuals think that admitting they're in pain is a sign of weakness. And others fear the side effects of drugs, particularly narcotics, used to treat pain.

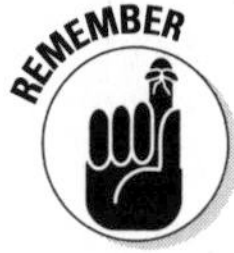

The consequences of these attitudes are all bad. Neglecting pain means a life of discomfort, when this pain could be greatly reduced with the help of a physician, other health-care professionals, and pain-relieving treatments and techniques. If you're an older person or someone who loves an older person, don't accept that older people are in pain solely because they're old. There may be other reasons for their pain.

According to the American Geriatrics Society, arthritis is the most common cause of pain in people over age 65. Circulatory problems, shingles, and other types of nerve damage, bowel diseases, and cancer are also other common causes of chronic pain in older people. In addition, muscle pain is also quite common. Conditions that contribute to muscle pain in older people are fibromyalgia and myofascial pain.

Admittedly, while it's not a given, pain is common during the later years. Two in three seniors in the United States say that pain prevents them from carrying out routine activities, such as cooking, housework, hobbies, and gardening. If you're age 65 or older, you may be wondering, "Why us? We finally have some time off from the daily grind of work, but now we have trouble getting around the grocery store and running the vacuum cleaner."

It may not seem fair, but many seniors have multiple medical conditions — arthritis, back problems, gastrointestinal problems, and other conditions that cause chronic pain.

Here's the good news: While chronic pain is far too common in older age, it is not inevitable.

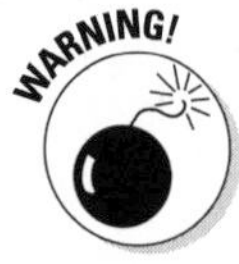

Many studies have shown that older people are often undertreated for pain, which means they're either given no pain medicine or are administered extremely low dosages that are ineffective. Some physicians are afraid to give narcotics to older people with severe pain from cancer, back pain, and other ailments because the doctors believe patients may get addicted.

In contrast, we agree with many experts who believe that severe pain should be treated with appropriate pain medications and that the risk of addiction is low unless the patient had a previous addiction problem.

Not only does the failure to treat chronic pain lead to discomfort, but it's also true that when neglected, chronic pain can cause other problems.

Possible ageist comments from docs and examples of responses

Here are some examples of ageist comments some doctors make and suggestions on how you might respond to them.

Ageist comment: You have to expect pain at your age! There isn't much we can do.

Possible response: My pain is severe. Please help.

Ageist comment: Older people have to take a lot of medicine.

Possible response: I understand that I need a lot of medicine. But I'm wondering if we could review all the drugs I take. Maybe I don't really need them all.

Ageist comment: I only prescribe narcotics for short-term pain. Do you want to become a drug addict?

Possible response: Of course I don't want to become a drug addict! But the other medications we've tried don't help! I'd like to try a low dose of a strong pain medicine for awhile so that I might get some relief.

Ageist comment: When you get older, you have less energy. You're not 20 any more!

Possible response: I was old two months ago and had a lot more energy then. Could there be some other reason for my sluggishness now? (Give the doctor an example, such as you could take daily walks two months ago, but can't now.)

Managing Pain with Medications

Taking medications for long periods of time to treat chronic pain is always a complex issue, regardless of how old you are. Aging adds other complications to the mix. Older bodies process drugs differently than younger bodies, and it often takes smaller dosages to reach an effective pain-killing effect in older people.

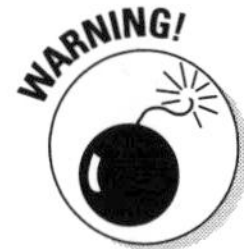

A number of ways to control pain are available in addition to or along with medicines. You can read about these techniques in many chapters of this book, but for specific tips, be sure to see the appropriate chapter for your condition. In addition, Chapter 15 discusses alternative and complementary approaches to pain control.

Even if certain pain drugs work well for you when you were younger, you need to be careful about taking the same drug as you age. This caution is also important for people who care for (or care about) an elderly person. For example, if you're in your 40s and you've had great success in managing your own arthritic pain with NSAIDs, you may be tempted to give them to your 80-year-old mother for her arthritis pain. Resist this impulse. Ask your mom to talk to her doctor first, particularly if she has any stomach problems. Depending on the level of pain that your mother has, the doctor may recommend trying another medicine first. (See Chapter 14 for a description of NSAIDs).

Never give away your opiate pain medication to another person. It's illegal under federal law and may be very dangerous to the person receiving the drug.

The American Geriatrics Society has developed guidelines for fighting off chronic pain (which they call *persistent pain*) in older people. The society convened a panel of experts to make the recommendations. They built their guidelines around two important types of drugs:

- **Acetaminophen (Tylenol):** This drug is the first choice for mild to moderate musculoskeletal pain.
- **Opiods:** Older people with persistent, severe pain require strong drugs, including opiates such as morphine or oxycodone.

When doctors decide on dosages for acetaminophen, opioids, or other drugs for older people, they usually "start low and go slow." In other words, they use the lowest dose possible and then build slowly until the patient's pain is relieved.

The good and bad about opioids

Opioids, also known as *narcotics* or *opiates,* generally have a greater pain-killing effect in older people than in younger patients. As a result, if you're an older person, you probably need a lower dose than someone who's younger, although the dose should be sufficient to provide pain relief. (See Chapter 14 for information on opioids.) However, *geriatricians* (doctors who specialize in aging) say that these drugs are prescribed too infrequently rather than too often. Undertreatment leads to breakthrough pain, which means that the drug isn't keeping the pain under control. If your doctor says that you or your older loved one should consider taking an opioid, he will work with you on the type of drug and dosage.

Some opioids, such as propoxyphene (Darvon, Darvocet), should never be taken by seniors. And some opiods, such as morphine, can cause confusion and even hallucinations in some older people, so the drug itself should be selected with care.

Narcotics have side effects. While opioids are recommended for severe pain in seniors, almost every older person who takes them has problems with constipation, and sometimes with urination as well. Therefore, older people who take these drugs regularly should get plenty of exercise, drink lots of fluids, and take laxatives if needed (under the watchful eye of a physician who can monitor their heart and sedation levels).

Identifying potential problems

Some health conditions that commonly strike older people can greatly affect their ability to take their pain medications safely and effectively. The result can be loss of pain control, as well as dangerous reactions from taking drugs incorrectly.

The loved ones in your life may not want to talk about these conditions, such as vision or hearing loss, because they're afraid of losing their independence. However, if they (or you) have any of the problems listed in this section, valuable techniques are available to help you adapt and keep your independence. In addition, if you're concerned about a loved one with these problems, assure him that talking them over with you and your health-care professionals can help him find techniques and treatments to adjust to the problems so that he can remain independent.

The following conditions can affect the ability to take pain medications:

- **Problems with vision:** By the age of 65, about one in three people has a vision-reducing eye disease. An older person may have difficulty reading, or she may not be able to read prescription labels and consumer materials about medications. She also may be unable to see the differences between pills. A resource for adapting to vision problems is The Vision Learning Center (`www.preventblindness.org`).

  Having a daily pill container filled by another person for the week may help a person with poor vision. Then the individual can simply take Monday's pills on Monday. (However, some pills need to be taken with food or have other restrictions, so this aid doesn't work in such cases.)

- **Hearing problems:** As you grow older, it often becomes more difficult to hear soft sounds and conversational speech. In fact, one-third of adults between the ages of 65 and 74 and about half the people age 85 and older have a hearing loss. As a result, listening to advice from doctors and others about prescriptions and treatments for pain control is difficult or impossible. Many people think that they can read lips accurately, but they still miss a great deal of what is said. A resource for adapting to hearing loss is the American Speech Language Hearing Association (`www.asha.org`).

- **Cognitive impairment:** Some older people have some form of dementia, and the older the individual, the more likely dementia is present. In fact, dementia is tragically common among people of advanced age, such as those over age 85. The Alzheimer's Association reports that in 2007, 5 million seniors in the United States had Alzheimer's disease. (Alzheimer's is just one form of dementia.)

  Studies have shown a correlation between memory problems and not taking medications according to directions or not taking them at all. The Alzheimer's Association (`www.alz.org`) has local chapters and offers assistance to people in these situations and their families.

- **Dexterity:** It's one of the most frustrating things about the aging process: As you grow older, your physical dexterity declines. This loss of dexterity can make opening child-proof or even standard packages or containers difficult or impossible. To help with dexterity issues, ask your druggist for easy-to-open packaging, pre-filled syringes, and pre-measured liquid dosages.

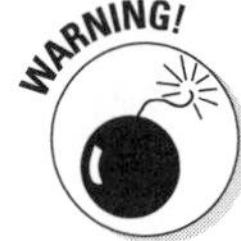

Antiaging drugs or techniques are completely experimental at this time and may have severe negative side effects.

Affecting older bodies differently

As we discuss in Chapter 14, many drugs are available to manage pain. However, older people are more likely than younger people to experience side effects from pain-killing drugs because aging increases sensitivity to most drugs. This is especially true for medications affecting the central nervous system. (See Chapter 2 to review how pain works in the central nervous system.)

A sad truth of science today is that very few drugs are tested on older people. Instead, they're studied in young people — often college students. A general understanding of how drugs work in the bodies of older people is very limited. However, some facts are known.

When you take a medication, your body circulates the drug in its fat and water. But this process has different results when you're older. For example, aging causes a decrease in blood flow in the liver, which is the organ in our bodies that metabolizes most drugs. This reduced vitality of the liver can have a substantial effect on the effectiveness and side effects of medications. In addition, while most drugs are metabolized by the liver, they're eliminated by the kidneys. But for people over age 75, kidney function is half what it was at a younger age. The result is that drugs eliminated by the kidneys hang around longer in older people.

Sometimes kidney or liver function may change very suddenly without the older person even being aware of it. If you or a loved one are over age 65 and you notice side effects, such as confusion or extreme fatigue, contact a doctor or pharmacist right away.

Guidelines for taking pain medicines

As you and your loved ones age, your bodies change in the way they process drugs. As a result, you and your doctor understand that effectively managing your pain medications is one of the most important things you can do for your health.

Use the medication log in Chapter 17 to keep track of all the drugs you take. Keep a copy in your purse or wallet, give a copy to your doctor, and make sure that your loved ones and caregivers have copies. Here are a few guidelines if you or a loved one is older and taking medications:

- If possible, use only one pharmacy to fill all your prescription medications so that your druggist will have an updated chart of all the drugs you take. She can also check for possible incompatibilities between the drugs you take.
- If you take two or more drugs, ask your doctor and pharmacist to run your medication list through a drug interactions database. (Four eyes are better than two!) You can also check for drug interactions yourself at `www.drugs.com`. (Click Interactions Checker.)

Deciphering Pain in Seniors with Memory Problems

Dementia is a tragic condition of declining mental abilities. If a loved one has a diagnosis of dementia, it means she may have difficulty reasoning and remembering. In fact, your loved one may not even fully understand physical problems, such as pain.

Older people with dementia may have many medical problems that can make diagnosis difficult. If you have a loved one with dementia, try to determine whether he's experiencing pain.

If you see any clues that pain is present in a senior with dementia, talk to a doctor or other health-care professional right away. Using the list of nonverbal cues that we include in Chapter 17, try to fill in the blanks, giving as much detail as possible. Here are some observations important for the older person's doctor or other health-care provider to know:

- Offer your best guess as to how you think the pain is experienced by the senior (for example, burning, aching, stabbing). Also, explain what you've observed that led you to these guesses.
- Describe *when* you observe the pain occurring, such as when the senior is getting up from a chair or lying in bed.
- Provide a history of all prescription and over-the-counter medicines your loved one takes. (Use the log in Chapter 17.)
- Give examples of displays of pain you've noticed, such as grunting or clutching a hip.
- Report on what — if anything — appears to relieve the pain.

Chapter 25

Pain at the End of Life

In This Chapter

- Discovering the total pain concept
- Understanding palliative care
- Coping with terminal pain
- Knowing your rights as a patient

This chapter is hard-hitting, and it's one that many people would prefer *not* to read. But if you or someone you love has chronic pain and a terminal illness, this chapter is important because it covers the difficult situation of having chronic pain that is amplified by end-of-life pain.

Pain associated with the dying process may or may not be related to the pain of an individual's chronic condition. For example, Nora struggled for a decade with fibromyalgia, and she now has a rare condition called primary pulmonary hypertension. It affects the blood vessels in her lungs and makes breathing difficult. Nora is faced with managing both her fibromyalgia pain and the pain from the primary pulmonary hypertension.

In order to manage her condition and the resulting pain, Nora has taken advantage of a concept called *palliative care,* which uses a team of doctors and other types of professionals (such as palliative-care social workers and chaplains) who meet regularly to plan and coordinate their patient's interdisciplinary care.

This chapter covers the palliative care approach and offers information about total pain, an idea particularly relevant for people with chronic pain who also have a terminal illness.

Managing Total Pain with the Palliative Approach

The concept of *total pain* dates back to Cicely Saunders, the founder of the first hospice in the United States. She opened St. Christopher's Hospice in 1967, with the wise perception that chronic pain in the face of death presents challenges to the patient, doctor, and other members of the health-care team. Saunders saw such pain as endless and meaningless, bringing a sense of isolation and despair to the patient. She described the concept of total pain as the suffering that encompasses a person's physical, psychological, social, spiritual, and practical struggles.

Saunders and her colleagues saw that people with constant pain experienced a worsening of chronic pain when they were diagnosed with a terminal illness, largely because of the many stressors associated with a fatal disease. Here are some examples of the types of distress that contribute to total pain:

- **Psychological pain:** Difficulty coping with a diagnosis and adapting to physical changes, such as the loss of hair or a limb.
- **Social pain:** Sorrow over the idea of leaving family and friends and the loss of a career and/or parenting.
- **Spiritual pain:** Questioning whether an afterlife really exists; anger at God.
- **Practical:** Organizing necessary care and finances as the illness progresses.

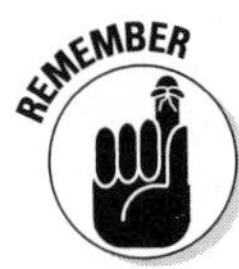

The palliative approach to managing total pain includes a team of experts who help you cope with sources of distress. For example, a grief counselor can help both you and your family cope with the distress of possible separation. A chaplain or other spiritual advisor can help you work through spiritual issues. And an estate attorney and/or financial advisor can help you put your financial affairs in order.

Palliative care focuses on the relief of the pain and the symptoms and stress of a serious illness. The goal of this type of care is to give comfort and support to the person receiving care. It's not an alternative to conventional medical care, but complements it. It is also not the same thing as "comfort measures only." It's a coordinated effort to give the best possible comprehensive care under the circumstances. Palliative and hospice care were recognized as a medical subspecialty in 2006 by the American Board of Medical Specialties.

Palliative care is not a one-size-fits-all treatment. The palliative care team devises and carries out treatment to meet the particular needs of each patient.

You or your loved one can receive palliative care in your own home, in a nursing facility, hospital, or other setting of your choice.

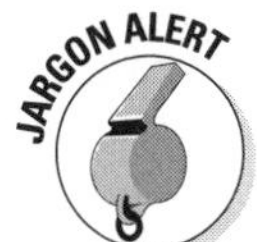

Palliative care is often confused with hospice care, but they differ. Specifically, hospice care involves helping ill individuals and their families during the last days or months of life and is often an important part of palliative care, which can involve caring for the individual over a longer period of time and is compatible with treatment that aims to cure the terminal illness.

One of the many advantages of palliative care is that it's patient-centered. If you're the patient receiving palliative care, you'll be the central force of your team. The team is all about you!

You also have a responsibility to be as informed as possible about your condition, your needs, and the desires you have for the future. For example, is it important that you never, ever go to a nursing home, even if a very good one is nearby? Is it important to you to never have invasive medical procedures? If so, it's up to you to make these wishes known to your family members, doctors, other members of your team, and particularly anyone who you choose as a *health-care agent* (a person you predesignate to make medical decisions for you if you can't make them).

Facing the Hard, Physical Truth about Dying

In addition to severe pain, people who are dying can suffer additional unpleasant and uncomfortable symptoms that impede quality of life. Yet many people at the end of life want to spend their precious remaining time with loved ones. Or, they may have some unfinished business to work out with family and friends. They may also want to set their financial affairs in order. When physical problems get in the way of such meaningful and significant activities, patients feel even more frustrated on top of the already- difficult circumstances.

Common physical problems that occur during the dying process are nausea, lack of appetite, difficulty breathing, weakness, fatigue, and problems with elimination. In addition, the fear of intolerable pain can cause great anxiety and irritability, and some studies have shown that the fear of future pain is a major source of stress. You can treat most of these problems, and your team can work to put these treatments in motion for you. For example, for fatigue, your team can focus on finding and treating possible causes, such as anemia and depression. For loss of appetite, your doctor can prescribe a variety of measures, such as the drug *megestrol,* a synthetic version of the hormone progesterone. It increases weight gain by increasing appetite for women with certain types of cancer.

Managing the pain of a terminal illness

As death draws near, the standard of treatment for pain control is the use of opioids, sometimes along with other analgesics. (See Chapter 14 for information on these drugs.) In addition to managing pain, opioids can help with anxiety and breathlessness, common problems at the end of life. If the individual can't take medication by mouth, drugs can be delivered in the cheek or under the tongue *(sublingually)*. In addition, skin patches or rectal suppositories are sometimes easier for patients to use at home. Other options, such as intravenous medication, can cause more discomfort for the individual and usually can't be done at home.

There is good news, however. Some newer delivery systems for drugs are now available, which can provide pain relief at the end of life with little or no drowsiness or hallucinations. (These procedures are mouthfuls and are called tunneled epidural catheters with continuous external infusion pumps and implanted internal intrathecal infusion pumps.) In addition, in some cases painful nerves can now be removed.

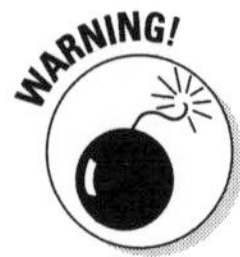

A major tradeoff with taking opioids is that, at the levels necessary to control severe pain, they can cause drowsiness, hallucinations, and other unpleasant symptoms.

End of life is a time when your wishes (or the wishes of your loved one) are extremely important, and you have hopefully conveyed them to the person who'll act in your behalf if you can't speak for yourself. The question to answer and convey to your health-care agent is whether you would rather have the pain than the side effects of the drug.

Lamenting loss of control

If your loved one has chronic pain and is approaching the end of life, loss of control is likely to be one of his most frustrating concerns. As a terminal illness advances and pain takes over, the individual loses more and more control. For most, this loss of control is a dreaded aspect of the end of life. In fact, many people fear the loss of independence more than death itself.

For example, you may need help with all your private needs, such as toileting, or you may need to be fed by hand. Many people become depressed and grouchy at this point. It's important for the patient to retain any kind of control still possible. If you're caring for someone in this situation, try to find things that he can still control. For example, let him decide what food to eat and what time of day to eat it, or give him a choice of TV shows to watch. Or arrange for him to administer his own dosages of painkiller when he wants it through PCA. (See Chapter 14 for information on PCAs.) These decisions may seem like little things to you, but they can help raise the spirits of the person who is dying.

Comparing hospice and palliative care

Many people confuse hospice and palliative care. Here is a comparison chart:

Issue	Palliative	Hospice
Several months or less to live	No	Yes
Pain control is very important	Yes	Yes
Compatible with treatment to cure, such as chemotherapy	Yes	No

Looking at Hospice Care

Most people want to stay home until they die, and, most of all, they don't want to be in a hospital or nursing home. However, sometimes there's no choice because the individual needs care — such as being hooked up to a heart monitor or infusion equipment — that can't be provided at home.

Understanding what hospice care is

Many people with terminal illnesses choose hospice care. In fact, the National Hospice and Palliative Care Organization estimates that approximately 36 percent of all deaths in the United States are under the care of a hospice program. Patients make this choice at the point when a cure is no longer possible for their condition. Hospice care provides palliative care along with other services to make the dying process as comfortable as possible. This type of care stresses peace, comfort, and dignity for the patient.

Hospice care recognizes death as the final stage of life, and the typical hospice patient has a life expectancy of only a couple of months. The care may be provided at home or at a facility specifically planned and organized to care for people at the end of life.

Most hospice programs require a doctor to verify that a patient's probability of survival is less than six months, a requirement for eligibility to receive Medicare or other insurance coverage.

You have two options when it comes to hospice care:

Types of care often needed at the end of life

The types of care needed to control total pain often include the following services. In addition, in most geographic areas, hospice-care programs provide or coordinate many of these services:

- Physician services, including pain management and other comfort care
- Nursing care
- Physical therapists
- Home medical equipment, such as hospital beds and oxygen
- Grief and related counseling for yourself and your loved ones
- Spiritual support
- Social services and support
- Personal care, such as assistance with bathing and toileting
- Assistance with errands, meals, housecleaning, and other domestic tasks
- Respite care, which fills in for caregivers so that they can take breaks

- **Home hospice care:** Most dying patients want to remain at home as long as they possibly can. Home hospice typically provides items to make this possible, such as medications, ventilators, walkers, and other durable medical equipment. In addition, nursing visits, home health-care visits, volunteer support, chaplain services, social workers, and so on allow the patient to receive care at home. A lot of the time, the family provides most of the care to the individual.

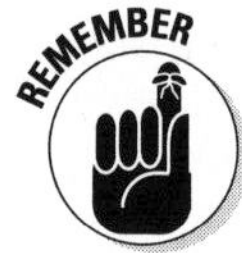

- **Hospice care in a hospital, nursing home, or other facility:** Some people with terminal illnesses require more care than can be provided at home. When this is the case, inpatient hospices in acute-care hospitals, chronic care hospitals, or nursing homes are an option. These programs try to provide a home-like setting.

Locating a reputable hospice service

Hospice care providers can vary a great deal. Some are based in home-like buildings, some are part of hospitals, and others provide only home-health care. They may be run by religious organizations, for-profit companies, or not-for-profits. Or, they may serve only people with acquired immune deficiency syndrome (AIDS), cancer care, or another area. So how do you find the best program in your geographic area? Here are some tips to help guide you:

- Visit the Hospice and Palliative Care searchable database at `http://caringinfo.org`. Click Caring for Someone and then Find a Local Hospice to locate hospice providers nationwide.
- Ask for opinions from people who've had personal experience with specific hospices. Ask your friends, your doctor, the discharge planner at your local hospital (she'll know all the services in your area), and social workers from local agencies.
- Find out whether the hospice is certified. Medicare requires certification for payment eligibility, and in some states, so does Medicaid. State health departments certify hospices.
- Find out whether it's licensed. Licensing is also usually handled by your state health department.
- Find out whether its employees are bonded. If so, you have some protection against any potential legal problems.

Understanding Your Rights

By bioethical standards, as patients, you or a loved one have the right to choose your treatment as long as you're competent. But what if you're *not competent* — in other words, you're not capable of making a decision in your own best interests, and this fact has been established legally in court by a relative, guardian, or other interested party. In this case, a health-care agent substitutes for you to say what you would say if you could make the decision yourself. So, it is important to pick someone for this position whom you trust to respect your wishes. See the contact information for the National Hospice and Pallative Care Organization in the next section for information about picking a health care agent.

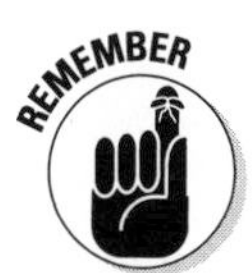

Understand that the health-care agent is not making the decision for you. She will tell others what you would value if you could make the decision. So, it is key that you let anyone who you arrange to stand in for you know exactly what your wishes are.

Following are examples of the types of questions you should discuss with your health-care agent:

- Would you want to be kept alive at all costs, even if it meant that you would have pain even more severe than the pain you have now?
- Do you want to receive ventilation if needed?
- Is it okay to perform surgery if necessary?

Resources

Many organizations provide important services to people at the end of life, as well as their loved ones. Here are three of the top national programs:

Hospice Foundation of America (HFA), 1621 Connecticut Ave. NW, Suite 300, Washington, DC 20009; phone 800-854-3402; Web site www.hospicefoundation.org. HFA programs assist individuals who are coping with issues of caregiving, terminal illness, and grief. Use HFA's interactive Locate a Hospice page to find hospice programs in your area.

National Hospice & Palliative Care Organization (NHPCO), 1700 Diagonal Road, Suite 625, Alexandria, VA 22314; phone 703-837-1500; Web site http://caringinfo.org. NHPCO represents hospice and palliative care programs and professionals in the United States. Go to the NHPCO-sponsored Web site to find information on designating health-care agents through advance directives and other legal matters relating to the end of life.

The Center to Advance Palliative Care, 1255 Fifth Ave., Suite C-2, New York, NY 10029; phone 212-201-2670; Web site www.getpalliativecare.org/providers. CAPC is a national organization dedicated to increasing the availability of quality palliative care services for people facing serious illness. The center sponsors the Palliative Care Directory of Hospitals to help consumers locate a hospital in their area that provides a palliative care program.

Part VI
The Part of Tens

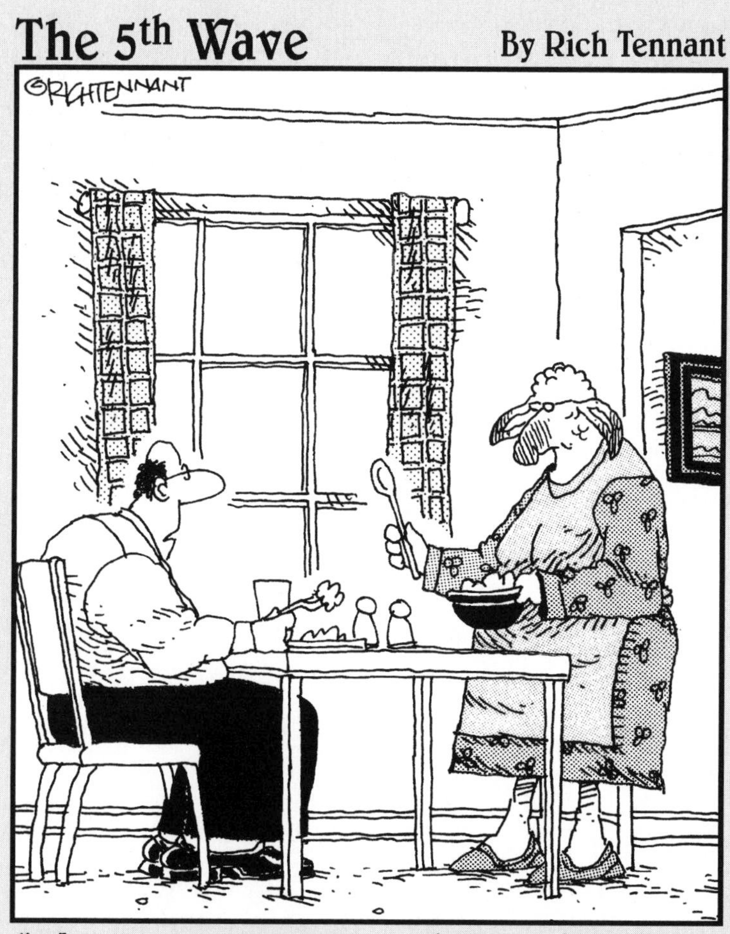

"Maybe you need to withdraw from the clinical trial."

In this part . . .

No *For Dummies* book is complete without this irreverent part. In this part, we give you ten ways to detect bogus cures. We also cover ten things to remember about chronic pain and sexuality and ten important sources of help for pain. Finally, we remind you of ten things you should avoid doing when you have chronic pain.

Chapter 26

Ten Ways to Detect Bogus "Cures"

In This Chapter

- Staying away from bogus arthritis and cancer remedies
- Shunning false anti-aging promises

Have you seen ads that offer intriguing promises like "Natural Secret Cures They Want to Hide from You" or "The One Cure for All Diseases"? If so, hopefully you tuned them out. Or perhaps you bought one of these products, thinking, "Maybe it'll work," and you were disappointed. Bogus remedies for chronic pain often make major money for sellers because so many people are eager for relief. But these products often have serious consequences for the purchaser. They waste precious dollars that could have been spent on legitimate medical treatments. They may prevent people from getting the medical treatment they really need. And these so-called remedies may even be harmful to your health.

So why do so many people fall for these sales pitches? For one thing, distributors are not just selling a product. Instead, they're primarily selling *hope* to people with serious diseases and chronic pain. Who wouldn't want to take the XYZ potion and obliterate all their pain and the disease itself, forever? Sounds great! But hold on! You're being scammed.

Quack cures for chronic pain and the diseases that cause them come in the form of drugs (pills, lotions, or other forms) and nutritional supplements (including some that you can buy at health-food stores). Miracle cures may be touted on "infotainment programs" on radio and television. Sometimes they're promoted by direct mail. However, the fastest growing sales medium for these products is the Internet. Information on fake cures is also published in books available for purchase on Amazon.com and other Internet sites.

Because ads for bogus cures are everywhere, you can't steer entirely clear of them. And sometimes it's tough to figure out when a remedy may be legitimate. In this chapter, we provide you ten important points to help you identify and avoid bogus cures. Hopefully, they'll prevent *you* from being victimized.

Many bogus cures use the *placebo effect,* in which drugs with no active ingredients seem to be effective, to make victims (you, your family, your friends) feel that they're getting better, when the truth is that many people feel better just because they're taking a pill or potion —regardless of what is in it. The fact is that this type of relief does not last.

Avoid Products Promising to Halt Aging

Remedies that claim to stop aging play on fears of growing old as well as the worry that current pain problems may worsen with aging You may think, "I hurt now, but what about in five years? How will I be able to stand it? Maybe taking an anti-aging miracle cure now is just the ticket." Sorry, but no, it's not!

"Anti-aging" medicine is a multibillion dollar industry in the United States today, so a lot of people are buying into staving off aging. However, *no* treatments have proven to slow the aging process. Consequently, no treatments can stop chronic pain by slowing down aging.

Here's a checklist from the World Health Organization of anti-aging potions to avoid:

- **Injections of human growth hormone (HGH):** Some dietary supplements are known as *HGH-releasers,* which purportedly stimulate the body's production of the hormone. HGH-releasers, which can cost $15,000 a year, are marketed as a cheaper alternative to shots. But no valid evidence supports that any type of HGH supplementation offers life-extension benefits.
- **DHEA:** DHEA breaks down into estrogen and testosterone in the body. Found in anti-aging dietary supplements that supposedly improve libido, strength, energy, muscles, and immunity to disease, DHEA also supposedly decreases fat. What a wonder drug! Feeling strong, energetic, muscular, sexy, healthy, younger, *and* thinner sounds pretty great. Too bad it isn't for real. No evidence supports DHEA as an anti-aging hormone.
- **Melatonin:** Often included in anti-aging supplements, melatonin may help you get to sleep if you have insomnia, but it won't slow down the aging process.

Stay Away from Products Promising to Cure Arthritis Overnight

Unproven arthritis remedies are easy to fall for because many symptoms come and go. Maybe today was a good day, and you attribute it to the anti-arthritis supplement that you took yesterday (or the copper bracelet you wore), when the truth is that it was really just a good arthritis day. Maybe the weather was nice, and your arthritis calmed down. Or something else helped you feel better. But your good arthritis day had nothing to do with the pill or the bracelet.

At present, no cures exist for any of the 100-plus forms of arthritis. We really, really wish there were. The authors of this book are a rheumatologist who treats many people in severe pain (Dr. Kassan), a pain researcher and avid golfer with arthritis in his wrists (Dr. Vierck), and a medical writer with arthritis throughout her body (Elizabeth Vierck). We'd love for those phony ads to be true! But they're just not.

Shun Amazing Cancer Cures

Quacks prey on people's fear of cancer. Their ads say things like "This Cancer Cure Really Works." They claim all you have to do is take their pills or potions or follow a special (and often very complicated) diet, and you'll be free of cancer and the pain that goes with it. Or they push special facilities, making such statements as "Visit our clinic in Mexico, and in two weeks you'll be cancer free."

When these cure-alls fail for desperate consumers, the hucksters then claim it was because of damage done by previous "conventional" therapy. Or it's that the consumer didn't follow their regimen to the letter. In other words, you did it wrong, and it's your fault that it didn't work. Don't believe any of this rubbish!

Laetrile is a famous example of a bogus cancer cure. Not only has it been found to *not* cure cancer, but it's also poisonous in high dosages. The sad truth is that by using unproven methods such as laetrile, people with cancer may lose valuable time when they could be receiving effective treatment and often ridding themselves of cancer.

Suspect Common Sales Tactics

Health quacks often use similar techniques proven to sell their bogus products. Stay away from products with the following claims:

- **Our product cures everything.** The distributor may claim that the product cures arthritis, cancer, stomach ulcers, and depression. About a hundred years ago, people bought potions that purported to cure everything, like Mrs. Winslow's Soothing Syrup (containing morphine), because there were few reliable drugs available at the time and almost no government oversight. Those cure-all potions were dangerous. They didn't cure disease then, and the current crop of "amazing" drugs still doesn't work now. Stick with mainstream medicine.
- **The product cures diseases not yet understood by medical science, such as fibromyalgia and other forms of arthritis.** The reality is that these medical problems have no known cures. Yet medically documented treatments really help. These treatments, discussed throughout this book, are the ones you should be using.
- **Promoters say they're valiant souls persecuted by evil people who want to prevent them from telling you the truth.** They may claim that universities or pharmaceutical companies seek to suppress their treatment out of professional jealousy or fear of losing profits. These promoters don't have credible scientists and medical professionals to back them up, so they invent conspiracy theories instead. Don't believe them. There *are* some bad guys out there, and they're the promoters of fake remedies.
- **Sales people give testimonials and no scientific proof.** When no studies support the use of a product, scam artists often revert to the use of testimonials that can't be verified for accuracy or effect. Usually, these testimonials are nothing more than an infomercial and don't give any useful scientific information. Typically, the claims range from vague descriptions of feeling better to miraculous transformations.

Be Aware of Safety Concerns of Supplements

Dietary supplements are regulated very little by the government compared to the scrutiny given to over-the-counter or prescribed medications, yet taking supplements can be akin to taking drugs — or worse.

Once in your system, many supplements interact with other medications and supplements and may cause serious harm. For example, the popular supplement St. John's Wort can be dangerous when taken with a number of commonly prescribed drugs. According to the National Center on Complementary and Alternative Medicine, part of the National Institutes of Health, some drugs that St. John's Wort may interact with include

- **Birth control pills:** St. John's Wort may cause breakthrough bleeding.
- **Antidepressants:** When combined with some antidepressants, St. John's wort may increase nausea, anxiety, headache, and confusion.
- **Warfarin and related anti-clotting drugs (anticoagulants):** When combined with St. John's Wort, warfarin is less effective.

To ensure the safe use of any health-care product, read labels and package inserts, follow product directions, and check with your physician about substances you're considering taking. In addition, make sure that no warnings have been issued about the product. The following Web sites list supplements that are questionable or have been found to have adverse effects. Check these sites out before you buy!

- Federal Trade Commission: `www.ftc.gov/bcp/menus/consumer/health/drugs.shtm`
- Food and Drug Administration: `www.cfsan.fda.gov/~dms/supplmnt.html`
- Arthritis Foundation: `www.arthritis.org/conditions/supplementguide`

Check Out Health Claims Before Sampling

To check a product out, follow these tips:

- If it's an unproven or little-known treatment, always ask a doctor, pharmacist, or other medical specialist if the product is safe.
- Talk to others. Be wary of treatments offered by people telling you to avoid talking to others because "It's a secret treatment or cure."
- Check with the Better Business Bureau or local attorneys generals' offices to see whether other consumers have lodged complaints about the product or the product's marketer.

- Contact appropriate health professional groups, such as the American Cancer Society and the Arthritis Foundation. Many groups have local chapters that provide various resource materials about your disease.
- Check with the FDA. It's part of the FDA's job to see that medicines and medical devices are safe and effective. For more information, call toll-free, 1-888-INFO-FDA (1-888-463-6332), or visit `www.fda.gov`.

Avoid Impulse Buying!

Never decide "on the spot" to try an untested product or treatment. Ask for more information and then consult a knowledgeable doctor, pharmacist, or other health-care professional. Promoters of legitimate health-care products don't object to your seeking additional information.

To learn whether the FDA or the FTC has taken action against the promoter of a product, visit `www.fda.gov/oc/enforcement.html` or `www.ftc.gov`. You can also check out `www.cfsan.fda.gov/~dms/ds-warn.html` for a list of dietary supplement ingredients for which the FDA has issued warnings.

Be Wary of "Cures" Sold on the Web

It's easy to run into ads for unproven remedies when surfing on the Web. We recently did an Internet search using the keyword "chronic pain," which turned up a front-page ad for a supplement that claimed to take away pain, elevate your mood, and cut your food cravings. Hey, sounds great! But such claims are unsubstantiated.

When searching on the Web, try using directory sites of respected organizations, rather than doing blind searches with a search engine. Also ask yourself the following questions:

- **Who sponsors the site?** Is the site run by the government, a university, or a reputable medical or health-related association? Is the information written or reviewed by experts in the field, academia, the government, or the medical community? If not, then claims provided on this site are suspect.
- **What is the purpose of the site?** Is the purpose of the site to educate the public objectively or just to sell a product? The intent may be hard to determine sometimes, but see how many places the Web page has where you can click to buy the product. The more places and the easier it is to purchase something, the less likely the site is objective.

- **What is the source of the information, and does it have any references?** Have any studies supporting the "cure" been reviewed by recognized scientific experts and published in reputable peer-reviewed scientific journals, such as *The New England Journal of Medicine?* Can you find the study in the National Library of Medicine's database of literature citations at `www.ncbi.nlm.nih.gov/PubMed`? If you can't find any legitimate studies, stay away from this so-called cure.
- **How reliable are Internet or e-mail solicitations?** While the Internet can be a rich source of reliable health information, it's also an easy vehicle for spreading myths, hoaxes, and rumors about alleged news, studies, products, or findings. To avoid falling for such hoaxes, be skeptical and watch out for overly emphatic language with ALL UPPERCASE LETTERS and lots of exclamation points!!!! Also, beware of such phrases, such as "This is not a hoax" or "Send this to everyone you know." Don't do it! Instead, move on.

Watch Out for Celebrity Promotions

Tommy Terrific, the famous hockey star, and Sandy Glamorous of television fame are promoting a brand new product that they swear will eradicate your pain. They emphatically repeat on TV that this product is an absolute must for you! It'll ease your chronic pain, and you won't have to take dangerous drugs like narcotics. Instead, call right now and order their amazing just-discovered cure from the jungles of Peru. You reach for the phone because you're confident that Tommy or Sandy wouldn't lie to you. They're so sincere! Well, maybe they aren't lying — sometimes celebrities actually believe in the product. That *still* doesn't make it okay for you. Ask your doctor first.

Always Report If Anything Goes Wrong!

If you have a negative reaction to any unproven remedy, be sure to report it to the federal government. Your action could prevent other people from having the same bad reaction. So be a good guy and help others. Call the Food and Drug Administration at 1-800-FDA-1088. You can also fax the FDA at 1-800-FDA-0178 or report online at `www.fda.gov/medwatch/how.htm`.

Chapter 27

Ten Things to Remember about Pain and Sexuality

In This Chapter

- Addressing your fears
- Checking your medications
- Talking to your partner

Maybe you're starting to feel some of that special spark once again, and your partner is hinting about some action, too. But darn it, you're just in too much pain for sex right now. Or maybe *you* are the one desiring intimacy, but you're worried that your partner is in too much pain, and you're afraid to initiate anything sexual. So you hold off.

Chronic pain, and some of the medications that treat it, can curb sexual enjoyment for both you and your partner. But sexual intimacy is an important part of a healthy relationship and quality of life for the individuals involved. So don't give up on sex! Read this chapter for helpful hints on re-igniting your relationship despite your pain problem.

In this chapter, you find ten things to keep in mind in order to ignite a healthy and pleasing sex life.

Address Your Fears

If you have chronic pain, you may have some fears about sexual relations. You're not alone. Many people with chronic pain develop these issues. Here are three top concerns and what you can do about them:

- **Fear of rejection:** It's common to worry that chronic pain makes you less sexy. For example, maybe you're less active now during sex than before your pain condition struck. You may think that your partner will be "bored" with the lower level of activity that you need in order to avoid pain. If so, talk about this fear together. Focus on new and creative ways that don't hurt so that you can enjoy sex together.
- **Fear of pain:** You don't want to hurt, and your partner doesn't want to hurt you either. (Yelling "ouch" during a heated moment can be a major letdown for both of you.) Make sure that you've taken your pain medication before launching any sexual activity. Regular exercise and relaxation exercises may also help reduce your anxiety about pain. In addition, many people find that it also helps to try different ways to satisfy their partner. Try experimenting with sexual positions that can cause less pain. Also, don't forget lubricants!
- **Fear of failure:** If you're having trouble becoming aroused or achieving an orgasm, consult your doctor. Several medications that may help are available for men and women that your physician can prescribe.

Figure Out What to Do about Specific Problems

Chronic pain can cause problems that ultimately affect your sexuality, such as a lack of sleep, stiffness, and difficulty moving around.

Make a list of problems that may affect your desire and ability for sex and then strategize on what to do about them. Strategize with your partner, if you have one. (More about that in the upcoming "Talk to Your Partner" section.)

A great resource for identifying problems that may be hampering your desire for sex is the Sexual Health page on MedlinePlus at `http://medlineplus.gov`.

Check Your Medications

Make sure that none of the drugs you're taking are causing sexual problems. For example, narcotics frequently lower the hormone testosterone's levels to the point that the following side effects exist: lack of interest in sex, inability to achieve erection or orgasm, clinical depression, and a general lack of energy. (These side effects are often alarming to the male chronic pain patient, and if you or your partner feel this way, it's important to mention them to your doctor. A simple blood test may demonstrate low testosterone levels that can be treated effectively with a testosterone patch, skin gel, or injections.)

Other medicines can also cause arousal problems, including the following:

- Some pain medications
- Blood pressure medicines
- Antihistamines
- Antidepressants
- Tranquilizers
- Appetite suppressants
- Diabetes drugs
- Some ulcer drugs, such as ranitidine

Some of these drugs may lead to impotence or make it hard for men to ejaculate, while others can reduce a woman's sexual desire.

If you're taking any of these categories of drugs and experiencing sexual problems, consider asking your doctor to prescribe a different drug without this side effect or to lower your dosage.

Pay Attention to Your Emotions

How you feel may affect what you're able to do sexually. Are you depressed because of chronic pain? Are you angry? Frustrated? Do you have a "Why me?" attitude toward your pain? All these emotions and attitudes can affect your sexuality.

Living with chronic pain often requires making adjustments to daily life. Many people find it useful to talk these issues out with a good therapist.

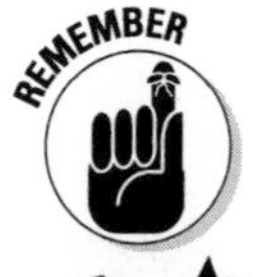

Don't blame yourself for sexual difficulties you and your partner are having. It takes two to have fun with sex, and it also takes two to fix it when it isn't fun anymore.

Rest can greatly help your emotional state. Take a nap before having sex so that you won't wear out when you least want to.

Talk to Your Partner

Sex can be difficult to talk about, even with someone you've been intimate with for a long time. Counselors suggest that you talk about sex when you're fully clothed and in a neutral setting. Of course, you should probably avoid having this discussion in a crowded public place. People nearby may find your discussion far too fascinating not to eavesdrop!

This discussion is the time for both of you to talk about your fears and desires. During your conversation about sex, begin sentences with "I," not "you." For example, saying "I feel loved and cared about when you hold me close" is much better than "You never touch me anymore!"

You may think that your partner has stopped touching you because of a lack of interest, or that you're no longer desirable. Instead, your partner's main concern may be fear of causing you more physical pain. Only when you talk it out can you find out what's going on with each other.

Let Go of Stereotypes about Sex

Many people have stereotypical ideas about sex, and these ideas can impede their sexual happiness. Here's the thing: The only rules about sex that everyone should follow are

- No one should get hurt, physically or emotionally.
- Sexual activity should be between consenting adults.

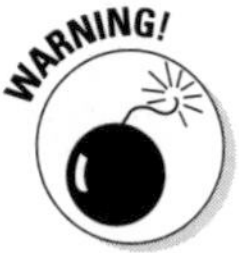

Another common and mistaken assumption is that sex should always be spontaneous. But spontaneity can be difficult when you have chronic pain. It's okay (really!) to plan your sexual activities together, whether it's best for you on Friday night after dinner when your pain is often at its lowest level or during an "afternoon delight" when you're both home.

Lots of people also think that certain things must happen during sex. For example, they think that it isn't real sex if no orgasm occurs. But that isn't true either. You can have intimate times together in many ways that are not mind-blowingly sexual, but that still feel great and make you and your partner happy.

Try new ideas and new positions that may be more amenable to a body in pain. For example, maybe the missionary position hurts you, so try having sex side-to-side or in another position. Be creative.

Get Help from the Experts

Sexuality experts can assist with sexual problems that result from chronic pain and also help you come up with ideas for sexual enjoyment. Obviously, you'll want a therapist sensitive to you and your partner's needs, so check out the resources listed in the "Educate Yourself about Sex" section, later in this chapter.

In addition, Widener University in Chester, Pennsylvania (`www.widener.edu`), and Hofstra University in Hempstead, New York (`www.hofstra.edu`), both have graduate programs in sex therapy. You may want to check with them to locate therapists who graduated from their programs.

Make Dates If You Sleep Separately

Chronic pain may mean that you and your partner sleep in separate beds or even in different rooms. The lack of proximity can create distance in your lovemaking activities, particularly if you're both on different schedules. But separate sleeping spaces don't mean that you can't get together often.

Make dates to meet in a comfortable place in the house when you know you'll be well-rested. Visit each other often in each other's bed, even if you're just relaxing and not doing anything sexual. These rendezvous will benefit your sex life if you make a habit of being close to each other often, even if you sleep separately.

Become Physically Fit and Work at Being Attractive

Keep a positive attitude about yourself. Being a positive person is attractive to others, while being too negative is a turnoff.

Also, looking attractive can help create a sexual spark — for you, because you feel good about yourself, and for your partner, because you look great. Sometimes people with chronic pain don't have the energy and strength to keep up their appearance. But making a special effort can pay off. It's easy to gain weight and get out of shape due to inactivity (especially when you feel that it hurts too much to exercise). But maintaining a healthy weight can greatly improve your appearance and desirability. Check out Chapters 18 and 19 to find out more about nutrition and exercise for people with chronic pain.

Educate Yourself about Sex

This tip is actually number 11, so you get a bonus! You should really check out the following terrific resources for information on sexuality.

Web sites:

- **Women's Health.gov:** This government agency provides lots of information on women's health topics, including sexuality.

  `http://4women.gov`

- **Drs. Laura and Jennifer Berman:** These well-known, sister sex therapists offer candid advice on improving your sex life, sexual health, and your relationship.

  `www.DrLauraBerman.com`

  `www.bermansexualhealth.com`

Books:

- ***Sex For Dummies*** **(Wiley), by Dr. Ruth K. Westheimer and Pierre A. Lehu:** This friendly, authoritative guide is by renowned sex therapist Dr. Ruth. Among other things, she debunks sex myths and covers new therapies to manage low libido, overcome sexual dysfunction, and enhance pleasure. Read it with your partner!
- ***The Power of Two: Secrets of a Strong & Loving Marriage*** **(New Harbinger Publications), by Susan, Ph.D. Heitler (Author), Paula Singer (Photographer):** This excellent book on marital relationships can help you have a positive conversation about sex with your partner.

Organizations:

- **American Association of Sexuality Educators Counselors & Therapists** (AASECT), P.O. Box 1960, Ashland, VA 23005-1960; phone 804-752-0026; Web site `www.aasect.org`. In addition to sexuality educators, sex counselors, and sex therapists, AASECT members include physicians, nurses, social workers, psychologists, allied health professionals, clergy members, lawyers, sociologists, marriage and family counselors, and therapists. The association has resources, including books, articles, and fact sheets, available for consumers.
- **American Association for Marriage and Family Therapy (AAMFT),** 112 S. Alfred St., Alexandria, VA 22314; phone 703-838-9808; Web site: `www.aamft.org`. The American Association for Marriage and Family Therapy is the association of marriage and family therapists in the United States and abroad. AAMFT members are mental-health professionals who treat and diagnose mental and emotional disorders and other arrays of problems, including sexuality issues.

Chapter 28

Ten or So Web Sources for People with Chronic Pain

In This Chapter

- Finding support groups
- Locating pain doctors and medical pain centers

Many free resources are available on the Web for people with chronic pain. This chapter describes organizational Web sites that can help you find out more about chronic pain. This information is organized into categories so that you can easily locate the help you need.

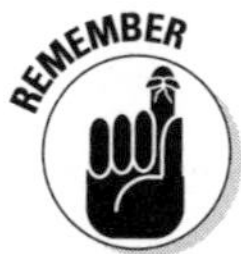

Keep in mind two important warnings on health information that's available on the Web:

- Although many reliable resources are on the Internet, including those we list in this chapter, sadly, far too many sites offer only incorrect and/ or outdated information, and many are downright hoaxes designed to sell empty promises. Make sure that you gather information only from reliable resources. Two good sites for checking out possible hoaxes are `www.quackwatch.org` and `http://hoaxbusters.ciac.org`.
- Don't forget that the information you obtain from any Web site is no substitute for a checkup and advice from an appropriate medical professional. If you have chronic pain and haven't told your doctor about it or found a doctor who can help you, please do it now.

Finding Information

Several helpful organizations offer you general information on chronic pain and the health conditions that cause it:

The American Pain Foundation (APF); phone 1-888-615-PAIN (7246); Web site www.painfoundation.org. The foundation's comprehensive Pain Information Library includes information on a broad array of topics of interest to people with ongoing pain, such as what kind of work you can continue to do if you qualify for Social Security disability payments, as well as background information on many diseases that cause chronic pain. The Web site also provides information on pain relief studies and therapies.

Danemiller Foundation; Web site www.pain.com. This Web site hosts not only substantial information for patients but also has a forum in which experts in pain medicine are available to answer questions posed to them.

The Mayo Clinic; Web site www.mayoclinic.com. The Mayo Clinic is a reliable and comprehensive source of a wide range of health information. You can look up diseases and conditions alphabetically and find background information and updates on research.

MedlinePlus; Web site http://medlineplus.gov. MedlinePlus brings together authoritative information from the National Library of Medicine, NIH, and other government agencies and health-related organizations. The Web site includes preformulated searches, which provide you with easy access to abstracts (summaries) of many medical journal articles. MedlinePlus also has extensive information about drugs, an illustrated medical encyclopedia, interactive patient tutorials, and the latest health news. This site is a great resource! Use it.

Finding Support Groups

Many people find valuable information, as well as understanding, by joining support groups whose members share their condition. Often, such groups are available locally, and their meeting times are listed in your local newspaper. If you can't find the information you need, call the reference librarian at your local library.

American Chronic Pain Association (ACPA); phone 1-800-533-3231; Web site www.theacpa.org. In 1980, after years of living with chronic pain, Penney Cowan placed a notice in her church bulletin, and she quickly found others living with chronic pain. As a result of Cowan's work, the first ACPA support group was born. Several hundred ACPA support groups now meet across the United States and Canada, as well as other countries. ACPA's Web site has a searchable database that enables you to find support groups in your area. You can then call its toll-free number for contact information or e-mail the organization at ACPA@pacbell.net.

Finding Doctors Who Specialize in Pain Management

When you have chronic pain, you need a caring and knowledgeable doctor. Maybe you already have one, and if so, she's a keeper! But if you need to locate a new doctor, consider online resources as one means for locating and/or screening the best physician for you.

American Academy of Pain Medicine (AAPM); Web site www.aapainmanage.org. AAPM provides credentialing to physicians, accreditation of pain centers, and other resources for medical professionals who treat people in pain. The academy has more than 6,000 members. Its Web site has a searchable database where you can find pain professionals and/or pain centers located near you.

American Board of Pain Medicine (ABPM); Web site http://www.abpm.org. The ABPM tests and certifies physicians in the field of pain medicine. Its Web site offers a searchable database of its qualified members (called *diplomates*). You can search for diplomates in your area and by specialty, such as anesthesiology or rheumatology.

International Spine Intervention Society; Web site www.spinalinjection.com. A physician organization in pain medicine dedicated to implementing guidelines for physicians practicing interventional pain.

Locating Medical Centers Specializing in Pain Management

Some medical centers concentrate on treating chronic pain only, and their services may be just what you need to get on the path to feeling better.

The American Pain Society; Web site www.ampainsoc.org. The society has a searchable database of pain treatment centers, which you can identify by location, services, classification, and setting (such as home or hospital-based).

Resources Outside the United States

Maybe the information you need isn't readily available in the United States, but you can access it online at a site in another country, such as Canada or England.

The Canadian Pain Society; Web site `www.canadianpainsociety.ca`. The Canadian Pain Society provides a bilingual Web site (English and French) offering free journal articles and a newsletter pertaining to pain and pain control, as well as links to Canadian resources.

The International Association for the Study of Pain (IASP); Web site `www.iasp-pain.org`. IASP's members include scientists, physicians, psychologists, dentists, nurses, and physical therapists dedicated to furthering research on, and improving the care of, patients with pain. The association's Web site provides free medical newsletters and clinical updates and resource listings by country.

Advocacy

You may be looking for an organization whose leadership and members understand the tough fight you and others must face to obtain relief from your chronic pain and who have some ability to get things done within local, state, and federal governments. If so, advocacy may be the answer for you. Consider the following Web sites.

Partners Against Pain; Web site `www.partnersagainstpain.com`. This alliance of patients, caregivers, and health-care providers works to advance standards of pain care through education and advocacy.

The American Pain Society; Web site `www.ampainsoc.org`. This go-to organization covers what's happening in the area of advocacy about chronic pain issues. The society has a three-part agenda guiding its national advocacy efforts. It focuses on enhancing funding from the National Institutes of Health for pain research, removing barriers to effective clinical pain management, and providing evidence and analysis to further the understanding of controversies surrounding opioid use and abuse.

Chapter 29

Ten Things to Avoid When You Have Chronic Pain

In This Chapter

- Knowing what not to do when you have chronic pain
- Discovering your rights as a health-care consumer

Most of this book tells you what you should do to better deal with your chronic pain. This chapter takes an entirely different approach, advising you about what not to do when you have chronic pain.

Don't Stop Caring for the Condition Causing Your Pain

Whether you have diabetes, arthritis, or one of the many other causes of relentless pain, it's important to work on controlling that medical condition as best you can. Sure, it can be an endless drag, with doctors' appointments, medications, physical therapy, exercise, proper nutrition, and so on filling your entire day. Enough already! Maybe you'd rather just collapse in a comfy chair in front of the tube and watch your favorite soap to find out whether Lois Loveless' eighth husband really was cheating on her while she had amnesia.

Forget about Lois and put yourself first instead. Once you get the hang of making these activities a regular part of your routine, you'll feel much better. And, *if* you still have pain, it will be much more manageable for you.

Don't Be a Couch Potato

A common cause of chronic pain is *deconditioning,* or getting badly out of shape, which can lead to more pain than whatever condition started this whole mess you're in to begin with. You need to know that deconditioning is often caused by couch potato-ism.

When you lie about watching TV or bemoaning your chronic pain (or both), your muscles lose their strength and endurance, your joints stiffen, your posture collapses, and you also lose cardiovascular strength — not good! (See Chapters 3 and 19 for lots of tips on avoiding deconditioning.) Take a walk, ride your bike, and do whatever you can (with your doctor's approval) to get moving again.

If You're Overweight, Lose Those Pounds

Are you a chocoholic? Is your secret passion gummy bears? Indulging every once and awhile is usually okay, but eating healthy food (see Chapter 18) and exercising (see Chapter 19) are both true essentials to maintaining a healthy weight, avoiding deconditioning (see preceding section), and controlling pain. As a general rule, do your best to maintain a healthy weight.

A great resource for discovering a healthy weight for you (and getting there) is *Dieting For Dummies* (Wiley) by Jane Kirby, RD, and the American Dietetic Association.

Avoid Pain Triggers

Hopefully, you've used a pain diary to figure out what triggers your pain. (See Chapter 17 for information on keeping pain diaries.) It's easy to think, "Oh, I feel so much better now, so I'm sure it's okay if I eat that extra piece of cake, play on the Internet for hours on end without a break, or stay up really late tonight." Then, wham! Irritable bowel syndrome kicks in, or the arthritis in your neck starts hurting from leaning over the keyboard, or maybe a massive migraine strikes. So, in advance, say no to pain triggers!

Don't Let Stress Pile on to Your Pain

Stress is the result of how you react to your world, and heightened stress equals heightened pain. Life is often stressful, but you can learn to relax. For example, adopt healthy breathing techniques. (When people are under stress, they tend to breathe shallowly.)

Or memorize a funny poem and recite it in your mind whenever you feel stress coming on (or you feel like honking madly at the slow driver in front of you, causing you to have a stress attack because you're late to your daughter's piano recital.) Singing or humming a rhyme is even better than reciting it. Try something along these lines:

Little Miss Muffet sat on a tuffet
Eating a Big Mac and fries
Along came a spider and sat down beside her
"Yuck," it said, "I prefer flies"

Many other good techniques are available to reduce stress, such as distraction and expressive writing. You can read about these techniques in Chapter 22.

Don't Neglect Your Sleep

Chronic pain is exhausting. If you don't usually get adequate sleep, you're not alone. The majority of people who wake up too early because of chronic pain are unable to fall back to sleep. In this case, don't go with the majority! You need to get enough Zzzzzs.

The first rule for getting adequate sleep is to maintain a regular time to go to bed and to wake up at the same time every morning, including on weekends. For other techniques, see Chapter 20.

Don't Let Depression Persist

Chronic pain can be depressing. The first step toward beating depression is to accept that you or your loved one needs help and then go find that help. (See Chapter 3 for a list of the signs and symptoms of depression.) The good news is that depression is highly treatable, and Chapter 22 helps you manage your pain with lifestyle changes.

In addition, here's another great resource:

National Mental Health Information Center; phone 1-800-789-2647; Web site `http://mentalhealth.samhsa.gov`. The center provides information about mental health via a toll-free telephone number, a Web site, and more than 600 publications that you can request online.

Don't Ignore New Pain Problems

You may be so used to your chronic pain condition that if a new type of pain pops up, you automatically think, "Oh, it's just another symptom of the same old thing." But just because you often get migraines doesn't mean you're immune from getting a brain aneurysm, which is a true emergency. Or, just because you have central pain syndrome doesn't mean that you can't develop peripheral neuropathy. Again, this situation is when your pain diary can come in handy. (See Chapter 17 for information on pain diaries.) If you're suddenly tracking new types of pain — particularly if the pain is severe — be sure to see your doctor.

Don't Forget Your Rights as a Health Consumer

You're the only one who knows how you feel, and you have to live with the results of your medical treatment. However, you may not know about your rights as a medical consumer. The President's Advisory Commission on Consumer Protection and Quality in the Health Care Industry adopted a list of consumer rights and responsibilities in 1998. Many health plans (hopefully yours) have adopted these principles, which are good to keep in mind.

Here are six key consumer rights that are important to the medical management of your pain:

- **Information disclosure:** The right to receive accurate, easily understood information to make an informed health-care decision.
- **Choice of providers and plans:** The right to a choice of health-care providers that's sufficient to ensure your access to appropriate high-quality healthcare.

- **Access to emergency services:** The right to access emergency health-care services if the need arises.
- **Participation in treatment decisions:** The right to fully participate in all decisions related to your healthcare. If you're unable to fully participate in treatment decisions, you have the right to be represented by a spouse, parents, guardians, adult children, or someone else.
- **Respect and nondiscrimination:** The right to considerate, respectful care from all members of the health-care system at all times and under all circumstances.
- **Confidentiality of health information:** The right to communicate with health-care providers in confidence and have the confidentiality of your individually identifiable health-care information protected. You also have the right to review and copy your medical records and request any needed amendments.

Don't Complain Too Much

Yes, maybe you're in your third year of constant pain, and that's a drag. And okay, maybe your spouse, kids, and colleagues were sympathetic for the first few months. But now you think, "No one pays attention to me any more!" Well, maybe you talk a little too much (or a lot) about your chronic pain.

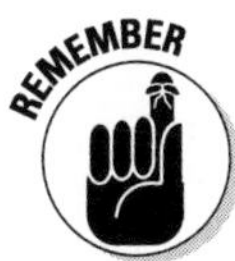

The hard truth is, people get tired of hearing the same old complaints, even if they're very real. Here's a good general rule: When talking to other people, unless you're in the middle of a medical emergency, keep the conversation off your pain and the condition causing it. Concentrate instead on the other person or talk about something positive in your life. (Come on, you can think of something!) Keep it up for a month or so, and this behavior will become a new good habit.

Index

• A •

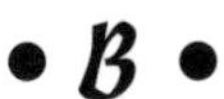

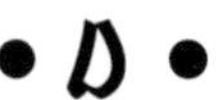

• E •

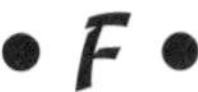

• G •

• H •

• I •

• J •

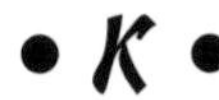

• N •

• O •

• S •

• T •

• U •

• V •

• W •

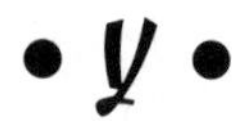

Notes

Notes

BUSINESS, CAREERS & PERSONAL FINANCE

0-7645-9847-3

0-7645-2431-3

Also available:

- Business Plans Kit For Dummies 0-7645-9794-9
- Economics For Dummies 0-7645-5726-2
- Grant Writing For Dummies 0-7645-8416-2
- Home Buying For Dummies 0-7645-5331-3
- Managing For Dummies 0-7645-1771-6
- Marketing For Dummies 0-7645-5600-2
- Personal Finance For Dummies 0-7645-2590-5*
- Resumes For Dummies 0-7645-5471-9
- Selling For Dummies 0-7645-5363-1
- Six Sigma For Dummies 0-7645-6798-5
- Small Business Kit For Dummies 0-7645-5984-2
- Starting an eBay Business For Dummies 0-7645-6924-4
- Your Dream Career For Dummies 0-7645-9795-7

HOME & BUSINESS COMPUTER BASICS

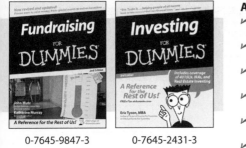

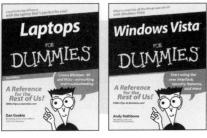

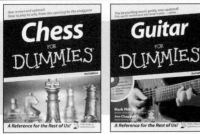

0-470-05432-8

0-471-75421-8

Also available:

- Cleaning Windows Vista For Dummies 0-471-78293-9
- Excel 2007 For Dummies 0-470-03737-7
- Mac OS X Tiger For Dummies 0-7645-7675-5
- MacBook For Dummies 0-470-04859-X
- Macs For Dummies 0-470-04849-2
- Office 2007 For Dummies 0-470-00923-3
- Outlook 2007 For Dummies 0-470-03830-6
- PCs For Dummies 0-7645-8958-X
- Salesforce.com For Dummies 0-470-04893-X
- Upgrading & Fixing Laptops For Dummies 0-7645-8959-8
- Word 2007 For Dummies 0-470-03658-3
- Quicken 2007 For Dummies 0-470-04600-7

FOOD, HOME, GARDEN, HOBBIES, MUSIC & PETS

0-7645-8404-9

0-7645-9904-6

Also available:

- Candy Making For Dummies 0-7645-9734-5
- Card Games For Dummies 0-7645-9910-0
- Crocheting For Dummies 0-7645-4151-X
- Dog Training For Dummies 0-7645-8418-9
- Healthy Carb Cookbook For Dummies 0-7645-8476-6
- Home Maintenance For Dummies 0-7645-5215-5
- Horses For Dummies 0-7645-9797-3
- Jewelry Making & Beading For Dummies 0-7645-2571-9
- Orchids For Dummies 0-7645-6759-4
- Puppies For Dummies 0-7645-5255-4
- Rock Guitar For Dummies 0-7645-5356-9
- Sewing For Dummies 0-7645-6847-7
- Singing For Dummies 0-7645-2475-5

INTERNET & DIGITAL MEDIA

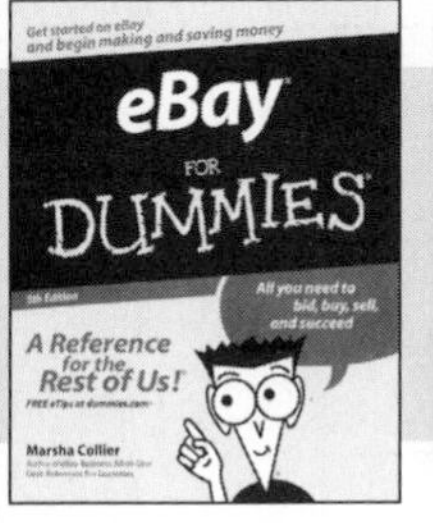

0-470-04529-9

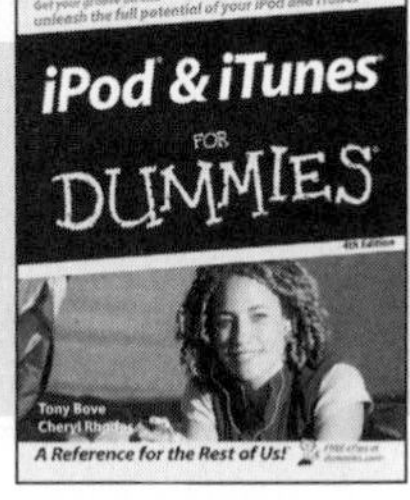

0-470-04894-8

Also available:

- Blogging For Dummies 0-471-77084-1
- Digital Photography For Dummies 0-7645-9802-3
- Digital Photography All-in-One Desk Reference For Dummies 0-470-03743-1
- Digital SLR Cameras and Photography For Dummies 0-7645-9803-1
- eBay Business All-in-One Desk Reference For Dummies 0-7645-8438-3
- HDTV For Dummies 0-470-09673-X
- Home Entertainment PCs For Dummies 0-470-05523-5
- MySpace For Dummies 0-470-09529-6
- Search Engine Optimization For Dummies 0-471-97998-8
- Skype For Dummies 0-470-04891-3
- The Internet For Dummies 0-7645-8996-2
- Wiring Your Digital Home For Dummies 0-471-91830-X

Separate Canadian edition also available

Separate U.K. edition also available

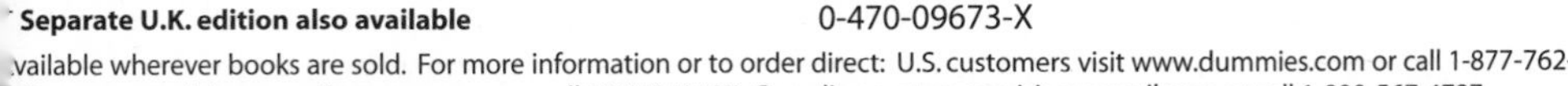
vailable wherever books are sold. For more information or to order direct: U.S. customers visit www.dummies.com or call 1-877-762-2974.
.K. customers visit www.wileyeurope.com or call 0800 243407. Canadian customers visit www.wiley.ca or call 1-800-567-4797.

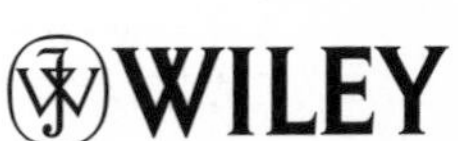

SPORTS, FITNESS, PARENTING, RELIGION & SPIRITUALITY

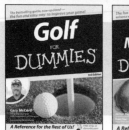

0-471-76871-5

0-7645-7841-3

Also available:

- Catholicism For Dummies 0-7645-5391-7
- Exercise Balls For Dummies 0-7645-5623-1
- Fitness For Dummies 0-7645-7851-0
- Football For Dummies 0-7645-3936-1
- Judaism For Dummies 0-7645-5299-6
- Potty Training For Dummies 0-7645-5417-4
- Buddhism For Dummies 0-7645-5359-3
- Pregnancy For Dummies 0-7645-4483-7 †
- Ten Minute Tone-Ups For Dummies 0-7645-7207-5
- NASCAR For Dummies 0-7645-7681-X
- Religion For Dummies 0-7645-5264-3
- Soccer For Dummies 0-7645-5229-5
- Women in the Bible For Dummies 0-7645-8475-8

TRAVEL

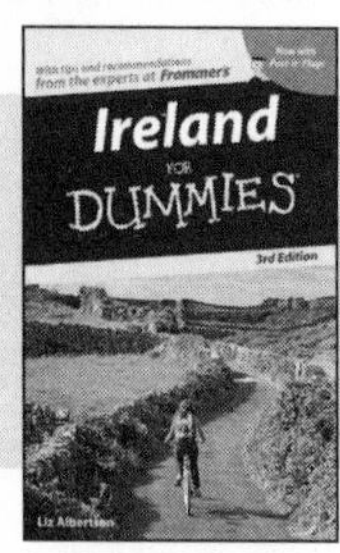

0-7645-7749-2

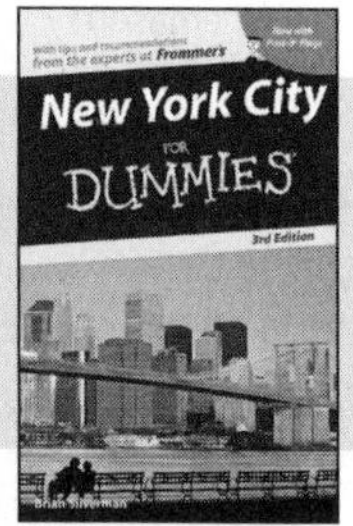

0-7645-6945-7

Also available:

- Alaska For Dummies 0-7645-7746-8
- Cruise Vacations For Dummies 0-7645-6941-4
- England For Dummies 0-7645-4276-1
- Europe For Dummies 0-7645-7529-5
- Germany For Dummies 0-7645-7823-5
- Hawaii For Dummies 0-7645-7402-7
- Italy For Dummies 0-7645-7386-1
- Las Vegas For Dummies 0-7645-7382-9
- London For Dummies 0-7645-4277-X
- Paris For Dummies 0-7645-7630-5
- RV Vacations For Dummies 0-7645-4442-X
- Walt Disney World & Orlando For Dummies 0-7645-9660-8

GRAPHICS, DESIGN & WEB DEVELOPMENT

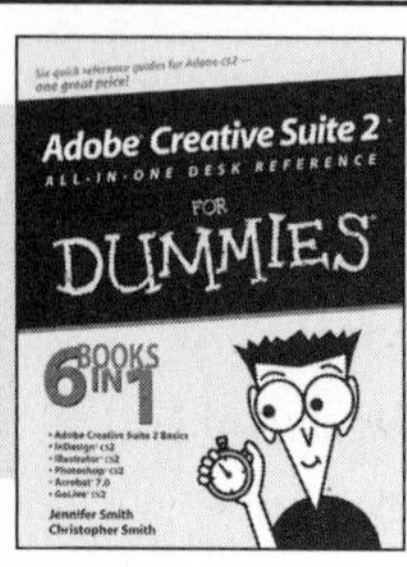

0-7645-8815-X

0-7645-9571-7

Also available:

- 3D Game Animation For Dummies 0-7645-8789-7
- AutoCAD 2006 For Dummies 0-7645-8925-3
- Building a Web Site For Dummies 0-7645-7144-3
- Creating Web Pages For Dummies 0-470-08030-2
- Creating Web Pages All-in-One Desk Reference For Dummies 0-7645-4345-8
- Dreamweaver 8 For Dummies 0-7645-9649-7
- InDesign CS2 For Dummies 0-7645-9572-5
- Macromedia Flash 8 For Dummies 0-7645-9691-8
- Photoshop CS2 and Digital Photography For Dummies 0-7645-9580-6
- Photoshop Elements 4 For Dummies 0-471-77483-9
- Syndicating Web Sites with RSS Feeds For Dummies 0-7645-8848-6
- Yahoo! SiteBuilder For Dummies 0-7645-9800-7

NETWORKING, SECURITY, PROGRAMMING & DATABASES

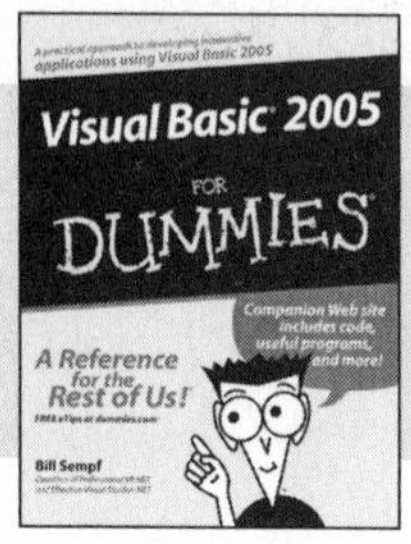

0-7645-7728-X

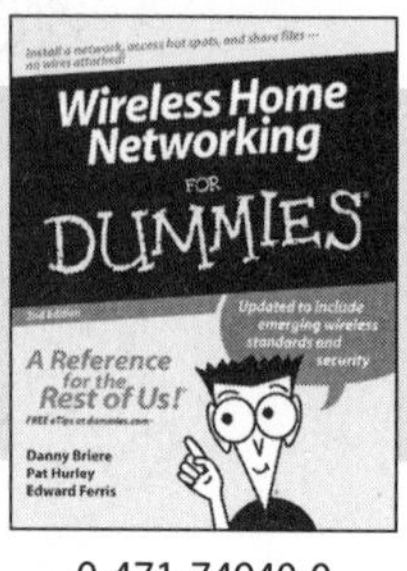

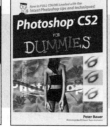

0-471-74940-0

Also available:

- Access 2007 For Dummies 0-470-04612-0
- ASP.NET 2 For Dummies 0-7645-7907-X
- C# 2005 For Dummies 0-7645-9704-3
- Hacking For Dummies 0-470-05235-X
- Hacking Wireless Networks For Dummies 0-7645-9730-2
- Java For Dummies 0-470-08716-1
- Microsoft SQL Server 2005 For Dummies 0-7645-7755-7
- Networking All-in-One Desk Reference For Dummies 0-7645-9939-9
- Preventing Identity Theft For Dummies 0-7645-7336-5
- Telecom For Dummies 0-471-77085-X
- Visual Studio 2005 All-in-One Desk Reference For Dummies 0-7645-9775-2
- XML For Dummies 0-7645-8845-1

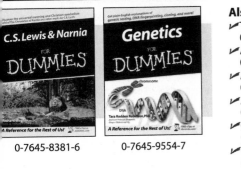

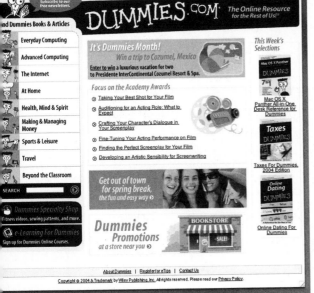

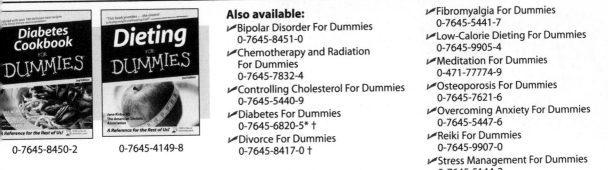

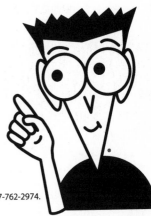

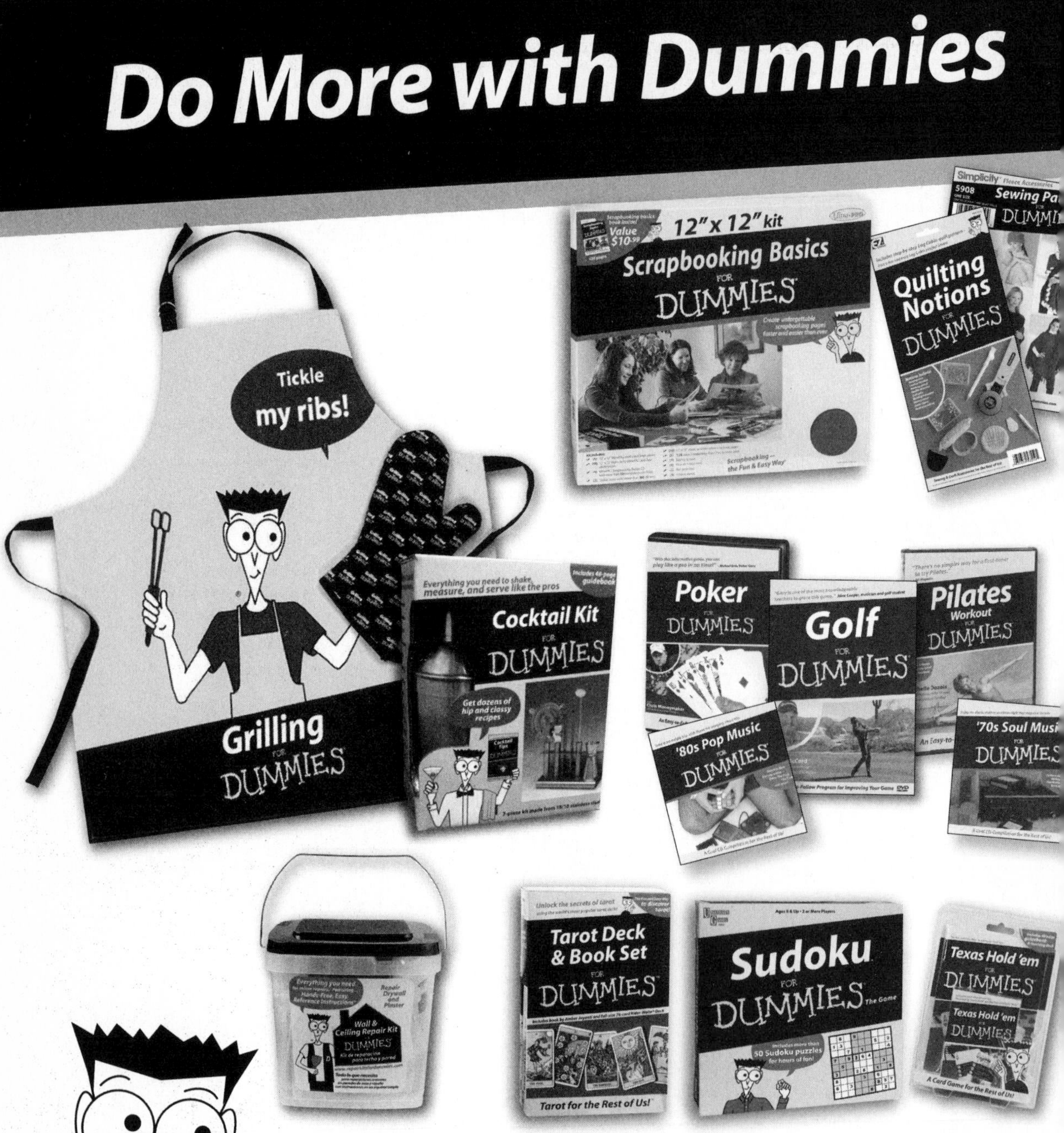

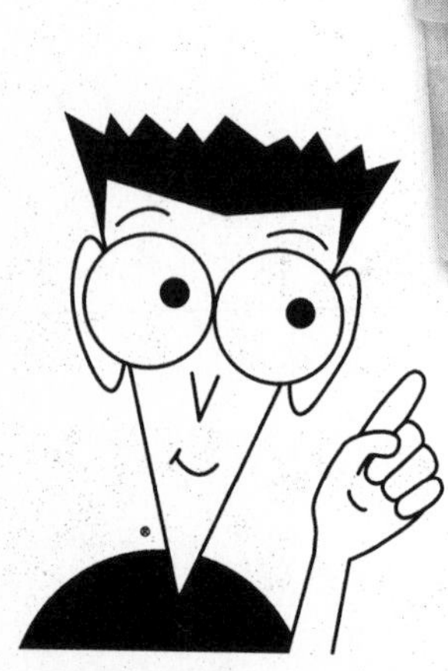

Gender Issues

Gender Issues in the Teaching of English

Edited by

Nancy Mellin McCracken
Bruce C. Appleby

Boynton/Cook Publishers, Inc.
A Subsidiary of
Heinemann Educational Books, Inc.
361 Hanover Street, Portsmouth, NH 03801
Offices and agents throughout the world

Library of Congress Cataloging-in-Publication Data
Gender issues in the teaching of English/edited by Nancy Mellin
McCracken, Bruce C. Appleby.
p. cm.
Includes bibliographical references.
ISBN 0–86709–310–2
1. Language Arts — United States — Sex differences. 2. English language — Study and teaching — United States — Sex differences.
3. Sexism in education — United States. 4. Sex differences in education — United States. I. Appleby, Bruce C. II. McCracken, Nancy Mellin.
LB1576.G37 1992 92-11979
428′.007 — dc20 CIP

Cover design by Twyla Bogaard
Printed in the United States of America
92 93 94 95 96 9 8 7 6 5 4 3 2 1

Contents

Preface

Dear Reader,

We have thought a lot about you as we worked on this book. How did you come to this page? Was it a conference panel or workshop you encountered recently that set you to wondering what more there is to be done about gender issues in English classrooms? Or have you been thinking, talking, and writing about these issues for years?

Because gender issues are experienced personally, we thought we might introduce ourselves and the book by writing how we each came to think about gender issues in our teaching and how we came to edit this book.

I (Bruce) first got involved with gender issues because of an experience in San Francisco in the mid-seventies. I was on a bus and next to me was sitting a well-dressed boy, about four years old, desperately hanging onto his mother and working with great effort not to cry. He had a button on his shirt which read "I didn't cry today." When I saw the sadness and distress in this boy's face and realized he was terribly upset about something, I was hit by how unfair the button was and by how unfair it was to him that he was not allowed to share or express his feelings. Because the women in my life were becoming involved in what was then called "the women's movement" and because their changes were bringing about welcome and needed changes in my life, I started a presentation soon after, a rumination which became "Big Boys Don't Cry."

I (Nancy), having been born female in post-World War II America, may have been born into an involvement in gender issues, but the roots of my research in this area began in a used bookstore one day in which I was escaping from a thorny puzzle in the dissertation I was writing. Tillie Olsen's book *Silences* beckoned to me from the shelf. On the flyleaf, I discovered the signature of a colleague who had recently died. She had raised five boys, served as dutiful hostess for her garrulous department chair husband, and taught part time quietly in our department for about fifteen years. She was not what I would have called then "a driving force" in the department, and I hadn't spent much time with her, but every now and then she would write me a note thanking me for giving some talk or other to one of her classes and enclose an absolutely stunning poem. The book seemed a posthumous gift from her. I read it breathlessly, and haven't stopped since, trying to learn about the "unnatural silences" in our lives and to find ways to turn those silences into whispers and shouts and songs.

When Bruce and I heard each other speaking at various conferences, we came to realize that we had similar, though certainly not identical, points of view about gender and the teaching of English. For example we both believe that gender is a social construct, or to use McConnell-Ginet's definition, "the complex of social, cultural, and psychological phenomena attached to sex." We both believe that women and men have been harmed by the expectations and limitations of gender as traditionally defined. As we have been involved with gender issues over the years, we have both come to see how our teaching and our relationships with our students and colleagues have changed for the better. We both noted that whenever we gave presentations about gender issues to English teachers at conferences, their response was always something like, "You're right. I've noticed that too in my teaching and in my life. I just haven't thought about it before. Where can I go to find out more about this?" Bruce had been building a file of bibliographies for years and was always eager to share but that's all we had—except our stories and those of our colleagues. And so we've put this book together.

Our views about gender issues and the teaching of English have been shaped by our individual experiences. In this book, we have tried to represent a range of views. The voices you will hear are the voices of women and men, high school teachers, college professors, and their students. The authors are all teacher-researchers, professionals whose questions about how gender differences might play themselves out in their classrooms and in their professional lives led to inquiry and reflection on how they might change. We have chosen original essays with strong voices that we hope will create a sense of the conversation in progress about gender issues in the teaching of English and help us persuade you to join that conversation—both on and off the page.

Acknowledgments

Happily unmarried, I am grateful to my students and colleagues who don't let me get by with much without challenging me. I am grateful to my friends, men and women who are interested in gender issues in life as well as in teaching. In particular, I thank Cass and Barb for sharing their beautiful minds and lives and ideas. — Bruce

To my children, Thomas Patrick and Meridith Mellin McCracken, who teach me daily about life choices; to my students and colleagues who have challenged my thinking about gender issues and teaching, especially Denise Provens and Susan M. James; and to my husband and colleague, Hugh Thomas McCracken. I would also like to thank the Project for the Study of Gender and Education at Kent State University for continuing research support. — Nancy

1

An Overview of Gender Issues in the Teaching of English

Nancy Mellin McCracken
Bruce C. Appleby

> Joining Mill's insights that traits and gender are connected and that roles and gender are not fixed by nature, we can adopt a GENDER-SENSITIVE ideal as opposed to either an illusory gender-free one or a vicious gender-bound one. Taking gender into account when it makes a difference and ignoring it when it does not, a gender-sensitive ideal allows educators to build into curricula, instructional methods, and learning environments ways of dealing with trait genderization and with the many and various other gender related phenomena—for example, the portrayal of women [and men] in the subject matter of the curriculum—that enter into education today.
>
> J. R. Martin, 1988

Why a book on gender and the teaching of English? In the seventies and early eighties, a number of works appeared urging us to attempt to erase gender in our language and in our teaching of language. The generic third person singular personal pronoun may stand as the emblem for this early effort to combat sexism in the teaching of English. We went from the generalized *he* to *he/she* or *they*. We learned to say *chairperson* rather than *chairman* or *chairwoman*. We made concerted efforts to include stories and pictures of women doing well-paid professional work and men parenting and working in the "helping professions." NCTE and other organizations adopted policies banning the use of sexist language in publications. To some, it might seem that the gender problem has been solved, but in fact, there has been little progress.

Blakesley's essay in this volume summarizes a large body of research indicating that, despite efforts to legislate grammatical equity, the English language continues to reproduce gender stereotyping. The language our children learn carries with it, like a virus, the historical sexist message. When children enter schools from kindergarten through graduate school, this message is gradually refined into ever more resistant strains.

In recent years a number of startling works have appeared pushing us to look again at the effort to combat sexism by attempting to erase all difference related to gender and teaching. These works come from at least five distinct research communities—educational research on sex equity in schools, developmental psychology, sociolinguistics, feminist philosophy, and literary and rhetorical studies, yet they all lead to the strong conclusion that gender is a difference that makes a difference in teaching, particularly in the teaching of English.

Research on gender and school performance such as that reported in Sadker and Sadker (1986), Klein (1985), Gilligan, Lyons, and Hanmer (1989), and Stake (1984) demonstrates that males and females continue to be socialized differently in schools with what we believe are strong implications for teaching and learning. Boys consistently receive more teacher attention, attribute low grades to forces beyond their control, and when they succeed at school tasks, graduate with self-esteem and career aspirations intact. Girls consistently receive less teacher attention, take personal responsibility for low grades, and when they succeed at school tasks, graduate with measurably lower self-esteem and career aspirations.

In addition to educational research on gender differences in school performance, feminist philosophers have provided important insights in recent years. Jane Roland Martin (1985) has been particularly influential. Martin argues eloquently that if women were socialized exactly as men, then identical educations for both sexes would be effective, but since men and women are clearly socialized differently, they have different strengths and weaknesses that must be taken into account by educators if the end result is equal opportunity to achieve. French feminist philosophers from Simone de Beauvoir to Helene Cixous have made the case that, to the detriment of all students but especially to those socialized as females, the very core of our thinking, our logic, is restricted to a hierarchical, limited pattern commonly genderized as male. Curriculum research and theory cited by Miller in this volume has explored ways in which hierarchical structures related to gender, class, and race prevent schools from being places where most people are learning most of the time.

Appleby's essay in the first section of this book reviews significant ideas in the work of developmental psychologists from Chodorow's *The Reproduction of Mothering* (1978), Gilligan's *In a Different Voice* (1982), and Belenky, Clinchy, Goldberger, and Tarule's *Women's Ways of Knowing* (1986). A significant theme in each of these works is that for too long psychologists from Piaget to Perry and Kohlberg have generalized from work with males to conclusions about males and females, accepting certain male patterns as the human pattern of psychological development. When Gilligan and Belenky and their colleagues redid developmental studies with women, they found different patterns of moral development and cognitive style. The difference is described as a difference between a morality of "response" versus a morality of "rights," and "separate" versus "connected" knowing.

In classroom research, teachers have noted that some students learn very efficiently in the compartmentalized subjects and lessons typical of our educational system, while others have to talk long about each new idea, and insist on asking, "But what is this for?" and making other (seemingly irrelevant) personal connections. Gilligan, Lyons, and Hanmer's (1989) research suggest that girls, who typically learn by making these personal connections, are at a serious disadvantage in schools organized to produce efficient, silent, separate knowers. Of course, there are many boys (although perhaps a real minority) whose style of learning is like that of the girls studied by Gilligan and her colleagues. Unless their teachers allow them ample opportunities for expression of their cognitive styles, both groups of "connected knowers," boys and girls, learn to doubt the worth of their participation in class. Research continues to show that as academically successful girls progress through higher grade levels in school, they gradually retreat—unlike successful male students—into a silence born of the conviction that their comments are irrelevant. Clearly, gender plays a role in both teacher-student interactions and in student-student interactions in classrooms. The results of this unexplored variable appear to include failure for many potentially successful students.

Related research from linguistics on male and female styles of conversation suggest important developmental differences in the language usage of boys and girls and men and women. Deborah Tannen's latest book, *You Just Don't Understand* (1990) is a fascinating discussion of this research. What she and others have discovered and documented is that from their early schoolyard days, boys learn to use talk to *report* on their accomplishments, or to establish control of the action, while girls use talk to establish *rapport*, to create and sustain close friendship. As a result when boys talk in pairs or groups, they don't discuss personal events or feelings, and they don't try to connect one person's discourse to the next person's. Boys' conversations sound like a series of unrelated paragraphs. When girls talk in pairs or groups they often discuss personal events and feelings, and they offer sympathy and support to one another. They also contribute to one another's stories, sometimes talking right along with the speaker or filling in details to indicate their understanding. Girls' conversations sound like collaboratively written stories with a chorus. The implications for English teachers at all levels seem obvious: since there are such clear differences in styles and functions of language usage by males and females, any class dominated by either pattern is not likely to support the linguistic growth of as many as half of the students. Again, most American classrooms are structured to favor the style of conversation that has been genderized as male: students are asked to report their knowledge, one person at a time, in a competitive series. Since boys in our culture have almost no experience with collaborative, connected discourse inside or outside of school, they are at a disadvantage when asked to write well-organized essays that incorporate more than one viewpoint. In this volume, Bowman's essay demonstrates the difficulty high school boys have in creating speculative dialogic discourse in response to literature. Sanborn's essay demonstrates conversely the failure many women college students encounter when they try to fit complex ideas and discourse structures into the prescribed single-focus academic essay form. Roen's research on teacher response to student writing indicates that even when college writers' essays do not reflect their gendered conversational styles, teachers clearly genderize certain elements of writing style as they evaluate student essays. Classrooms where students are encouraged to talk together to solve problems and compose collaboratively would provide the best educations by providing ready access to learning and practice with a variety of discourse forms and styles for all students, but such classrooms are still the exception. Efforts to increase collaboration and greater student control of language activities that are uninformed by gender research are unlikely to be effective, however. McClure's essay in this volume suggests numerous ways to transform traditional gender-blind English classrooms into gender-sensitive ones.

Feminist literary and rhetorical theory has provided direction for curriculum reform reflecting gender differences in the past twenty years. Who has not heard how women writers were not permitted to publish for most of our history, with the result that there are very few women writers in anthologies and many of those who are included have taken male names or neuter initials (George Sand, George Eliot, H. D., S. E. Hinton). Women writers, when they are anthologized, are introduced to the reader as wives or daughters or lovers of prominent men (Willa Cather was a lesbian, we learn; Emily Dickinson was a frustrated unmarried woman; Mary Shelly was a loving wife; Virginia Woolf led a literary circle with her husband, Leonard . . .). One result of this publishing history is that there are so few models for young girls who would be writers.

Perhaps less often considered is the fact that regardless of the gender of anthologized authors, the most anthologized pieces are representations of stereotypically male experience. The details of Hemingway's fly fishing characters are deemed worthy of careful study; the details of Virginia Woolf's dinner party hostesses are deemed trivial and unworthy of reading or writing. This is a vicious circle because without lots of models of women who become writers and live to raise their children, not many girls will think to become writers. Those who do will find almost no examples from which to learn how to write effectively about the subjects they have most closely experienced as young women (menstruation, for example, care of younger siblings, unwanted affection from older male family members, intense friendships with girlfriends, pride in being like mother . . .) And finally, those who do unearth the few models available and do work their craft to publishable quality are up against a publishing establishment that has consistently privileged male experience and the male point of view. British researcher Dale Spender's recent study of gender and publishing titled, *The Writing or the Sex* (1989) reports women account for only twenty percent of published books in English today. A seven-week survey of the *New York Times Book Review* during 1984 showed that eighty-six percent of the reviews were written by men about men. Besides the fact that this perpetuates a shortage of women writers, it perpetuates a cultural silence about issues of concern to girls and women.

English teachers need to ask how the girls respond to the male-authored literary works they read in class. Do they take the point of view of the male narrators and heroes, or do they try to peek into the female characters' minds, where they exist in the traditional school curriculum in works such as *1984, Of Mice and Men*, or *Julius Caesar*? What about the boys? Is there anything in the novels they are reading to challenge their gender stereotypes or to give them insights to girls' or women's experiences?

Even if Tillie Olson's (1965) estimated ratio of one in twelve anthologized female to male authors has narrowed in selected anthologies, the works by women authors selected for anthologies are not often ones which focus on the experiences of girls and women. Cooper's (1989) examination of Newbery and Caldecott winners from 1980–1987 reveals that despite the fact that the majority of authors and illustrators of the selected books are females, the books consistently portray men and women in traditional sex roles and feature male characters far more prominently than female characters. Even if more works are included by women authors representing girls' and women's experience, as long as the instructional apparatus surrounding the literature remains unchanged, small changes in the academic canon are not likely to have much impact. Comley's report in this volume on girls' male-centred responses to Hemingway's story "Indian Camp" and McCracken's students' responses to "Greasy Lake" indicate the extent to which textbook questions which guide readings in traditional, male-centered ways can silence young men's and even young women's responses to women's experiences in literature. Stover's analysis of gender issues in young adult literature provides an excellent resource for junior high and high school teachers who want to provide students with opportunities to explore literature that does not perpetuate gender stereotypes.

Finally, it is apparent that not only students are affected by a false gender-blindness. Teachers themselves as they engage in professional development run into powerful gender stereotypes that hinder them from both within and without. Essays by Greenwood and Miller in this volume explore the role of gender in the professional development of teachers with the clear implication that English Education professors, mentor teachers, and directors of graduate research need to reconsider the effect of excluding gender as a variable in studies of the teaching and learning of English. The essays in this book bring the current research on gender and education, and gender and language to bear on the teaching of English in high schools and colleges. If the classroom is a microcosm of our society, then gender is a powerful factor in English classrooms and the study of gender issues must inform both theory and practice in the teaching of English. We are always theorizing as teachers and each decision we make as English teachers—which story, taught to whom, by what methods, for what purposes, followed by what kind of writing assignments, evaluated how, by whom, and for what purposes—is a decision we make from a theoretical framework that includes gender, self-consciously or not. We can't decide what we do without having decided at some level what we value and what we believe about teaching and learning. The English curriculum needs a close look in the light of gender sensitivity if all our students, males and females, are to fully develop the potential to hear the voices of others clearly, and use their own voices to understand, shape, and share their worlds, and imagine other worlds. This collection is an effort to begin such an inquiry.

Works Cited

Belenkey, M., B. Clinchy, N. Goldberger, J. Tarule. 1986. *Women's ways of knowing: The development of self, voice, and mind*. NY: Basic Books.

Chodorow, N. 1978. *The reproduction of mothering: Psychoanalysis and the sociology of gender*. Berkeley: U. of California Press.

Cixous, H. 1981. The laugh of the Medusa. 245–264 in *French Feminisms*. E. Marks & I. deCourtiuron, eds. NY: Shocken.

Cooper, P. 1989. Women's way of writing. In M. Cooper and M. Holzmann, eds. *Writing as social action*, 141–156. Portsmouth, NH: Boynton/Cook.

deBeauvoir, S. 1952. *The Second sex*. NY: Knopf.

Gilligan, C. 1982. *In a different voice: Psychological theory and women's development*. Cambridge, MA: Harvard UP.

Gilligan, C., N. Lyons, T. Hanmer, eds. 1989. *Making connections: The relational world of adolescent girls at Emma Willard School* Troy, NY: Emma Willard School.

Klein, S., ed. 1985. *Handbook for achieving sex equity through education*. Baltimore: John Hopkins UP.

Martin, J. 1985. *Reclaiming a conversation: The ideal of an educated woman*. New Haven, CT: Yale UP.

Olsen, T. 1965. *Silences*. NY: Delta/Seymour Lawrence.

Sadker & Sadker. 1986. Sexism in the classroom: From grade school to graduate school. *Phi delta kappan*, 67 (7), 32.

Spender, D. 1989. *The writing or the sex? or why you don't have to read women's writing to know it's no good*. NY: Pergamon Press.

Stake, J. E. 1984. "Educational and Career Confidence and Motivation Among Female and Male Undergraduates." *American Educational Research Journal*. 21.3: 565–78.

Tannen, D. 1990. *You just don't understand: Women and men in conversation*. NY: Morrow.

Part I
Gender and the Teaching of Language

In this section we include essays that focus on gender issues and the teaching of language. Appleby reviews recent studies in developmental psychology and sociolinguistics and discusses their implications for both male and female students in English Language Arts classrooms. Blakesley's essay offers ample illustration that, despite concerted efforts to the contrary, the English language continues its long history of sexism. McClure offers a wealth of suggestions for helping students understand and make use of their language to question its stereotypes. As you read these essays, we'd like you to think about what differences it would make in your students' lives if they could better see how language shapes their perceptions of themselves and others as gendered beings. At the end of this section we have included a number of questions for you to think, talk, write about in order to help us "Continue the Conversation."

2

Psychological and Sociolinguistic Bases for Gender-Sensitive Teaching

Bruce C. Appleby

When I give talks on the topic of gender issues in the teaching of English—often titled "Women and Men and Language: Two Cultures"—I usually have the bibliographies printed up on pink paper, because I want to be gender appropriate.

Before World War I, in our culture, pink was the color chosen when giving a gift to a baby boy: pink was bold, made a strong statement, and was best worn by a strong person. Blue was a soft background color, good for backing up and supporting other colors. Apparently, this changed sometime after World War II.

I like this anecdote, for it points out how we are creatures of our culture and how we view the world through the glasses provided by that culture. From our point of view, as English teachers, this is most important because the way a culture expresses itself and the way a culture distinguishes itself is through its language. Gender has been and continues to be part of our language legacy and gender issues in the teaching of English have been and continue to be part of our teaching heritage.

When looking at a topic as potentially volatile and of such importance as gender and language, a definition of terms helps. As with other words whose definitions have changed in the last few years—words like *conference* (remember when it was exclusively a noun?), *chauvinism* (remember when it meant excessive patriotism?), *hegemony* (remember when you hadn't heard the word?), *problem* (remember when that word hadn't been matized?)—gender has taken on meanings beyond its use to denote the two sexes. For some, gender has become a word to substitute for "female" or "woman," so that what used to be "women's studies" is now referred to as "gender studies." Here, I refer to both male and female when I refer to gender.

The best definition of gender I have encountered is that of Leslie Flemming, who observed in 1988 that all writing on gender—whether the perspective be historical, anthropological, political, literary, or other—shows us that ". . . gender is a social construct, not something 'natural' or God-given, but constructed, patterned, by every society for its own purposes and according to its own ideology." Wolfram, in his excellent book *Dialects and American English* (1981), talks of "genderlects." Using McConnell-Ginet's definition, the label gender, as opposed to sex, is used to capture the "complex of social, cultural, and psychological phenomena attached to sex" (1978, 76). This definition offers sharp contrast with the demographic or physiological distinction between male and female.

We need, then, to look at gender and the issues it raises for us as teachers of English from two perspectives: the psychological and the sociolinguistic.

A Psychological Perspective

Chodorow's 1978 classic, *The Reproduction of Mothering*, argues that women's mothering experiences produce differences in the relational experiences of girls and boys as they grow up. Mothers are the child's primary caretakers in our culture. They are the socializers of our children. Males and females grow up with very different points of view toward what constitutes a relationship with the other sex. Females, as they grow into their self-identification as females, can maintain their primary object identification with the female/mother. Males must shift their primary object identification from the female/mother to the male, as they grow into their self-identification as males. Male personality comes to be associated with independence and being alone, on seeing the self as separate and distinct from any other person, with a great sense of rigid ego boundaries and differentiation from others. Female personality is based on retention and continuation of relationships with others. Growing girls come to define and experience themselves as continuous with others, with more flexible ego boundaries. The basic feminine sense of self is connected to the world. The basic masculine sense of self is separate from the world. It is in the dichotomy between the feminine sense of attachment, cooperation, and caring and the masculine sense of detachment, fairness, and justice that we find most of the linguistic—and hence pedagogical—differences between females and males. Carol Gilligan, particularly in *Mapping the Moral Domain* (with Ward, Taylor, and Bardige, 1988), helps us to understand that the male emphasis on justice and rights does not necessarily meld well with our pedagogy of collaboration and cooperation, as seen in the feminist pedagogy that now dominates our teaching, particularly the teaching of writing.

In Chodorow's 1984 study on the sexual sociology of adult life, she shows that for girls as they develop in Western culture, "feminine identification . . . is predominantly *parental* [emphasis in original] and females tend to identify with aspects of their own mother's role, developing through their ongoing relationship with their mother's affective relationships to others" (361). "A boy, in order to feel himself adequately masculine, must distinguish and differentiate himself from others in a way that a girl need not—must categorize himself as someone apart. Moreover, he defines masculinity negatively as that which is not feminine and/or connected to women, rather than positively" (359). Because many boys in our cultures are raised in a home where the father is absent or not involved in their raising, except to reinforce stereotypes, they grow up with an unattainable, romantic cultural stereotype of masculinity. "Masculinity and the masculine roles are fantasized and idealized for boys . . . whereas femininity and the feminine role remain for a girl all too real and concrete" (361).

Carolyn Heilbrun (1974) has stated that ". . . our future salvation lies in a movement away from sexual polarization and the prison of gender toward a world in which individual roles and the modes of personal behavior can be freely chosen . . . Androgyny defines a condition under which the characteristics of the sexes, and the human impulses expressed by men and women, are not rigidly assigned. Androgyny seeks to liberate the individual from the confines of the appropriate. . . . Androgyny suggests a spirit of reconciliation between the sexes" (ix–x).

As Tavris and Wade have pointed out in their book, *The Longest War: Sex Differences in Perspective* (1984), ". . . years of instruction about the proper roles of male and female, and about the social consequences of stepping out of line, are enough to keep both sexes doing what feels most comfortable (even if what is most comfortable is least satisfying). We are optimistic that the alliance the sexes will forge on the far side of change will be stronger, and will make more people happier, than the uneasy compromises of the longest war" (356–57).

Gilligan argues that the interpersonal focus in their lives leads women to develop more relativistic reasoning, particularly in moral and intellectual situations which have interpersonal implications. When we teach writing, we are then continually dealing with these interpersonal implications.

"In adolescence, when thinking becomes more reflective and more self-conscious, moral orientation may become closely entwined with self-definition, so that the sense of self or feelings of personal integrity become aligned with a particular way of seeing or speaking" (Gilligan, *Mapping the Moral Domain*). Those of us who have taught junior high have seen this phenomenon. There is no male more macho than the junior high boy who can stand for hours in front of a mirror, testing ways to show his body, to turn his head, to smile, and to present himself. This boy knows that he must carry his books on his hips, not on his chest, in order to be a man. In the same context, there is no female more feminine than the junior high girl who can wear what appears to be pounds of make-up as she tries to decide what look will best make her look the way she is supposed to look—whatever that may be this week or this month. My favorite image of adolescence is a young person standing with a 360 degree magnifying mirror hanging from the head. No matter where that person looks, what is seen is the self reflected. This young person is saying, "Since I am so unsure of myself and of how I look and since I am so self-conscious about it, when I look at the world, I see myself reflected and, of course, the world is always then looking at me." This child/adult knows "This pimple is the largest in existence. Everyone knows that I have the ugliest glasses in the world. These shoes are going to make me the laughing-stock of the whole school."

Gilligan points out that adolescence is the time when thinking becomes self-consciously interpretive. At the same time, ". . . the interpretive schemes of the culture, including the system of social norms, values, and roles, impinge more directly on perception and judgment, defining within the framework of a given society what is 'the right way' to see and to feel and to think, the way 'we' think" (Gilligan, *Mapping the Moral Domain*).

Let me digress to point out that "self-conscious" can mean being painfully aware of yourself and how you look or act or how you fear others see you as looking or acting. "Self-conscious" can also refer to the need to become aware, to "raise your consciousness" in the sense of becoming aware of the influences on you. Flynn (1984) feels we must encourage students (she means females; I mean all students, female and male) to become self-consciously aware of what their experiences in the world have been and how these experiences relate to the politics of gender. "The capacity for detachment in adolescence . . . is double-edged. It signals an ability to think critically about thinking [meta-cognition] but also has a potential for becoming . . . 'self-centered'" (Gilligan, *Mapping the Moral Domain*).

When we look at the differences between how we raise and treat children outside the home and when we look at the influences from the media, from the school, and from society in general, we come to realize that there are gender differences in many aspects of language and how it works. We have used, from Kohlberg's descriptions of adolescent development through Perry's schemes of intellectual development in college-age students, a male-dominated model of how people think and reason. Kohlberg, in his 1981 book *The Philosophy of Moral Development* and in most of his writings, tells of how people develop morally, basing his presentation on studies of males. Kohlberg sees moral development as being toward an objective and universal system of values based on rights. This becomes what many see as "either/or" thinking. On all of Kohlberg's scales, females are behind males, rarely reaching the highest stages of moral development.

Perry, in *Forms of Intellectual and Ethical Development in the College Years* (1968) again worked with male subjects to come to the conclusion that college students go through periods of dualistic and relativistic thinking before they affirm that identity is a process that is ever-changing.

Gilligan, most particularly in her 1982 *In a Different Voice*, shows us through her research with female subjects that women advance intellectually and morally on a different scale, a scale that emphasizes contextuality and local judgments based on obligations. This becomes what many see as "both/and" thinking. Howard Gardner has addressed these differences in *Frames of Mind*, but even then he does not look at the socially induced gender differences that can occur in his seven forms of intelligence.

Having looked at the research from women's studies and from traditional psychology, let me shift to what I call a masculinist point of view (as opposed to a feminist point of view).

Osherson in his 1986 book *Finding Our Fathers: The Unfinished Business of Manhood* points out that "men's early and ongoing relationships with their fathers shape the intimacy and work dilemmas they face in coming of age today" (87). Research has shown us that boys at about the age of three—when the mother is having to push them away and when they are starting to have peer relationships and a sense of their own identities—are searching for masculine models. Between the ages of three and five, boys begin to withdraw from mothers and femininity, becoming quite stereotyped in their thinking about what it means to be 'like Daddy' and 'like Mommy.' Little boys begin to segregate by sex, to focus on rules rather than relationships, and to emphasize games of power, strength, and achievement. Eventually, they repress their wishes to be held, taken care of, and cuddled, the wish, as Osherson puts it, to "Burrow among women" (89).

If you have worked with preschool and primary kids, as I have, you have seen how this behavior plays itself out. When the kids go out to recess, the girls go to their play groups and immediately get into the play. The boys go off to the fields and spend most, if not all, of their time arguing about the rules. Another and most important point must be made here, however. When the boys go off to play their rule-bound games of strength and achievement, all of them get to play, as long as they are willing to acknowledge the hierarchy of who stands where in the pecking order. Girls do get into their play quickly and do play together well in their small groups, but their groups are exclusive and do not include or invite those not already in the group. The small cliques that girls form are held together with tenacity and strength; if a girl is not in the group, she is not only not invited in, but she can easily became the object of scorn for the rest in the group. Margaret Atwood treats this kind of behavior with devastating accuracy in her novel, *The Cat's Eye*.

In addition, we must look at the differentiation between boys and girls in their emphasis on the concepts of what caring and justice mean in their play groups. And finally, I would point out the differences in how boys and girls react when someone is hurt during play. For the boys, the game must go on, so the injured player is removed from the field and the play continues. For the girls, the game must stop so that all can help and show their concern about the injured player.

We have recently seen an increase in the direct involvement of males in the raising of children in our country. For many, this involvement is still not as great as needed. However, there is still a problem of both gender and race which manifests itself in school. As *Policy Review* pointed out, "Fifteen million American children, one quarter of the population under 18, are growing up today without fathers. A black child is three times as likely as a white child to live without a father. The percentage of black children living without fathers has soared from 17.7% in 1960 to 58.4% in 1988." The articles by Page, Holland, and Parham and McDavis in the bibliography deal with this particular problem and the varying solutions being looked at in Washington, D.C., Miami, and Minneapolis. Specifically, these articles face the problems of the young black male in our culture and how the schools might help to alleviate these problems. A current (Fall 1991) court case in Detroit about the legality of boys-only academies with an all male staff within the public school system illustrates a possible solution to this cultural and educational problem. We still must face the concomitant issues when finding institutional answers to social problems of race, gender, and culture.

Carol Gilligan's books, *Mastering the Moral Domain* and *Making Connections*, show us how these distinctions between the early childhood experiences of males and females manifest themselves in the identity of self that occurs in adolescence and thus in school.

Let me also point out that discrimination by gender occurs mainly outside the home, perhaps mostly in school. As Pfeiffer pointed out in 1985, mothers do little behavior stereotyping and appear to treat their own little boys and little girls the same. Fathers tend to treat their children in more gender-stereotyped ways during playtime, though we know that outside a minority of homes (those homes where both mother and father are present and active in the raising of the children), fathers have less influence on child raising and on creating the home environment. "Parents tend to have gender-based conceptions more often about other people's children than about their own" (Pfeiffer, np.). It is interesting to wonder how this relates to teachers' treatment of children.

Belenky, Clinchy, Goldberger, and Tarule, in their important book, *Women's Ways of Knowing: The Development of Self, Voice and Mind* (1986), show how females develop socially and morally, particularly through the interpersonal strengths they have developed from childhood. In contrast to Perry's emphasis on autonomy and independence and achievement, Belenky *et al.* show us how women see and talk about growth and relationships as based on trust. Men approach relationships as a task. Males emphasize autonomy and achievement and females emphasize attachment and intimacy.

This male emphasis on achievement becomes so pervasive in all aspects of life that Komarovsky, in her 1976 study, *Dilemmas of Masculinity*, shows how "social role strain" affects a considerable majority of the men she studied. Seventy-two percent of the men she studied showed stress in carrying out their sexual roles. As I pointed out in "Big Boys Don't Cry" (1976), sex for the men Komarovsky studied (college seniors) was clearly an obligation, a proficiency test in which they were supposed to get straight A's. Having an open relationship with a woman appeared to those male college seniors to be one of the highest and most elusive personal achievements possible.

In the bibliography at the end of this book, I have included a large number of texts which look at these issues of how children are taught their sex roles from a masculinist point of view. Balswick's *The Inexpressive Male*, Farrell's *Why Men are the Way They Are*, Garfinkel's *In a Man's World*, Abbott's *Men and Intimacy*, Gilmore's *Manhood in the Making: Cultural Concepts of Masculinity*, and Raphael's *The Men From the Boys: Rites of Passage in Male America* treat specific aspects of how males are conditioned and raised. If you have time to read only one book, I would recommend Stoltenberg's *Refusing to be a Man: Essays on Sex and Justice*. He deals specifically with the gender issues that adolescent males must face.

A Sociolinguistic Perspective

If we accept the premise that men and women differ in their relational capacities and in their moral and intellectual development and if we accept Gilligan's perception that such differences are gender related and not gender specific, then we can look directly at how gender influences language and social interaction patterns in our classroom.

Males and females are very different in how they see small groups operating. A fact of small group work in speech communication research is that males account for 96 percent of the interruptions. Males interrupt females three times as often as they interrupt other males, but they still do nearly all the interrupting that goes on (West and Zimmerman 1975). Fishman (1983) found that women do much more of the conversational "work" than do men. Women ask two and one-half times as many questions as men ask; women consistently provide supportive utterances (*uh huh*, *yeah*, *mmmm*), timed so they rarely overlap the statements of the other in the conversation. Men, conversely, pause longer when talking with women than they do when talking with other men (West and Zimmerman 1975). Men so clearly control topic choice by their conversation behavior that Fishman concludes (1983), "The definition of what is appropriate or inappropriate conversation becomes the man's choice."

Paula Wodak, the Polish psychologist, titled an article she did, reporting on gender differences in small groups, "Women Relate, Men Report."

Women and men talk and listen differently. Deborah Tannen has written two brilliant and important works in this area: *You Just Don't Understand* (1990) and *That's Not What I Meant* (1986). Through these best-selling books, as well as her research publications, Tannen has documented the differences in "genderlect" between males and females and how we fail to realize that our conversational behaviors reflect different assumptions—different and equally valid—about how people carry on conversations.

Men "report"—they generally have conversations in which one person imparts information in a style that demonstrates the independence of the speaker. For most men, there are unspoken but heavily inculcated rules about pauses, taking turns, and displaying knowledge.

If men report (as Tannen and Wodak have shown), then women, according to Tannen, "rapport" in their conversations. Women speak to explore and express the intimacy of the relationship. They speak with high involvement and constantly show support for conversational partners. Overlapping speech for women is not an attempt to gain control of the conversation because both players are on the same team and working toward the same goals. For men, the other in a conversation is not a member of the team and overlapping speech is most often an indication of a need to dominate the conversation.

Consider, for example, a conversation where a woman is describing a upsetting problem she is having. Typically, a female listener will react with sympathy and empathy for the problem. The typical male response is to offer a solution to the problem. It took me many years to learn from my best friend that when she was posing a problem or describing an upsetting situation, she was not seeking a solution or a reassurance that things weren't so bad ("You think that's bad. Let me tell you what happened to me when . . .").

So, men and women talk and listen differently. The give-and-take-turns conversations of males show this, for men tend not to listen to what is being said to them, as much as they are waiting to refute it. Men listen and respond in a "rights and justice" mode; women listen and respond in a "connecting and care" mode. Look at the conversational turns described above and you can see how these differences manifest themselves in everyday conversation. Our task here is to consider what these differences mean in our classrooms.

Gender Problems in the Classroom

My major concerns are that we are incorporating into our classrooms, without serious question of the gender implications, practices which are doomed to failure before they start because we have not looked at the gender and language implications of such pedagogy.

One such implication has to do with journals. Cinthia Gannett of the University of New Hampshire has been keeping records for years on her college freshmen and how they approach journals. She is finding that females write more than twice as many words in their journals as do males. Females often keep personal journals in addition to class journals. Few males do. In the content of their journals, males tend to use their journals primarily to plan and to vent, rarely discussing personal relationships or issues. Females often write extended, reflective and descriptive entries which weave together social, academic, and personal lives. Recently, Gannett has published her findings in *Gender and the Journal* (SUNY Press, 1991).

When Cinthia first asked me what I thought of when I heard the word "diary," I gave a stereotypic adolescent male reply: "Sissy girls' stuff!" Her question took me back to my early adolescence and to my remembered feelings about my younger sister's diary. Male students tend to see little difference between diaries and journals and are comfortable with neither. Cynthia Bowman's chapter is this book offers startling information on how pervasive these differences can be.

I had a interesting situation along these lines last year with a student of mine, a bright and sensitive "non-trad" (college slang for non-traditional). My non-trad was in a class with a colleague and friend next door at the office, Lisa McClure. When Lisa mentioned how much she enjoyed Brad's journals, especially when he reflected on my class and the commonalities between how the two of us teach, I was amazed. Brad wrote next to nothing for me.

Lisa and I talked with Brad, an affable man working his B. A. so he could teach high school English, about the differences in his journals for the two of us and asked him to reflect in his journals on why he seemed to write so differently for each of us. (We assured him that we hadn't swapped his journals and read them). In his journal for me, he wrote "I've been taught NOT to express my emotions and feelings, especially to another man. Maybe it's okay to a woman I'm close to (mother, friend, lover), but not to a stranger and never to a man. Most of what I wrote for you is a lie."

If we don't acknowledge the differences between how men and women see, use, and employ journals, if we don't look at the social history our students bring to us, such as all the baggage that goes with notions about diaries for a male, then we are not going to be getting what we hope from our students and we won't be using journals to their maximum value.

Another area of major concern is in the use of small groups—for peer evaluation, for discussion, for collaborative work, and for reading groups: all major approaches to teaching being espoused by most disciplines. The research reported in the last section clearly demonstrates how we have been ignoring what is known about the gender differences in conversation and interaction when we use small groups in our classrooms.

And if these differences in how we are enculturated to speak and listen in groups weren't enough going against small group work in the classroom, consider the place of and attitudes toward competition. The recent and growing research on collaboration in writing (see Lundsford and Ede) is making us aware that our emphasis on competition for grades and for "place" in the classroom may be operating against that which we hope to teach. Certainly, more and more of us are questioning whether the competitive model is the best for training our students and ourselves to get along in the world.

In journals, in small group work, in collaboration, and in the very act of reading our students' writing, we experience strong gender differences in language. From psychology and sociology, we are gaining greater understanding of the social dimensions of language in our classrooms. Finally, we are perhaps slowly changing as we realize how we use and are used by language.

Carol Gilligan, in *Mapping the Moral Domain*, tells a wonderful story: Two four-year-olds, a girl and a boy, were playing together and wanted to play different games. The girl said, "Let's play nextdoor neighbors."

"I want to play pirates," the boy replied.

"Okay," said the girl. "You be the pirate next door."

When we look at this story and realize its full implications, we can then better understand the gender differences in language. Our problem is how we can promote abstract thinking higher and order reasoning, as we most emphatically do when we teach English, and yet maintain and sustain human connections. We want to strengthen the ability to understand relationships between people and we must better understand those relationships as they are manifested in language. As long as we continue to burden ourselves with the metaphors of gender differences, with the myths and the baggage we carry from our childhoods, we give in to that way of thinking that has permeated Western thought: dichotomizing and splitting attributes of human behavior as one or the other, as male or female, as masculine or feminine. By this thinking, we have split and placed at opposite ends of continuums reason and emotion, thinking and feeling, public and private, political and personal, and objective and subjective. We can no longer afford to align these arbitrary divisions with equally arbitrary distinctions between male and female.

Works Cited

Alishio & Schilling. 1984. Sex differences in intellectual and ego development in late adolescence. *Journal of youth and adolescence.* 13 (3), 213–24.

Belenky, M., B. Clinchy, N. Goldberger, & J. Tarule. 1986. *Women's ways of knowing: The development of self, voice, and mind.* NY: Basic Books.

Chodorow, N. 1978. *The reproduction of mothering: Psychoanalysis and the sociology of gender.* Berkeley: U. of California P.

———. 1984. Gender personality and the sexual sociology of adult life. In Jaggar & Rothenberg, eds. 358–67. *Feminist frameworks.* NY: McGraw-Hill.

Flemming, 1988. New visions, new methods: The mainstreaming experience in retrospect. In Aiken et al., eds. *Changing our minds: Feminist transformations of knowledge.* Cambridge: Harvard UP.

Flynn, E. 1988. Composing as a woman. *College composition and communication.* 39 (4), 423–35.

Gardner, H. 1983. *Frames of mind: The theory of multiple intelligences.* NY: Basic Books.

Gilligan, C. 1982. *In a different voice: Psychological theory and women's development.* Cambridge, MA: Harvard UP.

Gilligan, C., N. Lyons, & T. Hanmer, eds. 1989. *Making connections: The relational world of adolescent girls at Emma Willard School*. Troy, NY: Emma Willard School.

Gilligan, C., J. Ward, J. Taylor, & B. Bardige. 1988. *Mapping the moral domain: The contributions of women's thinking to psychological theory and education*. Cambridge, MA: Harvard UP.

Heilbrun, C. 1974. *Toward a recognition of androgyny*. NY: Harper & Row.

Keller, K. 1985. *Reflections on gender and science*. New Haven, CT: Yale UP.

Komarovsky, M. 1976. *Dilemmas of masculinity*. NY: Norton.

Lakoff. G., & M. Johnson. 1980. *Metaphors we live by*. Chicago: U. of Chicago P.

Martin, J. 1985. *Reclaiming a conversation: The ideal of an educated woman*. New Haven, CT: Yale UP.

McConnell-Ginet, S. 1978. Intonation in a man's world. *Signs: Journal of women in cultures and society*. 3 (3), 541–54.

Osherson, P. 1986. *Finding our fathers: The unfinished business of manhood*. NY: Free press/MacMillan.

Pfeiffer. 1985. Girl talk-boy talk. *Science, '85*. Washington, DC: American Assn. for the Advancement of Science.

Smithson, I. 1990. Introduction: Investigating gender, power, and pedagogy. In Gabriel & Smithson, eds., 1–27. *Gender in the classroom: Power and pedagogy*. Urbana, IL: U. of Illinois P.

Spender, D. 1989. *The writing or the sex: Or why you don't have to read women's writing to know it's no good*. NY: Pergamon Press.

Tannen, D. 1986. *That's not what I meant! How conversational style makes or breaks your relations with others*. NY: Morrow.

———. 1990. *You just don't understand: Women and men in conversation*. NY: Morrow.

Vogel, N. 1990. Gender difference: Both/and, not either/or. In Moran & Penfield, eds. *Conversations: Contemporary critical theory and the teaching of English*. Urbana, IL: National Council of Teachers of English.

Wodak, P. 1981. Women relate, men report: Sex differences in language behavior in a therapeutic group. *Journal of pragmatics*, 5, 262–65.

Wolfram, W. 1991. *Dialects and American English*. NY: Prentice Hall.

3

He/Man and the Masters of Discourse

David Blakesley

For over twenty years now, educators, publishers, and writers of both sexes have argued for the use of nonsexist language.* In the mid-seventies, national organizations like NCTE, MLA, and APA adopted formal policies stating that, for instance, they "should encourage the use of nonsexist language, particularly through [their] publications and periodicals" ("NCTE Guidelines" 1). Many text-book publishers followed suit. Also in the seventies, researchers like Ann Bodine, Wendy Martyna, Janice Moulton, Julia [Stanley] Penelope, and Donald G. MacKay provided ample evidence that sexist uses of language—institutionalized by prescriptive grammarians in the eighteenth and nineteenth centuries—constituted "a major roadblock on the path toward a language that speaks clearly and fairly of both sexes" (Martyna 1983, 25).

Despite the many people committed to "Winning the Great *He/She* Battle" (Nilsen 1984, 151), the use of sexist language continues to present a problem for editors, teachers, and all those who believe that gender bias is a legitimate social concern. Efforts to purge our language of sexism have met with limited success for numerous reasons. Although many studies confirm that our language is gender-biased, rarely do any discuss how reform can be motivated, and when they do, they often make prescriptive pleas for gender-neutral language. Prescribing correct usage has rarely, if ever, induced widespread language reform. In the case of sexist language, it directs our attention to stylistic propriety,

* The author would like to thank Donald C. Freeman for his helpful suggestions on early drafts of this essay.

such as whether "personhole cover" is acceptable for "manhole cover," which merely trivializes the very serious conditions that merit change in the first place. Arguments over euphony and clumsy locutions obscure the larger issue of gender equality. Another reason for the lack of reform derives from confusion over whether sexist language is a symptom or the cause of gender inequity. On the one hand, it is symptomatic of widespread cultural bias. On the other hand, people who use it, consciously or not, reinforce the attitudes being challenged.

I want to argue that people will use nonsexist language only after they identify with the compelling social reasons for doing so, and coaching this identification requires patient, sustained dialogue on gender as well as stylistic issues. Because of the volatility of gender issues, teachers of English should remain aware of, in Dale M. Bauer's words, "the rhetorical situation of the classroom—of the necessity for a mastery that is not oppressive, of an authoritative voice that is not the only authority" (1990, 395). Resistance to sexist language issues will arise in the writing classroom and should not be silenced, but interpreted and continually challenged by class dialogue. Enforcing the use of nonsexist language by executive decree merely nurtures resistance toward a critique of language usage and attitudes in question. Teachers, if they hope to rid the language of sexism, should explore gender issues with their students and invite them to choose how they want to relate to their world, not theoretically, but practically, in their writing and speaking.

Originally, proponents of language change in the seventies meant to foster greater sensitivity to the ways in which sexist language determines *and* reflects cultural practices. The writing classroom was an obvious place for this consciousness raising to occur. In 1975 NCTE's published guidelines told us:

> The dramatic changes in language now taking place pose a special challenge to NCTE members and staff. Whether the members work as teachers, authors, or editors, they not only help shape students' language patterns but are also viewed by the public as custodians of what is 'correct' in the language. The very newness of these changes offers English teachers a unique opportunity. Under their guidance, eliminating sexism can bring a new vitality to the English language. (7)

In these early stages of reform, teachers were asked to "shape" and "guide" students' language patterns, but the pedagogical means were vague and the challenge greater than some had first thought. Many handbooks, to their credit, now include nonsexist usage guidelines, but their presentations of the problem itself are so innocuous that few students realize its relevance to their writing, let alone their lives.

Research and experience (my own and that of others) confirms that sexist usage has not diminished, that the general public, aspiring authors in our profession, and students in English classes have not been persuaded to use nonsexist language when they speak and write. The "special challenge" posed by NCTE and others to eliminate sexism has unfortunately not been met, despite many convincing arguments by language theorists and the vitality of gender studies in academia.

The reasons for this lack of reform are complex and numerous. They include, for instance, a failure to distinguish between "prescriptive" and "descriptive" grammars. Prescriptive grammars try to legislate usage by establishing guidelines for writing standard English "clearly," which supposedly displays intellectual prowess. In the eighteenth century, prescriptive grammarians systematically defined "correct" grammar, which included the use of *he* and *man* as gender neutral terms. Much of what is today considered proper grammar arose from arbitrary (and sexist) conventions of usage. Descriptive grammars, however, explain how language is acquired, used, and understood by people, not necessarily by those people deemed masters of discourse. Numerous descriptive grammars now demonstrate that when people use *he* and *man* "generically," for instance, they do not always mean to include women in the reference, and even when they do, their readers may not. After two centuries of prescription, people have persuaded themselves that intended meaning equals real meaning. Other reasons for the lack of reform include conscious resistance by the media, especially conservative, "pop" language commentators, and the polemics of grammarians and teachers who perpetuate the conceptual traps of sexist language by not considering the impact their rhetoric has on people they hope to influence.

As teachers of English, we should be aware of how each of these patterns of resistance affects teaching. Because we often aren't, many students—women and men—perceive the issue of nonsexist usage as a threat, a private assault on gender identification, and then dismiss the issue as "feminist propaganda." Taught prescriptively, without considering the feminist critiques they derive from, guidelines for nonsexist usage are perceived as weapons for teachers to use in pointing out errors in student writing and thinking. As Alleen Pace Nilsen wrote in 1984, "It is not the role of English teachers to insist, or even request, that their students use sex-fair language. But English teachers do have an obligation to inform students of the controversy" (153). The controversy ranges far afield, reaching into the lives of individuals who, sympathetic or not, must decide how they want their words to be received.

Do college writers use and have they been taught (or told) to use nonsexist language? Jinni Harrigan and Karen Lucic's research (1988) demonstrates that students use nonsexist language infrequently and reluctantly; students also report that encouragement by faculty to use nonsexist language is unpersuasive (139). In my own study, I asked sixty male and female students to respond to a questionnaire that measured their tendency to use, for example, *he* when referring to generic antecedents, and asked them to recall whether they had been taught to use nonsexist language when they write (see Appendix). The first part of the questionnaire consisted of completion tests, such as "Before a judge can give a final ruling, ______," and "Everybody did ______ best." The completion test section replicates research described by Wendy Martyna in "What Does 'He' Mean? Use of the Generic Masculine" (1978). In her attempt to construct an accurate "descriptive grammar," Martyna studied the extent to which college students used "he" to refer to generic nouns and, further, how they comprehend the generic masculine when used in a clearly generic context, e.g., "When someone is near a hospital, he should be quiet." Discussing her findings in "Beyond the He/Man Approach: The Case for Nonsexist Language" (1980), she concludes that there are "striking sex differences in both the use and understanding of the generic masculine" (1983, 31). Martyna's findings confirm that the generic masculine often does exclude women. My questionnaire also included questions about the acceptability of certain pronouns in a given context and the generic use of *man*. The last section surveyed the respondent's background. I should emphasize that my purpose was not to demonstrate that, for instance, *he* used generically is sexist; Martyna's study demonstrates that it is. Rather, my aim was to demonstrate that the pleas of English teachers to use nonsexist language have for the most part neither worked nor been heard.

The completion test results show that both men and women tend to use the masculine pronoun to refer to a generic noun, *unless* the noun was stereotypically female-related. For instance, women completed the phrase, "Before a judge can give a final ruling ______," with *he* in 94 percent of the cases in which a pronoun was used. Men used the masculine pronoun 90 percent of the time. Women completed the phrase, "Once a secretary makes coffee ______," with *she* in 81 percent of the cases; men, 92 percent. These results were consistent with all responses to this section of the questionnaire.

The other completion test measured whether or not respondents would abide by the prescription that a singular pronoun should be used when the antecedent is an indefinite pronoun, such as *everybody*, in which case they would use the singular *he*, *his*, *she*, or *her* or the nonsexist form *her or she* or *his or her*. When the respondents did not use *they* or *them*, women showed a greater tendency to use nonsexist forms. For instance, the sentence, "Everyone should hand in ______ test," was completed with *their* by 42 percent of the women and 67 percent of the men. When they didn't use *their*, men used *his* in *every* case. Women, however, used *his or her* in 25 percent of the cases in which they did not use *their*. These results confirm what Martyna's study showed—that women use nonsexist forms more frequently than men—and also that both men and women use the third-person plural pronoun to refer to indefinite pronouns. Whether students use the plural pronoun to avoid nonsexist usage or because they reject or do not know of the "rule" concerning agreement remains unclear. (Ann Bodine's research [1975] has shown that the agreement argument of nineteenth-century prescriptive grammarians continues to be ignored, even in much published writing.)

Finally, respondents were asked whether they had been told to use nonsexist language when they write. Half of the men reported that they recalled having been told. All but one of the women reported that they *had not* been told. The disparity here is odd—men, though they rarely use nonsexist language, have heard of it, while women, who use it slightly more often, say they haven't. It may be that for men, being told to use nonsexist language generates resistance; they may simply associate their awareness of the problem of sexism in our culture with having been told to use nonsexist language. Women, and Martyna's research (1978) confirms this, use nonsexist language not merely as a consequence of having been taught it, but because they experience sexism repeatedly. Whatever the reason, the overwhelming fact is that few college students, women or men, use nonsexist language, and most claim they have never been told to.

My own experience as a teacher and journal editor tells me that more advanced writers—graduate students and professionals—continue to use sexist language when they write. As a teacher I have confronted the problem far too often in graduate seminars. As an editor I found that at least half of the submissions I reviewed contained sexist language. And, sadly, I frequently had to invoke the oft announced right to edit essays so that they conformed with published guidelines for the use of nonsexist language. In 1984 Nilsen reported a similar experience. At the time, one-third of all the articles published in the *English Journal* had to be changed to eliminate sexist usage, even though the journal had formally censured such usage since the mid-seventies (152). The habit of using sexist language in our early years is not easily broken.

People react slowly, if at all, to pleas for widespread language reform. The history of the English pronoun's development shows the change in language happens slowly, seemingly as a result of cultural forces we do not fully understand. Albert C. Baugh and Thomas Cable describe the failures of eighteenth-century grammarians to institute new rules of usage:

> They did not realize, or refused to acknowledge, that changes in language often appear to be capricious and unreasonable—in other words, are the result of forces too complex to be fully analyzed or predicted. Accordingly, they approached most questions in the belief that they could be solved by logic and that the solutions could be imposed upon the world by authoritative decree. (1978, 285)

Prescriptive grammarians in the eighteenth and nineteenth centuries tried to dampen structural changes in English by legislating correctness. Grammar, the formal structure of a language, came to mean "proper usage." As Lindlay Murray describes it in 1826, "English grammar is the art of speaking and writing the English language with propriety" (11).

One structural change bearing directly on the *he/man* issue arises from the shift in English from grammatical gender to natural gender, which was a major structural change in the language. The decay of inflections in Middle English resulted in the elimination of grammatical gender, doubtlessly before 1500, so that the use of *he*, *she*, and *it* depended upon the categorization of nouns as male, female, or inanimate. With the disappearance of grammatical gender, sex became the only factor in determining the gender of English nouns (Baugh and Cable 166). Following this event was the development of a new pronoun reference system in the sixteenth century. *Thou*, *thy*, and *thee* fell into disuse, *you* was substituted for *ye*, and *its* was accepted as the neuter form of the possessive pronoun (Baugh and Cable 1978, 242). Likewise, the Old English *hit*, *his*, *him*, *hit*—originally neuter—evolved into the Middle English *it*, *his*, *it*. *His* retained its status as a neuter pronoun (243). The Old English personal pronoun had forms for practically all genders, persons, and cases (58). But the shift to natural gender in Modern English led to a more gender-specific system of pronoun reference. Instead of using pronouns to replace nouns whose grammatical gender was unambiguous, "meaning came to be the determining factor in the gender of nouns, and all lifeless objects were thought of as neuter" (243). The loss of gender-specific inflections on nouns had led to the use of meaning as the basis for assigning nouns natural gender. All these changes occurred over a relatively long period of time and without conscious intervention by prescriptive grammarians to guide the change.

Over time and partly due to prescriptive grammarians, nouns were assigned gender based on cultural stereotypes. In 1826, for instance, Lindley Murray endorsed the use of suffixes like *-ess* to mark nouns as female, then argued that

> when we say of a woman, she is a philosopher, an astronomer, a builder, a weaver, we perceive an impropriety in the termination,

> which we cannot avoid, but we can say that she is a botanist, a student, a witness, a scholar, an orphan, a companion, because these terminations have not annexed to them the notion of sex. (36)

Murray's *English Grammar* poses as a "description" of the current state of English, but at the same time, because of the use teachers and students made of his text, descriptions like the following established precedent:

> Figuratively, in the English tongue, we commonly give the masculine gender to nouns which are conspicuous for the attributes of imparting or communicating, and which are by nature strong and efficacious. Those, again, are made feminine which are conspicuous for the attributes of containing or bringing forth, or which are beautiful or amiable. (35; also quoted in Penelope 1978, 803)

Assigning nouns natural gender based on sex-role stereotypes resulted from the habits of using gender-specific pronouns to refer to abstract nouns, a practice which stigmatized both sexes and belied the fact that English had natural gender, which all grammarians admitted. Although the practice arose as a result of social stereotypes that might one day change, grammarians retarded such change by making convention the rule. The student was told to adhere to convention in the interest of "perspicuity". The irony is that we now know that sexist language is not perspicuous, that when people use *he* or *man* generically they confuse us by not realizing that when we read *he*, for example, we do not always include women, even though the antecedent noun includes both men and women. People who resist nonsexist usage reform with appeals to correctness believe that its proponents wish to tinker with the grammatical structure of English. This appeal has little merit, however, because nonsexist usage guidelines challenge only those conventions that exclude people from the context of reference. If the aim is to teach students to write clearly, to write what they mean, teachers should help students realize that it will no longer do to stereotype or exclude people by using pronouns indiscriminately.

The most active opponents of nonsexist usage advertise themselves as language purists and view usage change as a threat not only to the integrity of English, but also to the American way of life. The most common objection is that language is a neutral tool, that words are less important than things. If there is indeed social inequity, society is the real cause, and people should spend more time trying to solve social problems than quibbling about something as esoteric as pronoun usage. This argument is not a new one. In *Rudiments of English Grammar* (1761) Joseph Priestley stated his distaste for narrow arguments over usage:

> We have infinitely greater things before us; and if these gain their due share of our attention, this subject, of grammatical criticism, will be almost nothing. The noise that is made about it, is one of the greatest marks of the frivolism of many readers and writers too, of the present age. (qtd. in Baugh and Cable 277)

Priestley mainly objected to the practice of grammarians who, citing proper uses of English, condemned even accomplished writers for disobeying rules that were, in Priestley's view, unnecessarily prescriptive. Many modern grammarians persist in this practice of stabilizing rules of usage that should neither be fixed nor considered universal.

Martyna (1980) has shown that the news media frequently portray the issue as "amusingly insignificant" (27). For a recent example, we have only to recall the attention paid to the efforts by the Sacramento, California, City Council to solicit nonsexist alternatives to *manhole cover*. The media's coverage of the incident tapped the resentment people have for "making a big deal out of nothing," which politicians are renowned for doing. Such incidents are numerous. (Casey Miller and Kate Swift have collected many of them in *The Handbook of Nonsexist Writing* [1980].) One way to silence or trivialize the issue of gender equality is to deflect attention to issues of usage and prescriptive attempts to regulate it, which only reminds people of muddling through writing courses in which comma splices constituted moral depravity. As English teachers, we need to be aware that the limited exposure our students have had to the issue of sexist language probably comes from popular representations of it in the media.

In addition to trivialization by the media, "pop" language commentators persistently refuse to take the issue seriously. In *New Words for Old* Philip Howard displays the common response, typifying both the tendency to depoliticize the issue of sexism and mock those who consider it an important problem:

> Such nonsense as chairpersons, or the proscription of mankind (to be replaced by personkind?), or the invention of an artificial neuter singular pronoun to avoid having a masculine pronoun doing duty for both sexes is not just loony, but also mischievous. It is loony, because, as the lawyers engagingly put it, in such cases the masculine embraces the feminine. . . . While the lunatic fringe of Women's Liberation strain at such semantic gnats as neuter pronouns, it swallows the whole male chauvinist camel of real injustice to women. . . . Injustice exists in real life, not in dictionaries. (1977, 94–5)

The central point here—that "the masculine embraces the feminine"—is arguable, but Howard surrounds it with words that make it appear uncontestable. He describes those who do contest it as "loony," "mischievous," "a lunatic fringe." Then, once he has dismissed the issue, he moves to higher ground: "Injustice exists in real life. . . ." The rhetoric here is representative of many such arguments against nonsexist usage. First, the issue itself has already been settled, so its not worth fretting over. Second, those who contest it are feminist propagandists. Third, language is a neutral tool. Fourth, we have more serious matters to contend with than questions of usage. All of these assumptions, having been repeated so often, masquerade as common sense, and because they do, many students likely believe them. As teachers, we have to realize that asking students to critique common sense requires rhetorical savvy. The idea that the masculine "embraces" the feminine has to be made a contestable issue, which means exposing students to situations when the masculine excludes the feminine. Students must also learn that feminism itself is a means of critiquing how and why people are "placed" in the world according to gender. The belief that language is a neutral tool—that we use words, words don't use us—is so deeply ingrained in our consciousness that undermining the assumption is extremely difficult. Doing so requires sustained discussion of the ways people view the world through and with language, and how it is possible to name the world in more, or less, liberating ways. The final assumption, that we have more important matters to deal with, must be exposed as a form of socialization that represses rather than liberates social critique.

Arguments against nonsexist usage are political because they seek to incorporate difference into a centralized, patriarchal discourse. One side believes it has a legitimate argument with political consequences, the other side calls the whole business silly. William E. Connolly points out that efforts to remove contestability from the terms of political inquiry sterilizes conceptual analysis. These efforts appear

> either as a desire to rationalize public life, placing a set of ambiguities and contestable orientations under the control of a settled system of understandings and priorities, or as a quest to moralize public life thoroughly, bringing all citizens under the control of a consensus which makes politics marginal and unimportant. (1983, 139)

Pleas for nonsexist usage are politically motivated, clearly. Arguments against it are equally political, but these politics are denied in the interest of preserving the illusion of neutrality and protecting allegiances that already exist. The task for proponents of nonsexist usage is to help people understand and critique consensus politics, which preserves and fortifies sexist language. People will begin to use nonsexist language only after ideological critique helps them break down the hierarchies implicit in the culture's patriarchal unconscious. Until then, we should expect that guidelines for nonsexist usage will remain unobserved.

Feminist critiques expose the social hierarchy that normalizes inequity, but they also aim to construct through dialogue an alternative consciousness, helping people to describe and understand their experience in new ways. One problem, however, has been that in seeking to displace patriarchal thought, some feminist critiques slip too readily into the mode of discourse that sustains and validates patriarchal thinking. As Elaine Showalter puts it, "[f]eminist criticism has worried too much already . . . about communicating with the white fathers, even at the price of translating its findings into the warp of their obscure critical languages" (1987, 119). It is useful to bear in mind that forms of critical writing condition attitudes toward knowledge and experience that may undermine innovative perspectives and valuable scholarship. Mainstream critical discourse, says Olivia Frey (1990), seeks to "get it right," to establish cognitive authority (509). This quest for power has traditionally sought to regulate knowledge and reserve it for those who can successfully speak the discourse of domination. The question I want to address is whether polemic is the best means of persuading people that sexist language is unfair to both sexes. In fact, I want to argue with Frey and others that conventional critical discourse undermines the values and attitudes necessary for changing the minds of those who already view feminism as threatening and nonsexist language reform as trivial. Patriarchal rhetoric serves well those who want to anesthetize doubt, but it does not serve well those who wish to cultivate it.

Julia Penelope's *Speaking Freely: Unlearning the Lies of the Fathers' Tongues* (1990) exemplifies the anger and resentment that fueled the feminist critiques of the early seventies. On the one hand, her book is an impressive historical study of the ways in which the structure of English controls the way women think and act. "Most women," she writes "remain mostly unconscious of how English forces us to repeat the structures that deny us stature and agency in the world and of the role of language in our oppression" (xiv). These structures need to be studied, and the ways in which they act to preserve what Penelope playfully calls PUD (Patriarchal Universe of Discourse) need to be elaborated if we are to fully understand how thoroughly English cultivates sexism. Penelope is writing to women who feel they have been trapped in a male-dominated universe and who remain trapped because they have learned to be passive. She hopes to persuade women to seize the power traditionally reserved for men. She concludes that in the interest of conceptual exploration and restructuring "we [women] will have to improve our ability to use the structures of PUD in our dealings with men. That is we must become better liars, better verbal acrobats, in order to sustain ourselves in the world as men have made it" (235).

What is most troubling about Penelope's book is her willingness to use the structures of PUD in her dealings with women, as well as men, which makes us wonder who she is really writing to. Early in the book, she speaks for men when she says that "men perceive both language and women as property that they have the right to control and restrain and the obligation to protect" (xv). In the same vein, she writes, "Because being a woman is the worst thing men can think of, we are most accessible to insult and the basis of men's worst insults" (xiii). Some men may indeed think as Penelope claims they do, but this early in the book, the generalizations she makes are so offensive to men and women that I'm convinced she is writing to those people who already share her anger and resentment and thus feel the need to displace personal demons onto others. Such a rhetorical stance will only strengthen the resolve of those people who share her view. Those who don't, or those who haven't made up their minds, will remain either unconvinced or will, worse yet, turn against the issue.

Surely the structures of English do unfairly categorize both sexes, yet these structures are not limited to the linguistic sort Penelope understands so well. When she speaks of language she speaks as a linguist. Her concerns are syntactic processes, lexical cohesion, semantics, grammar, etc. It is surprising that, given her aim of identifying "immediately and *in context* uses of language that are dishonest, misleading, and manipulative" (xxxiii), she ignores some of the more common and oppressive devices of rhetoric, especially those that valorize authority and equate power with knowledge. For instance, to rally support and unify her readers, Penelope needs a scapegoat or sacrifice and, not surprisingly, she chooses men. At the same time, however, she wants to distance herself and women in general from the discourse of mastery that patriarchy values. Her desire for mastery and need of a sacrifice mirrors a symbolic order that must be challenged and transformed before people will begin to understand its limitations. Penelope calls this order PUD and cites the need to master it for the sake of conversion, even though its affects—exclusion and alienation—are what she resents most. All this adds up to the likelihood that her argument on behalf of nonsexist usage will not speak to those who need to listen.

There are ways of discussing nonsexist language that encourage inquiry rather than enmity, and we would be wise to enact them. In "The Other 'F' Word: The Feminist in the Classroom," Dale M. Bauer points out that "[r]ather than opposing the public and private voices or opposing masculine and feminine, we need to see how to negotiate that opposition in order to speak a multiplicity of voices into the cultural dialogue" (388). Her argument rests on the idea that "the classroom is a place to explore resistances and identifications, a place also to explore the ambiguous and often ambivalent space of ethics" (387). Students, like all people, must deal with a range of possible identifications, and can, when made aware of them, learn to pick and choose, to recognize the feminist voice as one means of challenging patriarchal systems of authority. There will be resistance to this feminist voice, and teachers need to realize that some students will refuse to acknowledge having become spokespersons for the patriarchal system that oppresses them. We can, however, try to demonstrate to students ways in which we subject ourselves to various means of placement and show them that we, too, struggle with positions that compete for our allegiance. To be convincing, we'll have to be honest and willing to talk with students about alternative identifications. Students do realize, I think, that they are often forced in school to extinguish their ambivalence about who they are and what they want to be. The difficulty they face is in acquiring perspectives and terminologies that make these multiple identities explicit and subject to critique.

To convert the classroom into a forum for exploring ways in which gender places us, I encourage students to compose dialogues representing various perspectives on particular issues they find important. (The process is fully described in William A. Covino's *Forms of Wondering: A Dialogue on Writing for Writers* [1990].) Briefly, the aim of such dialogues is not to resolve an issue, but to demonstrate its complexity by placing differing explanations in opposition. Students may explore an issue, for instance, from the perspectives of a feminist, a politician, an administrator, a teacher, a particular writer, a parent, a friend, and so on. Dialogue requires composing the voices of different perspectives and possessing them, and lets students feel firsthand the possibilities and limitations of assuming particular stances. Because I want my students to explore ways in which gender places us, class discussion focuses on issues that make gender differences explicit. Students learn that they perceive and construct reality through language, and they begin to appreciate the complexity of gender issues, an idea patriarchal rhetoric has traditionally sought to simplify or extinguish.

A dialogic classroom can make students more receptive to arguments on behalf of nonsexist usage. The words we choose define us, and once we realize that we do have choices, we're more likely to challenge received ways of speaking and writing. When we realize we may have been using the words of others without reflection, we're more apt to change our ways for the sake of equity, which is, ideally, what democracy should encourage.

In "Women and Writing: A Re/turn" (1990), Elizabeth Meese argues persuasively that "we have come to regard the matter of complicity with respect to power/knowledge more complexly, so that clear, 'pure' expressions of outrage are now more difficult to forge" (375). Indeed, they are not only more difficult to forge, they have become less and less persuasive in regard to the issue of sexist language. If we hope to see nonsexist usage become the norm, we will have to move beyond insisting or requesting that students obey the rules or else.

Questionnaire

Your responses to the following prompts will remain anonymous and will help a researcher study the writing habits of college students. To complete the questionnaire, please move quickly from beginning to end and do not go back to change any responses. Thank you for your cooperation.

Age of Respondent ___________ Circle one: female male

Class standing ______________

Please finish the following sentence openers with endings of your own.

When a teacher begins class, ________________________________
____.

Before a judge can give a final ruling, _________________________
____.

Once a secretary makes coffee, _____________________________
____.

Even though the coach was respected, _______________________
____.

The professor's book was accepted for publication, so __________
____.

***

Use a pronoun to complete the following:

Everyone should hand in ______ test.
None of the students would admit that _________ cheated.
Everybody did ______ best.
No egotist will voluntarily criticize _____________.
Since everyone in the room spoke Sanskrit, I addressed _________ in that language.

The phrase, "All men are created equal" includes

	True	*False*
any man	____	____
any woman	____	____
all people	____	____

Read the following phrase, then check the appropriate space:
"All men are mortal"

	yes	*no*
Refers to 1) women only	____	____
2) men only	____	____
3) all people	____	____

***

Read the following sentence, then decide which pronouns will make the sentence acceptable.

If a college student wants to succeed, ________ must study hard.

	Acceptable?	
	yes	*no*
"he"	____	____
"they"	____	____
"he or she"	____	____
"she"	____	____
"it"	____	____
"s/he"	____	____

***

Read the following sequence of sentences, then decide for yourself whether you think the sequence is acceptable. Check the appropriate box.

	Acceptable?	
	yes	*no*
1) All men are mortal. Socrates is a man. Therefore, Socrates is mortal.	____	____
2) All men are mortal. Sophia is a woman. Therefore, Sophia is mortal.	____	____
3) All men are mortal. Sophia is a man. Therefore, Sophia is mortal.	____	____

Read the following sentence, then answer true or false.

Any writer who tries her hardest will be successful.

	True	*False*
Refers to 1) any male writer	____	____
2) any female writer	____	____
3) all writers	____	____

***

1. When you write a paper do you always use "he" to refer to a "hypothetical" person or to humanity in general? ______ yes ______ no
   If you answered no, do you ever use "she" to refer to a hypothetical person? ______ yes ______ no
2. Have you ever been told to use any of the following forms of pronouns in your writing?

	yes	*no*
"he or she" instead of "he"	____	____
"he/she" instead of "he"	____	____
"s/he" instead of "he"	____	____

"his or hers" instead of "his" ____ ____

3. Have you been told to avoid using "they" or "their" when referring to singular pronouns like "anybody" and "everyone"? ____ yes ____ no

4. Have you been told to use nonsexist language when you write?
______ yes ______ no If yes, when? __________
If yes, at what level of schooling? __________
If yes, were you told by a writing teacher? __________
If yes, was your teacher a male or a female __________

That concludes this study. Thank you for your time.

Works Cited

Bauer, Dale M. 1990. "The Other 'F' Word: The Feminist in the Classroom." *College English* 52: 385–96.

Baugh, Albert C., and Thomas Cable. 1978. *A History of the English Language*. 3rd ed. Englewood Cliffs, NJ: Prentice-Hall.

Bodine, Ann. 1975. "Androcentrism in Prescriptive Grammar: Singular 'They,' Sex-Indefinite 'He,' and 'He or She.'" *Language in Society* 4: 129–46.

Connolly, William E. 1983. *The Terms of Political Discourse*. Princeton, NJ: Princeton UP. 213–247. Rpt. as "The Politics of Discourse." *Language as Politics*. Ed. Michael Shapiro, 139–67. New York: New York UP, 1984.

Covino, William A. 1990. *Forms of Wondering: A Dialogue on Writing for Writers*. Portsmouth, NH: Boynton/Cook.

Frey, Olivia. 1990. "Beyond Literary Darwinism: Women's Voices and Critical Discourse." *College English* 52: 507–526.

Harrigan, Jinni A., and Karen S. Lucic. 1988. "Attitudes About Gender Bias in Language: A Reevaluation." *Sex Roles* 19: 129–40.

Howard, Philip. 1977. *New Words for Old*. New York: Oxford UP.

MacKay, Donald G. 1983. "Prescriptive Grammar and the Pronoun Problem." In *Language, Gender and Society*. Eds. Barrie Thorne, et al, 38–53. Rowley, MA: Newbury.

Martyna, Wendy. 1978. "What Does 'He' Mean? Use of the Generic Masculine." *Journal of Communication* 28: 131–38.

———. 1983. "Beyond the He/Man Approach: The Case for Nonsexist Language." In *Language, Gender and Society*. Eds. Barrie Thorne, *et al*, 25–37. Rowley, MA: Newbury.

Meese, Elizabeth. 1990. "Women and Writing: A Re/turn." *College English* 52: 375–76.

Moulton, Janice. 1981. "The Myth of the Neutral Man." *Sexist Language: A Modern Philosophical Analysis*. Ed. Mary Vetterling-Braggin, 100–15. Totowa, NJ: Rowman and Littlefield.

Murray, Lindley. 1826. *English Grammar*. New York.

NCTE. 1975. "Guidelines for Nonsexist Use of Language in NCTE Publications." Urbana, IL: NCTE.

Nilsen, Alleen Pace. 1984. "Winning the Great *He/She* Battle." *College English* 46: 151–57.

Penelope, Julia. 1990. *Speaking Freely: Unlearning the Lies of the Fathers' Tongues*. New York: Pergamon.

———, [Stanley]. 1978. "Sexist Grammar." *College English* 39: 800–11.

Priestley, Joseph. 1971. *Rudiments of English Grammar*. 1761. New York: Garland.

Showalter, Elaine. 1987. "Critical Cross-Dressing: Male Feminists and the Woman of the Year." In *Men in Feminism*. Eds. Alice Jardine and Paul Smith, 116–32. New York: Methuen.

4

Language Activities That Promote Gender Fairness

Lisa J. McClure

As the first two chapters in this book indicate, language is a primary factor through which gender biases are explicitly and implicitly perpetuated. However, most of us are often unaware that our language reflects our thinking. In fact, students inundated with popular culture that perpetuates traditional views are often unaware that there are imbalances or that such imbalances are destructive. When asked, for example, to modify their use of the so-called generic "he," many students, male and female, respond with "Doesn't 'he' mean both 'he' and 'she'?" Some male students will almost belligerently retort, "I mean 'he'!" Of initial primary importance, then, is the recognition that imbalances do indeed exist and that language is a carrier of those imbalances. Students who do not recognize the imbalances will continue them. Thus, an exploration of gender issues in language is an avenue for teaching students both about gender fairness and about language.

Language study is a large part of many public school curriculums. Although much of that study occurs in the form of grammar exercises, more and more teachers are beginning to put the study of grammar into a new perspective for themselves and others, and many are beginning to help students improve their language skills through an exploration of language rather than the mere practicing of it. Essentially, students become ethnographers, collecting samples of the language around them and analyzing it, thus exploring how language functions in context. Furthermore, some teachers are choosing anthologies or readers which include readings to help students develop an awareness of language and the crucial role it plays in their lives.[1] In this way, they are practicing many language skills while learning more about language itself. The sequence of activities presented here is intended first to lead students through an exploration of how men and women use language alike and differently and then to analyze those likenesses and differences in order to better understand how sexist language and stereotyping, among other types of language biases, affect their thinking and their lives. Nevertheless, these activities can be used individually as well as sequentially, in whole or in part, as they are or in variations.

Students could begin their exploration of gender issues in language with study of language as it is used in their school and community. They first collect samples of language, both in isolation and in conversation. Students could collect samples of men talking to men, women to women, women and men talking to one another, and women talking to themselves and men talking to themselves. Conversations from school could include male teachers and female students, female teachers and male students, male and female teachers talking together, and female and male students talking together. Conversations in the community could involve older people talking to younger people of like or different genders, parents of like or different genders talking to their children, and community leaders talking to groups of like or different genders. Monologues and dialogues could be taped and the tapes transcribed by students. Students collecting the taped samples should also keep a log or journal noting non-verbal behavior such as arm movements and facial expressions of both speakers and non-speakers; additionally, they should make notes of speech and voice qualities. They could then analyze the data they've collected according to topics, language used, amount of time talking (i.e., turn-taking) versus perception of amount of time talking, voice, body language, and so on.

Turn-taking and interruptions in conversations among groups of like and different genders provide an especially enlightening discussion. Much research has been done in this area (see articles or books such as those by Spender, Pfeiffer, and West and Zimmerman).[2] In *Man Made Language* (1980), Dale Spender notes, for example, that women often perceive themselves as talking more than they actually do. Another interesting issue to raise would be the now quoted "men report, women relate" characterization of men and women in conversation; students could develop a method by which they would analyze the conversations they've taped according to statements which represent "reporting" and those which represent "relating." Selections from Tannen's *You Just Don't Understand* (1990) would provide informative and humorous reading for this discussion. If students are interested in group dynamics among their age group, they could explore how adolescents interact in groups of like and mixed genders (see, for example, Aries, Eckert, and Eder). Finally, students might explore the interactive relationships of parents and children by analyzing their conversations with their parents and other adults at school and in the community (see Philips, Thorne, and Greif). Regardless of which aspect of conversation they decide to focus on at this time, students should begin making lists of similarities and differences in female and male use of language in the various contexts; they may even want to make some tentative generalization or hypotheses about men's talk and women's talk.

Students could then collect samples from their reading material. (If collecting samples from the school and community is too cumbersome or represents a threat to some people in the community, teachers may wish to begin with this activity.) Students might initiate this search by compiling a simple tally of male and female authors in their literature anthology, perhaps categorizing them further according to genre or mode of discourse. Then, they could collect samples of the language authors used in the various genres or modes; e.g., they could collect samples from narratives written by men and by women, or they could collect samples of introductions to essays written by women and by men. While the earlier investigations were into the likenesses and differences in female and male languages in conversation, here students are looking at the written languages of women and men. They might explore such question as: Do men and women structure sentences differently? Do women and men use different vocabularies or the same vocabularies in different ways? Do female essayists use language in the same way male essayists do? What language do men use to portray the women in their texts, and what language do women use to portray men in their texts? They might even look at the conversations between female and male characters in the text and compare them to the real-life samples they collected earlier. Do female authors seem to represent men accurately in the conversations of male characters in their texts? Do male authors represent women accurately? At this time, students could add to their list of likenesses and differences in men and women's use of language. They could compare some of their earlier conclusions about how women and men talk to what they've discovering about how women and men use written language. They could also test their discoveries against what other researchers have discovered. (The pieces by Bleich, Lakoff, and Tannen would provide good starting points for such discussions, although the Bleich article may be difficult for some high school students.)

By this time, students have collected a large sampling of men and women talking and writing. And they have begun to analyze that data in terms of how women and men use language—separately and jointly, orally and in writing. When differences are noted, students can then ponder why such differences exist and how those differences might engender sexist beliefs and stereotyping; then, they could make suggestions about how we might go about counteracting generalizations which may have been initially based on some evidence but which have grown into stereotypes. A subsequent activity might be to create dialogues between a man and a woman, one which clearly illustrates stereotypes and one which is bias-free. Writing a newspaper or magazine article about their findings would be another activity through which they could share what they've learned. All of the activities involved in this research get students to *use* (not merely practice) reading, writing, speaking, and listening in context. Transcribing the tapes, for example, can be an exercise in reproducing conversation with appropriate punctuation. Collating data and making generalizations about the data (generalizations which they can then support with the data) require language negotiation skills and logical thinking skills—the working back and forth between generalizations and specifics our students need so much practice in. Writing articles for newspapers or magazines will make them consider audiences as well as how to present their views. In each case, then, students are using language to study language.

More importantly, such analyses lead students to ponder stereotypes and biases in language use, how they come to be and how they are perpetuated, thus laying the groundwork for future investigation into gender issues. One outcome or discovery students may make in these explorations is the recognition of the wide-spread use of sexist language. Sexist language itself could become the theme for a study or exploration of language. Whether or not students have observed sexist language in the earlier activities, the survey David Blakesley discusses in "*He/Man* and the Masters of Discourse" (this volume) will make students aware of how pervasive (and unrecognized) the use of sexist language is, and the results of the survey could also serve as data for further study. Students could first be given the survey themselves; after collating the data generated from their responses, they could each conduct surveys in the school or community and collate that data separately. Comparing their responses to the community's responses would be a good way to check the effectiveness of previous activities in their study of gender issues in language. Are the students now more sensitive to language? Do their responses reveal an awareness of how language reflects their thinking? Has their language changed as a result of their explorations? How does their language differ from the language of others in their community? Can they draw some conclusions about their community's use or non-use of sexist language? Are older people more or less apt to use sexist language than younger ones? Are females more or less apt to use sexist language than males? Are some types of workers more or less apt to use sexist language than other types of workers? Are some people more apt to use sexist language in some contexts or situations and not in others?

Once they've learned to recognize sexist language, students could continue their language exploration through additional surveys in which they tally the use of sexist language by people in various situations. In *Building Gender Fairness*, Stitt (1988) suggests activities for gathering data during classroom interactions (teachers with female students versus teachers with male students) and then analyzing that data according to verbal and non-verbal behaviors (145–67). Do teachers talk differently to male and female students? Do they, for example, praise female students for being neat and pass off the messiness or poor behavior of male students with comments like "boys will be boys"? Do they ask female students simpler, more factual-type questions than they ask male students? Is there a difference in voice quality when talking with students of different genders? With whom do they make eye contact? How do they deal, verbally and non-verbally, with misbehavior in male and female students? Stitt's analyses of verbal and non-verbal interactions could be applied to the tape recordings or scripts from the earlier samplings students took of males and females in conversation, or students could observe the behavior and language of those around them (particularly interesting to them may be the interactions of adults and young people).

Students could also review reading material and the media for uses of sexist language. They could collect samples of language from their textbooks, from the local newspapers, from the magazines they read regularly, from their favorite novel or story, from their favorite television show or music album, and so on. They could also return to the earlier samples collected from their literature anthology. How is language used? Are there differences in how men and women use language in the various media? How are men and women portrayed, or talked about, in the various media? What words are used to talk about men? What words are used to talk about women? Do some media perpetuate biased views through the use of sexist language? The lyrics of currently popular songs and the scripts of current television shows could provide particularly fruitful resources for a discussion of sexist language and other gender issues. Some students might compare the language of characters in various shows, currently, for example, Roseanne Arnold in *Roseanne* to Susan Dey in *LA Law* or the language of the various male and female lawyers in *LA Law*? Other students might study the language of sportscasters as they present male versus female sports results. Others may compare the language of *Sports Illustrated* to the language of *Woman's Day*. The possibilities for researching sexist language and for comparing the language of men and women in the media are numerous. (The essay by Miller and Swift (1990) would be a good resource for this discussion.)

Having discovered the sexist language that exists in their community and in their reading and viewing material, students can then explore the effects of sexist language on members of their family or community. Students could begin by developing a questionnaire to interview adults about the effects of gender bias or sexist language in their lives. They might include questions like: Have you ever been the victim of sexual bias? How do you feel about sexist language? When is language sexist? Have you ever been the victim of sexual harrassment on the job? What did you do about it? How did it make you feel? Have you ever been told to speak or write differently from what comes naturally to you? and so on. Each student is then responsible for interviewing four adults, two male and two female. Students collate the material and examine their findings, looking for common themes and experiences and identifying both positive and negative effects.[3] They can then report their findings in the form of magazine or newspaper articles. They may even want to compare their results with some of the published materials on sexist language (see, for example, August, Carter, Freed, Nilsen, Nilsen *et al.*, Rosenthal, and *Alice in Genderland*). This activity is probably the riskiest and most sensitive of the activities suggested in this chapter, and yet it could prove to be a most important and effective one, if handled carefully. As with the previous ones, this activity is one in which students must use language to study language. Students must first decide the issues to include in the survey; then they must determine how to phrase the questions to yield responses from which they can legitimately draw conclusions; they will use oral language skills in interviewing people as well as in discussing their findings with other class members; they will use math and logical thinking skills in collating the data and drawing conclusions; they will use reading skills in whatever library research they are assigned or choose to do; they will use writing skills in presenting their results.

Another activity with which students could continue their exploration of sexist language is the writing of their own handbook or guidelines on the non-use of sexist language or on effective alternatives to sexist language. They could begin this study by reviewing some of the already published guidelines: the Modern Language Association, the National Council of Teachers of English, and the American Psychiatric Association among others have published such guidelines (see also the articles by Frank, Maggio, Sorrells, and Nilsen). Students could use the published guidelines as models for developing their own guidelines for publications in and for their school (e.g., Guidelines for Non-sexist Language at Carbondale Community High School). Students would need to decide, based of course on *their* research, what language was acceptable and what was unacceptable; then, they would need to decide how to avoid the unacceptable language and write guidelines for doing so. This discussion might lead them into a debate about the rationale for or the feasibility of attempting to eliminate sexist language; different teams could take various points of view on the subject, conduct research, and then present their findings to the class, either in the form of group reports or debates (among the numerous articles on this issue, those by Alter, Blaubuergs, Cannon, Carter, Freed, McFadden, Nilsen *et al.*, and Switzer will give students a good start on this topic). A variation on the handbook activity would be for students to write guidelines for the selection of textbooks and other teaching materials for their school. (The articles by DeShazer, Federbush, Fiske, Harrison, Nilsen *et al.*, Stitt, and Worby will give students some ideas about how to review educational materials for gender bias and sexist language.)

Another discovery students may make as they explore the differences in how men and women use language is sexual stereotyping. An activity to explore personal biases or stereotyping in language is suggested by a Southern Illinois University graduate student. In the midst of an argumentative paper assignment, Jackie Pieterick spends a couple of days on an exercise which encourages students to "begin to look critically at their sources of information and their own preconceptions" (np). Students are divided according to gender, males sitting on one side of the room and females on the other. Students then brainstorm stereotypes; males call out stereotypes of females and females call out stereotypes of males, while recorders write their suggestions on the board. No discussions or arguments are permitted at this time. The next day, students are asked to exchange seats; males move to the female side of the room and females to the male side. Then, students are asked to role play, arguing against the stereotypes they suggested—that is, female students must role play men arguing against the stereotypes females have of men, and male students must role play women arguing against the stereotypes males have of women. No matter how the activity turns out, they learn from it. Students who are able to role play, in constructing their cases against the stereotypes (the stereotype *they* named), begin to recognize the fallacies in their thinking; they also learn how to filter through the emotional parts of their arguments and come up with solid evidence to back their assertions. Students who are unable to role play because they cannot conceive of how another thinks recognize that differences do exist; the discussion can proceed from there by investigating how such differences lead to stereotyping and biases, and how language is used to perpetuate them. (Pieterick, by the way, uses this activity to lead into a discussion of supporting generalizations and making unfounded or unwarranted assumptions. Therefore, although the activity itself is about gender and language, the purpose is related to other activities.)

Whether issues of gender bias become the focus of classroom

activities as in many of the activities suggested thus far or they become the means for acquiring other knowledge or learning other skills as suggested by Pieterick's activity, students will gain from these experiences. Activities which provide students with the opportunity to explore the issues of gender not only make students aware of the inequities that exist in their language use but also encourage them to take steps toward eradicating those inequities. Furthermore, all of the activities mentioned thus far in this chapter require students to *use* language in a variety of ways.

Some teachers may prefer, however, not to turn their entire language curriculum over to gender issues. They may choose instead to get at gender issues through more traditional types of classroom activities, such as vocabulary exercises or grammar study. Certainly, for many teachers there is a place in the curriculum for a formal study of how language functions, taking a more traditional approach through a study of vocabulary, grammar, and mechanics. The following examples, which of course could be integrated into the preceding sequence at various places, will illustrate how gender issues in language can be dealt with through more traditional activities.

An activity to get students to explore inequities in language is suggested by Pattie Cowell in "Valuing Language: Feminist Pedagogy in the Writing Classroom" (1987). She pairs terms like "bachelor" and "spinster," "master" and "mistress," and "courtier" and "courtesan" for language study, asking students to compare the connotations of each pairing (147–49). (Additional terms to explore could be drawn from Nilsen's "Sexism in English: A 1990s Update" [1990].) By exploring the connotations of such pairings students begin to recognize the inequities in how language represents women and men. Merely making students aware of these inequities prompts them to explore the effects of language on their own thinking and behavior. Students could do further explorations into the etymologies, tracing the histories of such words. Additionally, instead of using a conventional dictionary for developing dictionary skills, students might be exposed to some of the specialized dictionaries relating to gender issues and feminism (Capek's *Women's Thesaurus* [1987] is an excellent example of a specialized dictionary, and the new *Random House of Webster's College Dictionary* [1991] includes notes on sexist and other politically offensive usages). Students could even create their own dictionary of non-sexist language. Vocabulary and dictionary skills would certainly be enhanced by these activities.

Teachers who choose or are encouraged to conduct grammar exercises may discover exploring the differences in male and female languages to be an excellent way of studying grammar. Instead of analyzing sentences from handbooks, students might analyze the sentences they collect from observing men and women in conversation or from their literature anthology and other reading material. They could look at the vocabulary used or at the structure of sentences; whatever the current emphasis of their grammar study (e.g., conjunctions, complex sentences, avoiding run-ons and comma splices), students could apply that knowledge to their investigations into the differences in male and female language. Teachers who are concerned about students learning the standard written English they will be required to use in many situations could have students translate the oral statements of women and men in conversation into the standard English used in texts. And, of course, students could also practice eliminating sexist language from their own speech and writing as well as that of others. Activities such as these can teach students the same basics taught in the handbooks, but when real language (i.e., language in context) is used instead of the prepackaged, noncontextual examples of the handbooks, language becomes interesting and vital to the students.

Teachers who attempt to balance their curriculums through the use of such language activities as these, which are designed to explore gender bias and promote gender fairness, may find that students have gained a far greater understanding of how language functions and that students feel much stronger in their own use of language. Although little research has been done to justify a claim that such language study will improve specific language skills, activities which explore language *as it functions* give students the broader picture of language in context, enabling them to make choices in the language that they use and thus leading to overall language growth. If a goal of the English curriculum is to help students gain more personal power over language, surely language activities such as these will help them use language more effectively.

Notes

1. In preparing this chapter, I used *Language Awareness* (edited by Eschholz, Rosa, and Clark, 1990) because it has a good section on "Sexism and Language" and because it happens to be the text our university is using at this time. However, there are may current anthologies and readers which have included selections on language and on gender issues.

2. Although many of the readings mentioned in this chapter were written for an audience of professionals, most are accessible to high school students, though of course some more so than others.

3. This activity is a slight refocusing of an activity suggested by Stitt in *Building Gender Fairness* (137–38).

Works Cited

Alice in Genderland: Reflections on Language, Power and Control. 1985. Sheffield, England: The National Association for the Teaching of English.

Alter, Lance. 1976. "Do the NCTE Guidelines on Nonsexist Use of Language Serve a Positive Purpose?" *English Journal* 64.9: 10–13.

American Psychiatric Association. 1977. "Guidelines for Nonsexist Language in APA Journals." *American Psychologist* 32: 487–94.

Aries, Elizabeth. 1976. "Interaction Patterns and Themes of Male, Female, and Mixed Groups." *Small Group Behavior* 7.1: 7–18.

August, Eugene R. 1990. "Real Men Don't: Anti-Male Bias in English." In *Language Awareness*, edited by P. Eschholz, A. Rosa, and V. Clark, 289–300. New York: St. Martin's Press.

Blaubuergs, Maija S. 1980. "An Analysis of Classic Arguments against Changing Sexist Language." In *The Voices and Words of Women and Men*. Ed. Cheris Kramarae, 135–47. Oxford: Pergamon.

Bleich, David. 1985. "Gender Interests in Reading and Language." In *Gender and Reading: Essays on Readers, Texts, and Contexts*, edited by Elizabeth A. Flynn and Patrocinio P. Schweickart, 234–66. Baltimore, MD: The Johns Hopkins University Press, 1985.

Cannon, Garland, and Susan Robertson. 1985. "Sexism in Present-Day English: Is It Diminishing?" *Word* 36: 23–35.

Capek, Mary Ellen. 1987. *A Women's Thesaurus: An Index of Language Used to Describe and Locate Information by and about Women*. New York: Harper & Row.

Carter, Margaret. 1981. "What's Wrong with Using Generic Terms?" *Illinois English Bulletin* 78.3 (Spring): 23–30.

Cowell, Pattie. 1987. "Valuing Language: Feminist Pedagogy in the Writing Classroom." In *Teaching Writing: Pedagogy, Gender and Equity* edited by C.L. Caywood and G.R. Overing, 147–49. Albany, NY: SUNY Press.

DeShazer, Mary K. 1981. "Sexist Language in Composition Textbooks: Still a Major Issue?" *College Composition and Communication* 32: 57–64.

Eckert, Penelope. 1990. "Cooperative Competition in Adolescent 'Girl Talk.'" *Discourse Process* 13.1

Eder, Donna. 1990. "Serious and Playful Disputes: Variation in Conflict Talk Among Female Adolescents." *Conflict Talk*. Ed. Allen Grimshaw, 67–84. Cambridge: Cambridge University Press.

Frank, Francine Wattman, and Paula A. Treichler. 1989. *Language, Gender and Professional Writing: Theoretical Approaches and Guidelines for Nonsexist Usage*. New York: Modern Language Association.

Freed, Alice F. 1987. "Hearing Is Believing: The Effect of Sexist Language on Language Skills." In *Teaching Writing: Pedagogy, Gender and Equity*, edited by C.L. Caywood and G.R. Overing 65–79. Albany, NY: SUNY Press.

Greif, Esther Blank. 1980. "Sex Differences in Parent-Child Conversations." *Women's Studies International Quarterly* 3.2-3: 253–58.

Guidelines for Nonsexist Language in NCTE Publications. 1990. Urbana, IL: National Council of Teachers of English.

Lakoff, Robin. 1975. *Language and Woman's Place*. New York: Harper & Row.

Lakoff, Robin. 1989. "Talking Like a Lady." *The Written World: Reading and Writing in Social Contexts*. Ed. Susan Miller, 533–542. New York: Harper & Row.

McFadden, Cyra. 1990. "In Defense of Gender." In *Language Awareness*, edited by P. Eschholz, A. Rosa, and V. Clark. 320–21. New York: St. Martin's Press.

Maggio, Rosalie. 1988. *The Nonsexist Word Finder: A Dictionary of Gender-Free Usage*. Boston, MA: Beacon.

Nilsen, Alleen Pace. 1979. *Changing Words in a Changing World: Pop! Goes the Language*. Tempe, AZ: Arizona State University.

———. 1987. "Guidelines against Sexist Language: A Case History." *Women and Language in Transition*, 37–64. Albany, NY: State University of New York Press.

———. 1990. "Sexism in English: A 1990s Update." In *Language Awareness*, edited by P. Eschholz, A. Rosa, and V. Clark, 277–87. New York: St. Martin's Press.

———. 1984. "Winning the Great HE/SHE Battle." *College English* 46: 151–57.

Nilsen, Alleen Pace, Haig Bosmajian, H. Lee Gershuny, and Julia P. Stanley. 1977. *Sexism and Language*. Urbana, IL: National Council of Teachers of English.

Pfeiffer, John. 1985. "Girl Talk-Boy Talk." *Science, '85*. [Also in Eschholz, Rosa, and Clark. 277–87].

Philips, Susan U., Susan Steele, and Christine Tanz, eds. 1987. *Language, Gender, and Sex in Comparative Perspective*. Cambridge, MA: Cambridge University Press.

Pieterick, Jackie. 1990. "The Rhetoric of Gender." Unpublished lesson plan.

Random House Webster's College Dictionary. NY: Random House, 1991.

Rosenthal, Jack. 1990. "Gender Benders." In Eschholz, Rosa and Clark, 303–305.

Sorrels, Bobbye D. 1983. *The Nonsexist Communicator: Solving the Problems of Gender and Awkwardness in Modern English*. Englewood Cliffs, NJ: Prentice Hall.

Spender, Dale. 1980. *Man Made Language*. New York: Routledge and Kegan Paul.

Stitt, Beverly A. *et al*. 1988. *Building Gender Fairness in Schools*. Carbondale: Southern Illinois University Press.

Switzer, Jo Young. 1990. "The Impact of Generic Word Choices: An Empirical Investigation of Age-and-Sex-Related Differences." *Sex Roles* 22.1 & 2: 69–81.

Tannen, Deborah. 1990. *You Just Don't Understand: Women and Men in Conversation*. New York: William Morrow.

Thorne, Barrie, Cheris Kramarae, and Nancy Henley, eds. 1983. *Language, Gender and Society*. Rowley, MA: Newbury House.

West, Candace, and Don H. Zimmerman. 1975. "Sex Roles, Interruption and Silences in Conversation." *Language and Sex: Difference and Dominance*. Eds. Barrie Thorne and Nancy Henley, 105–129. Rowley, MA: Newbury House.

CONTINUING THE CONVERSATION: GENDER AND COMMUNICATION

In a curriculum that includes syntax and stylistics, usage and spelling, where would lessons on gender and language fit? One model is to add it on. Another—better, we think—is to integrate it with the teaching of literature and writing. How could you begin to include some of Lisa McClure's suggestions in your own classes?

What controversies revolving around language do you see every day in your school? What kinds of talk and what kinds of differences in talk do you see exemplified in the conversations of male and female teachers? Administrators? If you and a colleague of the opposite sex were to try to study teacher talk, what questions would you ask and how might your conclusions about the talk differ depending on the point of view and background you bring to the same questions?

Do you see differences in conversational style, particularly in presenting ideas, at teachers' meetings? Do you see Tannen's conclusions about gender differences in speaking and listening exemplified in how disagreement is dealt with in meetings? If you often attend meetings with your students' parents (e.g., conference night, freshman orientation) do you notice any differences in the ways mothers and fathers approach you? Do you respond differently to mothers and fathers?

Can you think of examples of how gender differences in style of listening and speaking have caused miscommunication, particularly miscommunication that has led to hurt feelings and damage to relationships? Although Tannen presents information on personal communication, how do the same kinds of differences show up in more public communication? In your own classroom?

Note how your students talk to each other, how their talk does or does not exemplify stereotypes, and how you respond to their talk. In particular, note how you may be acting out gender stereotypes in the way you respond to and talk with your students.

Part II
Gender and the Teaching of Literature

This section focuses on gender issues and the teaching of literature. McCracken and Comley present interesting and challenging ideas about how we read in ways limited by gender. Stover presents a provocative look at how one can study gender issues with young adults through the use of literature. Bowman's essay on the use of reading response with high school students presents both a method for studying gender differences in reading and for diminishing those differences. As you read, think about your own responses to literature. In what ways has your reading been limited by gendered responses? In what ways has your formal study of literature limited your response, and the responses evoked in your classrooms?

5

Re-Gendering the Reading of Literature

Nancy Mellin McCracken

In this essay, I suggest that we cultivate a particular kind of reading, gendered reading, both for ourselves and for our students. By gendered reading, I don't mean anything more esoteric than reading literature as the gendered persons we are. This might seem an unnecessary suggestion. Don't we all already read as gendered persons? Actually, I think we do, but in an odd way: in the current literature curriculum, for the most part, boys read as boys and girls read as boys. No one, not even the girls, gets much practice reading as girls. So my suggestion is that we teach girls and boys to read as girls just as they now read as boys, that we seek to re-gender the reading of literature.

One of the reasons why both boys and girls have learned to read as boys is that most of the stories they read in school are written by men. This is an old problem, though, and it is close to being solved. When Virginia Woolf was asked to speak on women and fiction in 1928, just seven names came to her mind:

> a few remarks about Fanny Burney; a few more about Jane Austen; a tribute to the Brontes ... some witticisms if possible about Miss Mitford; a respectful allusion to George Eliot; a reference to Mrs. Gaskell and one would have done." (3)

When Tillie Olsen wrote her famous essay *Silences* in 1965 things had improved somewhat; her review of literary anthologies indicated that "one in twelve" entries was written by a woman. Still, the relative silence on the part of women had at least two ill effects: 1) there were no models for women writers, and 2) there was very little opportunity for young women readers to gain insights into the minds of other females, the available fictional characters having been created almost exclusively by men. Virginia Woolf asks us to

> [s]uppose, for instance, that men were only represented in literature as the lovers of women, and were never the friends of men, soldiers, thinkers, dreamers; how few parts in the plays of Shakespeare could be allotted to them: how literature would suffer! . . . no Caesar, no Brutus, no Hamlet, no Lear, no Jacques—literature would be incredibly impoverished, as indeed literature is impoverished beyond our counting by the doors that have been shut upon women. (1957, 87)

Adrienne Rich writes about the secondary effect of these silences in literature on aspiring women writers:

> [T]he girl or woman who tries to write . . . goes to poetry or fiction looking for *her* way of being in the world, since she too has been putting words and images together; she is looking eagerly for guides, maps, possibilities; and over and over in the . . . literature she comes up against something that negates everything she is about: she meets the image of Woman in books written by men. She finds a terror and a dream, she finds a beautiful pale face, she finds La Belle Dame Sans Merci, she finds Juliet or Tess or Salome, but precisely what she does not find is that absorbed, drudging, puzzled, sometimes inspired creature, herself, who sits at a desk trying to put words together. (1979, 39)

Of course, now things are not so bad as they once were. Today we have ready access to literature by and about women writers. We have, for example, Celie's letters in *The Color Purple* (1982), Annie Dillard's *The Writer's Life* (1989), Eudora Welty's *One Writer's Beginnings* (1983).

Recent scholarship has enabled reprinting of once popular writers such as Rebecca Harding Davis and Nora Zeale Hurston. We now have the 2457-page *Norton Anthology of Literature by Women* (1985) edited by Gilbert and Gubar, and Henry Louis Gates is editing the *Norton Anthology of African American Literature* (forthcoming), with plentiful selections of women's writings. The most popular high school American literature anthologies now include more women and other underrepresented groups than they did even a decade years ago. Bonnie Davis's 1988 survey of the major high school American literature anthologies found on the average women's writings represented three in ten of the works included. The current fifth edition of X. J. Kennedy's Literature (1991) similarly contains approximately three works by women for every ten works in the main fiction section of the anthology. Of course this is still not ideal, but clearly at least the possibility for young men and women to begin to learn to read about the lives of others as seen through the eyes of both men and women is far greater than it once was.

Teaching Literature by Women

Granted that nontraditional literature, including that written by women, is readily available now, but it is still not easy to know how to teach it. What is particularly difficult for teachers who were initiated into formal literary study is that if the initiation has been successful, the graduate will have emerged with an acquired taste for "high" literature. Most of us have completed programs designed to systematically turn our heads away from the local, the immediate, the "merely" personal toward what we have come to believe are "universal themes"—themes such as "Man Against Man," "Man Against Nature," "Conquering the Great Frontier" (see Olsen, 186–93). Yet, as Alice Walker reminds us in "In Search of Our Mother's Gardens," since women's creative work has had to survive in a hostile environment, if we would seek it, we must look both "high—and low" (1985, 2379). In a society that forbade women an education for most of their history, and forbade women of color the leisure to pursue even the decorative, nonliterary arts available to white women, we must look for women's creative genius in songs, in quilts, in the amazing gardens Walker's mother planted every year, and in writings of the genres traditionally deemed "low" art, if art at all: diaries, letters, personal essays, and novels and stories written around intricate, intimate landscapes often within small private settings—kitchens, for example.

Most of us eventually get past the old notion that if it's not written on a grand scale, or touching one of the four or five recognized great themes, or at least written by a male author important enough to warrant a graduate seminar, it's not worth teaching. Even so, this newly discovered literature is still difficult to teach. Our old graduate school notes won't work with these "new" texts. Where can a middle class, white, male teacher, for example, acquire the authority to teach, say, Toni Morrison? Fortunately, guidance exists. The critics and writers of what Walker calls "womanist" writing have left us clear advice on how to go about reading these texts. These authors agree on two key points: (1) that it is best to begin reading ourselves freshly—using all we have learned about response to literature as we read—unjaded by the traditional and gender-limited critical readings in which we have been trained, and (2) that it is vital to our understandings of this literature that we share our readings. This fresh reading along with the willingness to share readings with colleagues and students can enliven our teaching—especially if we are honest about it.

An Example

Recently in a workshop, I presented the first three pages of Morrison's *Beloved* (1987) to a group of twenty teachers, half of them women and half of them men, all white, rural, and middle class. None of them had read the novel, or indeed, anything by Morrison before. I gave them the following directions—adapted from Bleich's heuristic for response to literature.

1. What is the most important (interesting, puzzling) word or phrase in the passage you have just read?
2. What personal associations come to mind when you say that word or phrase? Think of particular persons, places, objects, events, and write them here.
3. What emotions do you experience in connection with those personal associations (happiness, sadness, nostalgia, curiosity, anger, hunger . . .)?
4. Why did you select the word you did in answer to question #1 above? Why do you feel it is the most important word in the passage?
5. Suppose that the author of the passage has the same (or quite similar) associations for the word you selected. How can you use those associations to help you construct a meaning from the passage? Try to describe what the work means to you at this moment based on the passage you have read so far. When you are finished you will share your writing with other readers. Your answer cannot be wrong so long as you answer all five questions.

Beloved is written mostly from an African-American woman's point of view, but there is so much going on in the first three pages that there was plenty for all the teachers to respond to. Several of the men, for example, were young fathers and chose to respond to the text's image of a spiteful baby. Two of the women chose the word *beloved* and responded with memories of church rituals—one a wedding, the other a funeral. In just twenty minutes of reading and writing and fifteen minutes of discussing their readings, these teachers came up with all the themes raised in a recent series of lectures by Morrison scholar Barbara Christian—albeit in question form: the role of church, slavery and the underground railroad, Caribbean culture, ancestral ghosts, numerology, sexuality, family structure, and betrayal. Using their questions about these themes as well as about the author, these teachers created a list of topics, divided the list among themselves and spent the next twenty minutes researching in the very small, rural campus library in which we were meeting. When the group met back together to share their cursory findings, they found they had enough answers and enough questions to set the agenda for two weeks of classwork with their own students. All, incidentally, were fascinated by Morrison's writing and eager to finish reading *Beloved* right away.

The point is that the way to acquire authority in reading unfamiliar women's literature is really just to read it, respond to it personally, and share your responses with other good readers. Then study what you can and invite your students to join you. Some words from woman authors below suggest the immediacy with which their writing is to be read, and what it might mean to read this literature as women.

Learning to Read Again

Virginia Woolf describes a method for reading contemporary women's literature, about which one has read no criticism and for which there are no readily available author's notes in a Norton Anthology:

> It seems to be her first book . . . but one must read it as if it were the last volume in a fairly long series, continuing all those other books that I have been glancing at. . . . For books continue each other, in spite of our habit of judging them separately. And I must also consider her—this unknown woman—as the descendant of all those other women whose circumstances I have been glancing at and see what she inherits of their characteristics and restrictions. . . . (1957, 84)

Poet Audre Lorde, in her essay "Poetry is not a Luxury," also suggests a way of reading:

> Right now, I could name at least ten ideas I would have found intolerable or incomprehensible and frightening, except as they came after dreams and poems. This is not idle fantasy, but a disciplined attention to the true meaning of "it feels right to me." We can train ourselves to respect our feelings and to transpose them into a language so they can be shared. (37)

Barbara Christian arguing against the infringement of literary theory on the relationship between reader and text, writes,

> I consider it presumptuous of me to invent a theory of how we *ought* to read. Instead, I think we need to read the works of our writers in our various ways and remain open to the intricacies of the intersection of language, class, race and gender in the literature. And it would help if we share our process, that is, our practice, as much as possible since, finally, our work is a collective endeavor. (337)

Adrienne Rich has similar advice for re-gendered reading embedded in her argument for a "a radical critique of literature, feminist in its impulse," which, she says, would take the work first of all as a clue to how we live, how we have been living, how we have been led to imagine ourselves, how our language has trapped as well as liberated us, how the very act of naming has been till now a male prerogative, and how we can begin to see and name—and therefore live—afresh." (1971, 35)

Some Possible Effects of Gendered Reading

Because we understand the power of literature as a way of knowing, it is important to look at the effects of reading of literature in light of what is known about gender. Some points to consider: A report published recently in the *New York Times* (Jan 6, 1991) summarizes a recent study for the American Association of University Professors of self-esteem in 3000 adolescent boys and girls:

> Girls emerge from adolescence with a poor self-image, relatively low expectations from life and much less confidence in themselves and their abilities than boys. . . . [W]hen elementary school boys were asked how often they felt "happy the way I am," 67 percent answered "always." By high school, 46 percent still felt that way. But with girls, the figures dropped from 60 percent to 29 percent.

Stake's longitudinal study of educational and career confidence and motivation in college women and men suggested that "the men's achievement-related motivation and confidence increased with greater assimilation into the campus environment, but that the women showed more positive changes when they were less well assimilated" (1984, 565). Having eliminated other likely explanations for this difference, Stake wonders if "perhaps the campus experience was influencing the students toward traditional, sex-stereotyped attitudes and goals" (576).

It seems likely that as men and women acquire greater degrees of cultural literacy, men will derive support for their efforts at autonomous, competitive achievement, while women will derive further anxiety as they aim in the opposite direction of the self-sacrificing wife and mother. Could learning a re-gendered reading of literature help students resist the pressure of sex-stereotyped attitudes and goals?

In most literature courses, we ask students to ignore their gender roles as they read, to immerse themselves in the literature, following the central point of view where it leads them, and reflecting on that experience, seeking the high artistic universals. What I am proposing here is that we invite students to read with their full gender experience intact, to resist the central point of view when it contradicts that experience, and to seek artistry both in the particulars and the universals. I intend that students give the fullest possible readings to the literature. But aren't I in danger of the fallacy identified long ago by I. A. Richards as the critical "hobbyhorse"? Don't I risk seeming to encourage reductionist readings, say, of *Merchant of Venice* as an anti-Semitic tract and *Huckleberry Finn* as racist ideology? Yes, this proposal is risky, but it seems to me a risk worth taking.

In *Protocols of Reading* Robert Scholes (1989) offers an interpretation of *The Education of the Virgin*, a painting of the child Mary learning to read from a large book in the hands of a teacher. If the young woman in the painting is Mary, the mother of Jesus, and if the book is the New Testament, then, Scholes says, Mary is literally reading her life, "the book of herself." Echoing Roland Barthes, Scholes says that in just this way all of us reading are reading our lives:

> This is what we all do, all the time, when we read, and what we should do. To read at all we must read the book of ourselves in the texts in front of us, and we must bring the text home, into our thoughts and lives, into our judgments and deeds. We cannot enter the texts we read, but they can enter us. (4)

Reading Scholes's interpretation of the painting, we might envision a contemporary Mary reading the book of herself in the poems and plays and stories that she reads with us in class. If she is in secondary school she will look long to find a text that she can use to write the text of her life. If our contemporary Mary is studying modern American fiction, for example, from the ever popular HBJ Heritage Edition of *Adventures in American Literature*, she will read sixteen stories. Twelve of these will have men or boys as the main characters. Four of these stories will have no female character at all. Each of the female characters she does meet will dwell in tightly restricted, traditional feminine roles (McCracken 1991). From Hemingway's "Big Two-Hearted River" she will learn that there are two kinds of girls: the unimportant kind that the boys go out with and call names like "the Blonde Venus," and the kind that boys go out with and defend with their honor like "Hop's real girl." From Fitzgerald's "Winter Dreams" she will learn that there are two kinds of girls: those who are "destined . . . to be inexpressibly lovely and bring no end of misfortune to a great number of men," and those who are ". . . sweet and honorable and a little stout," and of little interest to men. From Sherwood Anderson's "Sophistication" she will learn that the hero "wanted to love and be loved . . . but he did not want at the moment to be confused by her womanhood." From Faulkner's "The Bear" she will learn to sanctify "that brown liquor which not women, not boys and children, but only hunters drank, drinking not of the blood they had spilled but some condensation of the wild immortal spirit."

The stories that will enter her life written by men offer few clues about how she might rewrite them differently in the text of her life. They present their ideas about the lives of women as direct reflections of life. Even the wonderful stories written by women won't challenge these limited and limiting ideas. From Porter's "Granny Weatherall," for example, she will learn that the central event in the life of a woman, what stays even after the faces of her children have slipped from memory is being jilted by a man. From Welty's "A Worn Path" she will learn that the central event in the life of a woman is the selfless journey to keep her grandchild alive.

If our Mary is studying Introduction to Literature as a college freshman, reading, say, X. J. Kennedy's *Literature* anthology, she will meet different texts, but not many different stories she can use to rewrite in the text of her life. Both the fourth and fifth editions of this popular textbook include women writers in the main fiction section at a ratio of one to three, but without a re-gendered reading, the texts that she reads will continue the story of her life as a forced choice between being an uninteresting, good girl and beautiful but hated bad girl; a wife and mother or loony spinster. She will find Kincaid's mother's advice to her daughter to "Try to walk like a lady, and not like the slut you are so bent on becoming," and she will hear versions of that message echoed in Updike's Queenie, Faulkner's Emily, and Steinbeck's Elisa. She will learn of the scorn meted out to those who don't live the role of doting wife and mother as she reads Thurber's "Unicorn in the Garden" and Mansfield's lonesome "Miss Brill," and Singer's "Gimpel the Fool." There are interesting exceptions, to be sure, for example in Toni Cade Bambera's "Blues Ain't No Mockin Bird," Kate Chopin's "The Storm," Tess Gallagher's "The Lover of Horses," and Anne Tyler's "Average Waves in Unprotected Waters." These stories all have strong female characters that we are not required to hate or scorn or pity, but given the training in reading our Mary has had so far, she is likely to read them just like all the others.

A Case In Point

I want to illustrate an effect of gendered reading with a case from my own recent teaching of the short story "Greasy Lake" by T. Coraghessan Boyle. I have taught this story to a gender-mixed class of college freshman and a roomful of English teachers, all but one females. The results, (McCracken, in press) were the same with both groups. A lot goes on in this story: There is a decomposed body floating in the lake, a bloody brawl in which the narrator believes he has killed his opponent, a narrow escape, and an attempted gang rape, which the author describes in vivid detail:

> [S]he was already tainted. We were on her like Bergman's deranged brothers . . . panting, wheezing, tearing at her clothes, grabbing for flesh. . . . Before we could pin her to the hood of the car . . . a pair of headlights swung into the lot. There we were, dirty, bloody,

> guilty. . . . the first of the Ur-crimes behind us, the second in progress, shreds of nylon panty and spandex brassier dangling from our fingers, our flies open, lips licked. (1991, 67)

After the story was read, I asked both groups to first tell in a brief sentence what mainly happened in the story, and second to consider the fact that the narrator said several times that he and the boys were "bad" in its popular slang sense ("They were slick and quick and they wore their mirror shades at breakfast and dinner. . . . In short, they were bad." [65] and decide whether the boys in the story really had been "bad."

The results of this discussion are surprising. The students and the teachers unanimously read the story as a tale about boys growing up. Just over two-thirds of both the students and the teachers decided the boys had not been "really bad," but were just boys being boys and getting into more trouble than they'd bargained for. I would argue that this is a culturally male-gendered reading of the text, prompted in part by the author's verbal trick of making the rape appear and disappear in the same instant. Just in the middle of the scene quoted above, the narrator says,

> We were bad characters, and we were scared and hot and three steps over the line—anything could have happened. It didn't. Before we could pin her to the hood of the car. . . . (67)

Unless one is reading entirely from this male narrator's view, it is hard not to ask, "What didn't?" Assault happened. Attempted gang rape happened. Apparently the narrator's assertion that nothing happened is so powerful that a first-time reader, student or teacher, instantly forgets what has just been read.

The reason for this reading of the story is not just lack of critical attention. Even the editors of the anthology in which it appears insist that the boys are just being boys: "Are Digby and Jeff really 'bad'? Well, no, and neither is the narrator. They're just engaging in the kind of behavior they think is expected of them." (Kennedy, Instructor's Manual, 1991, 16). Clearly this male-gendered reading is a common one in our culture, and it is important to understand.

When Twain has Huck answer the question if anyone was killed in an accident, with the line, "No,m. Just a nigger." contemporary readers don't miss the fact of the death—nor the devastating racism that underlies the comment. It seems that students and teachers—and probably even anthology editors—hear the *racist* lie in literature, at least when it is starkly put, because we have learned to read with sensitivity to race. We have learned, partly from Twain himself, I think, but also from Baldwin, Wright, Hughes, Ellison, Walker, Morrison, and others to hear, sometimes, from Jim's point of view.

Yet when Boyle writes about three man jumping on a single girl whose boyfriend they have just knocked unconscious, "grabbing for flesh. . . . shreds of nylon panty and spandex brassier dangling from our fingers, our flies open . . ." and has the narrator tell us "anything could have happened. It didn't," most readers, two-thirds in my sample, do not hear the lie—nor the sexism that underlies it. It appears that we and our students have a good way to go before we learn to hear the sexist lies that permeate our literature. There is some urgency here.

If the incidence of rape among college age students is now one in four, as suggested by research funded by the National Institute of Mental Health (Warshaw 1988), and if, as the study also suggests, the men who rape and the young women who are their victims acknowledge that force was used to have sex with the women against her will, but fail to label this use of force rape, then the young woman reading Boyle's story, like young Mary reading the Bible, may well be reading "the book of herself," and she should read, as Scholes (1989) says, "as if her life depended on it." How then does it happen that she does not? Mainly it is her habit of reading. As a reader, she has become unsexed—like Lady Macbeth, but unwittingly. When she reads Boyle's story, she is identifying with the male narrator. She is also reading in a school context in which she has come to believe her reader role is to seek the universal elements of fiction: setting, character, plot, and the universal themes (e.g., Man Coming of Age, Man Against Man, Man Against Nature). A central question we must answer is how can we elicit a culturally female gendered response from readers to the sexist actions described in literature but diminished or entirely suppressed by narrators and editors.

Re-Gendering Reading

As usual, Louise Rosenblatt offers good advice. Writing in 1938, she noted the gender stereotypes in literature and reminded us that as teachers of literature we have the choice to:

> help the student retain his [sic] living sense of the experiences through which he has just passed or, by pedantic "literature study," lead him to dismiss them as unimportant. By helping to focus the student's attention upon the actual emotions through which he has entered into the lives of others, the teacher can reinforce the power of literature to develop social imagination. (187)

One way we might do that is to provide students with different stories where the girls are given space to express their feelings. Perhaps one of the reasons readers fail to respond to the attempted rape in "Greasy Lake" is lack of experience hearing women's voices in literature.

Alice Munro's "The Found Boat" in the same anthology would be good to read before reading "Greasy Lake." In that story, we hear from the young girls' point of view. Reading *Beloved* would be good. Reading Amy Tan's *The Joy Luck Club* would be good. Joyce Carol Oates's "Where Are You Going, Where Have You Been?" would help tune readers' responses to the young woman's perspective on what counts as having happened in the case of attempted rape.

Where can you find good literature by women of different class and cultural perspectives to help balance the culturally dominant male-gendered stories that fill your anthologies? Besides the recent inclusions in all the major school anthologies, there is the new *Norton Anthology of Literature by Women*. Stover's essay in this section will help anyone trying to re-gender reading through young adult literature. NCTE's pamphlet "Guidelines for a Gender-Balanced Curriculum in English Grades 7–12" recommends other collections and single works as helpful for gender-balancing the literature curriculum at the secondary and college levels.

A number of essays in *English Journal* offer valuable insights on re-gendering the literature curriculum. Ray, for example, suggests that we "encourage students to liberate the female characters they encounter from the stereotypes to which they are confined. . . ." (1985, 57). Dehler uses women's diaries as part of her literature curriculum to expose her students to women's points of view. Roemer teaches a unit on feminism including Zora Neale Hurston's novel, *Their Eyes Were Watching God*, to help her students bridge the gender gap and to help her young women students find their experiences reflected in literature. Moore pairs works by male and female authors to help balance the literature curriculum. Pairing Wright's *Black Boy* with Angelou's *I Know Why the Caged Bird Sings* proves especially useful in allowing students to look from different perspectives. Finally, Barker describes his gradual shift to a gender-balanced curriculum in his American Literature Classroom. His four-part plan is a fine one:

1. include more female writers
2. examine the treatment of women in male-authored texts
3. design study activities that focus on gender differences and relations
4. focus discussion and writing topics on areas in which female students are authorities (1989)

He elicits animated discussions from his classes using primary sources as varied as Gilman's "Yellow Wallpaper" and "The MTV Half-Hour Comedy Hour":

> Women should rule the world. You outnumber us, you live longer than us, you're more mature than us, you're smarter than us. But you

don't rule the world. You know why? "Cause we can knock you out!" (1989, 42)

For teachers at the college level, there is a large body of feminist criticism to consult as well as frequent essays in *College English*. Highly recommended are Gilbert and Gubar's volumes, Flynn and Schweichart's *Gender and Reading: Essays on Readers, Texts, and Contexts*, and Lauter's *Reconstructing American Literature: Courses, Syllabi, Issues*.

"Why All the Suffering? and Where Are the Women?"

In *Making Connections*, developmental psychologist Carol Gilligan suggests an antidote to gender imbalance in the teaching of literature. She says,

> I will begin with Shakespeare, who turned at the beginning of his last play to the question of a daughter's education. Miranda, witnessing the terrible scene of storm and ship-wreck that opens *The Tempest*, cries out that she cannot bear to see such suffering. "Had I been any god of power," she says, she would have taken action to stop it. At which point Prospero decides that it is time for her education. "Pluck my magic garment from me," he tells her, "Ope thine ear,/Obey, and be attentive." But first he asks whether she remembers a time before they came to the island. "Tis far off," Miranda says, "And rather like a dream than an assurance . . ." [but] Had I not/Four or five women once that tended me?" More, Prospero says, "but; how is it that this lives in thy mind? (1990, 7)

Gilligan notes that "Miranda's questions—Why all the suffering? and Where are the women?—are essentially irrelevant to the story that Prospero proceeds to tell." Yet Miranda's questions are just the questions, I believe, we must keep helping our students to ask when we proceed to teach them literature. We simply cannot afford to have students for whom and to whom literature does not speak. In *Actual Minds, Possible Worlds*, Jerome Brunner concludes that as educators our primary task must be to

> . . . create a new generation that can prevent the world from dissolving into chaos and destroying itself. . . . to create in the young an appreciation of the fact that many worlds are possible, that meaning and reality are created and not discovered, and that negotiation is the art of constructing new meanings by which individuals can regulate their relations with each other. . . . (149)

As long as we continue to limit our students'—and our own—reading to literature written from a single, male-gendered perspective, and require all the men and all the women to read from that same perspective, we can't begin to move toward Brunner's goal. Only as we add literature written from multiple perspectives and teach ourselves and our students to read as both men and women will we start to reap the individual and cultural benefits long attributed to the reading of literature.

Works Cited

Adventures in American Literature, Heritage Edition Revised. Eds Francis Hodgins and Kenneth Silverman. NY: Harcourt, 1985. (All refs. to short fiction are from this edition)

Barker, Andrew P. 1989. "A Gradual Approach to Feminism in the American Literature Classroom." *English Journal* 78.6: 39–44.

Bleich, David. 1975. *Readings and Feelings: An Introduction to Subjective Criticism*. Urbana, IL: National Council of Teachers of English.

Boyle, T. Coraghessan. 1991. "Greasy Lake." In *Literature: An Introduction to Fiction, Poetry, and Drama*, edited by X. J. Kennedy, 99–106.

Bruner, Jerome. 1986. *Actual Minds Possible Worlds* Cambridge, MA: Harvard UP.

Christian, Barbara. "The Race for Theory." "*Doing Theory*", 335–45.

Davis, Bonnie. 1989. "Feminizing the English Curriculum: An International Perspective." *English Journal* 78.7: 45–49.

Dehler, Kathleen. 1989. "Diaries: Where Women Reveal Themselves." *English Journal*. 78.7: 53–54.

Dillard, Annie. 1989. *The Writing life*. New York: Harper.

Fetterly, Judith. 1978. *The Resisting Reader: A Feminist Approach to American Fiction*. Bloomington: Indiana UP.

Flynn, Elizabeth and Schwiechart. 1986. *Gender and Reading: Essays on Readers, Texts, and Contexts*. Baltimore: Johns Hopkins UP.

Gilbert, Sandra M., and Susan Gubar. 1985. *The Norton Anthology of Literature by Women*. New York: Norton.

———. 1987. *The War of the Words*. In *No Man's Land: The Place of the Woman Writer in the Twentieth Century*, Vol. 1. New Haven, CT: Yale UP.

———. 1989. *Sexchanges*. In *No Man's Land: The Place of the Woman Writer in the Twentieth Century*, Vol. 2. New Haven, CT: Yale UP.

Gilligan, Carol. 1982. *In a Different Voice: Psychological Theory and Women's Development. Cambridge, MA: Harvard UP.*

Gilligan, Carol, Nona P. Lyons and Trudy J. Hanmer, eds. 1990. *Making Connections*. Cambridge, MA: Harvard UP.

Kennedy, X. J. 1991. *Literature: An Introduction to Fiction, Poetry, and Drama*, 5th ed. And Instructor's Manual. New York: Harper Collins.

Lauter, Paul. 1983. *Reconstructing American Literature: Courses, Syllabi Issues*. Old Westbury NY: Feminist Press.

Lorde, Audre. 1984. "Poetry Is not A Luxury." *Sister Outsider*. Trumansburg, NY: The Crossing Press.

McCracken, Nancy. 1990/91. "Penelope Talks Back to Her Anthology." *Ohio Journal of English Language Arts*. 31.2: 14–17.

———. In press. "Rosenblatt and the Ethics of Reading." In *Readers, Texts, Teachers II*, Edited by W. Corcoran, M. Hayhoe, and G. Pradl. Portsmouth NH: Boynton/Cook.

Moore, Lisa. 1989. "One on One: Pairing Male and Female Writers." *English Journal*. 78.6: 34–38.

Morrison, Toni. 1987. *Beloved*. New York: New American Library.

Olsen, Tillie. 1965. *Silences*. New York: Delta/Seymour Lawrence.

Ray, Karen J. 1985. "The Ethics of Feminism in the Literature Classroom: A Delicate Balance." *English Journal*. 74.3: 54–59.

Rich, Adrienne. 1971. "When we Dead Awaken: Writing as Re-vision." In *On Lies, Secrets, and Silence: Selected Prose 1966–1978*. New York: Norton.

Richards, I. A. 1929. *Practical Criticism*. New York: Harcourt.

Roemer, Julie. 1989. "Celebrating the Black Female Self: Zora Neale Hurston's American Classic." *English Journal*. 78.7: 70–72.

Rosenblatt, Louise. 1938/1968. *Literature as Exploration*. New York: Noble.

Scholes, Robert. 1989. *Protocols of Reading*. New Haven: Yale UP.

Stake, Jayne E. 1984. "Educational and Career Confidence and Motivation Among Female and Male Undergraduates." *American Educational Research Association*. 21.3: 565–78.

Walker, Alice. 1982. *The Color Purple*. New York: Harcourt.

Walker, Alice. 1985. "In Search of Our Mothers' Gardens." In *The Norton Anthology of Literature by Women*, edited by Gilbert and Gubar, 2374–382.

Warshaw. Robin. 1988. *I Never Called It Rape*. New York: Harper.

Welty, Eudora. 1983. *One Writer's Beginnings*. New York: Warner.

Woolf, Virginia. 1929/1957. *A Room of One's Own*. New York: Harcourt.

6

Father Knows Best: Reading Around "Indian Camp"

Nancy R. Comley

Reading is not an innocent act. We come to a text laden with cultural, social, ideological, and literary baggage, all of which influence our responses to that text. Concomitantly, our subjectivity is structured by the texts we read, and this is an ongoing, never-completed process. In recent years, feminist theory and criticism have made us aware of how our conceptions of gender are shaped by what we read. As a result, strategies for reading against a male-authored text have been proposed, notably by Judith Fetterley in *The Resisting Reader* (1978). Greater representation of women writers has occurred in some quarters of academe, but the question of who's in and who's out of the canon remains a hotly debated issue. The choice of texts and the approaches proposed for them are particularly important at the introductory level, for it is here that students should be receiving basic training in the critical skills they will need for reading and writing throughout their academic careers and beyond. It's here too that their awareness of a literary canon is sharpened as well. Included in the skills we teach should be the lessons we've learned from reader-response and feminist criticism, along with a balanced representation of men and women writers.

As a demonstration of these needs, let us look at some student responses to Ernest Hemingway's story "Indian Camp." This story was chosen not only because it is a good story, but because it is a very masculine story. Though its events center on childbirth, women are virtually written out of the story; the Indian woman in labor is presented as a mere site to be acted upon. I wished to compare not only the responses of men and women readers, but also of readers at different levels of reading sophistication: freshmen (primarily) in a second-semester composition course that uses literature to generate writing, and juniors and seniors in an upper-level course in literary theory and criticism. I taught the latter course, and I asked a male colleague, a Hemingway fan teaching the composition course, to assign "Indian Camp" and to ask his students to respond to it in their journals. The theory class encountered the story as the first in Hemingway's *In Our Time*, which we were using to talk about interpretation of narrative. This class was asked to keep journals and to respond to the reading in them, but there was no specific written assignment connected to the story. The comments from this group are drawn from class discussion.

The composition class also kept journals and was asked to respond in writing to "Indian Camp." Both classes were given copies of the original opening of the story, cut by Hemingway, and reprinted in Philip Young's edition of *The Nick Adams Stories* as "Three Shots." The criticism class also considered this opening from a narrative point of view: that is, what did Hemingway gain or lose by cutting it? Though the composition class was told that "Three Shots" was originally part of "Indian Camp," all but three of the students read it as a separate story, and thus had much to say about its abrupt ending.

Originally, "Indian Camp" opened with Nick, a boy of perhaps nine or ten, undressing in his tent at a campsite in the woods. He is thinking about his behavior on the previous night, when he was scared of being alone in the silence of the woods while his father and his uncle were out on the lake fishing. He had become "afraid of dying," and had fired a prearranged signal of three rifle shots to recall his father. By the time they arrived, Nick had fallen asleep, and though his Uncle George was annoyed at his cowardice, his father was understanding: "He's pretty small . . . . we're all yellow at that age."

The next morning, Nick was instructed by his father that "There is nothing that can hurt you" in the woods. This section ends that evening with the sound of a boat arriving and his father's call to dress. "Indian Camp" now begins with two Indians, Nick, his father, and his uncle rowing across the lake to the Indian camp where "There is an Indian lady very sick." In a shanty is an Indian woman who, as Nick's father explains to him, "had been trying to have her baby for two days." When she screams with pain, Nick is instructed that this "is called being in labor . . . All her muscles are trying to get the baby born. That is what is happening when she screams." But when she screams again, Nick asks, "Oh, Daddy, can't you give her something to make her stop screaming?" His father replies that he hasn't any anaesthetic, "But her screams are not important. I don't hear them because they are not important." Nick must serve as an intern while the woman is held down and the doctor performs a Caesarean "with a jack-knife . . . sewing it up with nine-foot, tapered gut leaders," delivering a healthy baby.

In the bunk above the woman her husband has been lying all during her labor with a badly cut foot, and when Nick's father, "exalted and talkative as football players are in the dressing room after a game," turns his attention to him, saying, "Ought to have a look at the proud father. They're usually the worst sufferers in these affairs," he discovers the awful truth of his statement. The Indian husband, apparently unable to endure his wife's screams of pain, has slit his throat from ear to ear. Nick, who had his eyes averted during the caesarean operation, gets a full view of this. His father then apologizes for bringing him along. On the way back across the lake to their camp, the following dialogue ensues:

> "Do ladies always have such a hard time having babies?" Nick asked.
> "No, that was very, very exceptional."
> "Why did he kill himself, Daddy?"
> "I don't know, Nick. He couldn't stand things I guess."
> "Do many men kill themselves, Daddy?"
> "Not very many, Nick."
> "Do many women?"
> "Hardly ever."
> "Don't they ever?"
> "Oh, yes. They do sometimes."

Nick finally asks, "Is dying hard, Daddy?" to which his father replies, "No, I think it's pretty easy, Nick. It all depends." The story concludes with Nick sitting "in the stern of the boat with his father rowing" and feeling "quite sure that he would never die."

When the original opening is restored, "Indian Camp" becomes more obviously a story of a boy's fear of death that moves from fear of the dark and a death that might lurk there, to the experience of a violent death brought on by a violent birth. Without the opening, the reader is simply launched into the violence and Nick's experience of it, an experience which is not fully articulated. Nick's feelings must be interpreted through his actions, his looking away from what his father is doing to the woman, and by the nature of the questions he asks his father later. Given the original opening, one might say that Nick is trying to be a little man, trying to make up for being a coward the night before. As one composition student put it, "Nick seems to have become more comfortable with death." Death is a remote thing to most children, and Nick, now being carried away from the scene of violence by his father, can indulge himself in the fantasy of never dying.

Nick has also absorbed a lesson in sexual difference. Birth can be a violent, painful process for women but it doesn't kill them; however, a birth can cause a man to kill himself. In order not to die, the lesson is to avoid women; or at least, not to marry them and get them pregnant. Nick, at his age, can safely see himself avoiding such a situation.

But the reader might ask what Nick is to make of his father's "scientific" lesson that a woman's screams in childbirth are "not important," when they so obviously were to one who apparently lacked a rational, scientific mind. Does the woman's being Indian account for the doctor's cursory treatment of her, as if she were not a sentient being? The doctor is thrilled at having done "one for the medical journal," and is "exalted" as a football player after a winning game. Hemingway is careful to stress the male athleticism of the event, which is devoid of feminine experience. In this scene of childbirth, there is no elation or relief registered on the woman's part: "She was quiet now . . . She did not know what had become of the baby or anything."

There was little question on the composition students' part that Nick had undergone a "learning experience," and their interpretation of that experience did not break down along lines of gender, at least not in the way the criticism students' responses did. The latter group aligned themselves in two sexual camps: the women leaped on the doctor's statement, "Her screams are not important," while the men replied that this was simply a professional statement meant to instruct Nick. The women readers were quick to point out the irony: that the woman's screams were certainly important to her husband. And they also noted that all the other Indian men "had moved off up the road to sit in the dark and smoke out of the range of the noise she made." In the composition class, differences based on gender were barely noticeable: three women, but no men, registered some shock in their journal responses at the violence in the story. But these were only three women out of twenty. It wasn't, then, so much a question of difference as an issue of non-response to the violence of "Indian Camp." The composition students' responses can be categorized by the particular clichés they relied on. Though there is some overlap, these categories are: the (beautiful) miracle of birth; father as protector and teacher; handling death; and violence. Here are some examples from the first group, the miracle of birth:

> This was a continuation of the story Three Shots. I like this part better because it has a great deal of meaning. We see a woman in labor which is the most beautiful process in life. The baby's father kills himself because he can't cope with his problems. We find ourselves with this kind of situation now a days. —Pilar

> "Indian Camp" seems to be another learning experience for Nick. He sees the pregnant lady's husband after the husband slit his throat. At the same time he experiences the miracle of birth but the birth seems more difficult than the death. . . . We also see the comfort the father provides to Nick at the end when they are rowing back and Nick feels he will never die. — Alan S.

> As in "Three Shots," the concept of death is predominant in the writing. However, another theme, also holding significant bearing is the concept of birth and life. Nick, who had such trouble with death in "Three Shots," is forced to deal with it again, however this time, it is after he's been exposed to the beauty of life. Nick seems to deal with everything quite well, despite the difficult situation. As usual, his father is very comforting and happy to answer Nick's questions. At the end of the story, the reader senses a feeling of content as Nick has learned to handle the delicate balance between life and death. — Allen G.

Pilar provides an extreme example of the clichéd response that makes the teacher wonder whether she and the student read the same story. Note how her cliché regarding birth as beautiful takes over the difficult labor: "We see a woman in labor which is the most beautiful process in life." In Alan S.'s response, ambivalence is present. He joins the cliché "the miracle of birth" with an awareness that "the birth seems more difficult than the death," as indeed it was, though Alan does not go on to explore this ambivalence and thus explode his cliché: this birth caused a death. Allen G.'s response could as easily be discussed under "handling death," but it has been filed here because of his reference to "the beauty of life." If anything, this birth has been singularly unbeautiful, except for the healthy child produced. Nick has purposefully kept his eyes averted throughout: he doesn't *see* the birth (and neither do the students). Indeed, his first question to his father is "Do ladies always have such a hard time having babies?" And his next question is "Why did he kill himself, Daddy?" Nick now has death indelibly associated with birth, only it's men who are at risk rather than women. This anomaly is kept submerged. Allen notes, "As usual [as if Dad were a figure in an ongoing TV series], his father is very comforting and happy to answer Nick's questions."

The father as protector and teacher was a popular theme:

> My reaction to the story is pretty simple and clear cut. There was no difficulties in this story except for why the Indian father killed himself. Nick represented a pretty smart kid who knew a great deal more than what his father thought. I liked this short story because it was a typical father and son togetherness. — Jenny

> Nick's father is teaching Nick about life, starting with birth, the beginning of life. — Nicole

> Nick watches nature occur and sees the true reality of life. A baby is born and a man dies. . . . Nick's father continues to be a protector but also acts as a teacher. He explains to his son how a baby is born and discusses death with him as well — the two main themes of the story. — Yael

> Nick's father tries to control the way Nick sees the whole situation. In both stories Nick's father is like a protector. Here, he puts his arm around Nick to try and shield him from all the emotional tragedy and gloominess around him. — Rena

> Nick experienced life and death in one day. He must have thought life or birth was harder than dying. That's why he didn't worry about death at that moment. The way I can relate to the story is the way Nick's father was protecting Nick. — Maria

We might compare Jenny's response to Pilar's, because the story hardly presents "a typical father and son togetherness." Why would a protecting, comforting father ask a young boy to be his intern at such a birth? Of course, he does apologize later, but only because Nick saw the dead Indian father. This "protector" has thrust his young son — a child afraid of the dark — into violence he is not ready to understand. The story might be read as a father's terrible mistake in trying to "educate" his son. But if any students harbored such a thought, they substantially repressed it, which probably accounts for their positive readings of the father. Not only are fathers not supposed to make such mistakes, but also those writing their responses after discussion of the story in class might well have been influenced by the sympathetic view of the father that emerged from that discussion, as we see in Michelle R.'s response later in this chapter. We note in Maria's response, "The way I can relate to the story is the way Nick's father was protecting Nick," her instructor's injunction, "How do you relate to the story?" (Also phrased as "Which character can you identify with?") In a class where the women significantly outnumbered the men, perhaps "*Can* you relate to the story?" would have been a fairer request.

The "handling death" group's responses were based on a comparison of the Nick of "Three Shots" and the Nick of "Indian Camp," and their desire to see a progression from one story to the other — a learning experience:

> "Indian Camp" was a bit more interesting. . . . Nick seems to have become more comfortable with death than he was in the first story. — Jack

> In this story, Nick is in a situation in which he sees both life and death. He sees the woman being so strong in order to have her baby, while the father is weak and takes his own life. . . . Nick experiences people helping other people, the Indians are less knowledgeable, so they needed help. He sees that people can care about others. He sees that everybody is not like Uncle George.—David

> I think that because of this violence Nick was forced to grow up in this story. . . . He witnessed the birth of a child and the death of a man. In a way he has witnessed the full life cycle within a few minutes . . . . seeing what he did changed Nick's thoughts, he was no longer afraid of dying and felt he would never die.—Naomi

> We are meeting again the problem of death, but this time, Nick is experiencing the death of other people, i.e. the husband. He is not faced with the problem of thoughts of his own death. This story is told through Nick's eyes, and once again we see the transitivity from dark to light, from death, to life.—Allon M.

Jack's response is most reminiscent of the euphemistic emptiness of TV series talk: to "become more comfortable with death" is the ultimate learning experience. And Naomi agrees: "he was no longer afraid of dying." With David, the saccharine clichés of "sharing and caring" come to mind. Allon has a more literary approach: Nick is able to distance death from himself through someone else's death, "and once again we see"—again, as if this were an ongoing TV show. But in terms of the story, Allon has his sequences reversed, for the story moves from life to death.

The writers who responded to violence in the stories were few, as I've noted. Above, Naomi cited the violence as a force making Nick "grow up." Of the following, two women questioned their responses:

> I was also kind of shocked that the story had the part where the father killed himself. After all he wasn't the one having the baby. . . . I don't know if there is one character I could relate to. But by being a lady, I guess I eventually would be able to relate to the Indian woman and the pain of childbirth.—Tina

> This was a sad story especially when the Indian was found dead at a time when he should have been rejoicing at the birth of a healthy son. After finding out that the baby was alive I was happy, then shocked to find out the father's suicide. If anything, I feel that Nick would have been more frightened of dying after witnessing these events. . . . —Michelle S.

> When Nick entered the shanty he was met by screams—this scared the hell out of him and his father's answer was strange—"No, I

> haven't an anaesthetic, but her screams are not important." At first I thought this odd but after class I understood that he tried (father) to make it less than it was—for his son. I couldn't help but notice the strong contrast between birth and death—suicide. Nick was hit by both of them at once.—Michelle R.

Tina is perhaps hard on the Indian father, but is pragmatic in a way only inexperienced young adults can be. Michelle R. wrote more in her journal than any other student. She let her pen pull out her thoughts and looked forward to the thinking she did through writing. She is an active reader, and she begins by comparing "Three Shots" and "Indian Camp" as two separate stories. She defines Nick's father as "protector and teacher" and literally reads the Indian's death as a "turning point" which enables Nick, faced with reality, to stop imagining death and thus "accept it." She does wonder about the doctor's comment regarding the woman's screams of pain, but class discussion apparently urged a masculine (rational) reading of the text. Michelle comes away with such a reading, which, though somewhat at odds with her original response, constitutes for her an authoritative reading because it is sanctioned by her instructor.

And here, by way of summary, are two concise readings of the text:

> In my opinion, the difficult birth of the baby signifies that life is difficult, and the death of the father signifies that all things come to an end.—Lisa

> I found it easy to relate to the boy's fear, because it's a fear I think we all possess at some point. Our survival instinct is probably the flipside of our fear of death.—Jon

Overall, there is a desire for a quick closure of meaning, which results in a mini-summary, of which these two responses are extreme examples. In all the student responses one hears echoes of various discourses. In Allon M.'s, for example, a literary discourse drawn from earlier instruction in New Critical methods is present in "the transitivity from light to dark." There are echoes, too, of their instructor's suggestions for responding to the story: as we have seen, could they "relate" to it was clearly one of his questions. But most of the echoes here are not so much from earlier English courses as they are from *TV Guide*'s little blurbs for situation comedies or other half-hour weekly shows. In each thirty-minute segment, a situation must be presented, developed, and concluded. There is no chance for development of character or for complexity of situation. (Complexity is to be distinguished here from the mare's nest of relationships that typifies the American soap opera.)

The student writers were too young to have caught the initial flowering of *Father Knows Best*, but they have witnessed its various offspring, one of the most popular of which is *The Cosby Show*. No matter what the problem on such shows—and it's seldom much of a problem—Dad usually gets it resolved quickly. As Ella Taylor notes in *Prime Time Families*, "Narrative resolution . . . comes in the form of a learning experience, a lesson in social adjustment for the children" (1989, 161). Faced with a kind of violence that did not fit in their particular frame of knowledge, the student readers naturalized it. In this process, we take strange, and in this case, shocking information and we make it conform to a discourse we understand. And so Hemingway's story was transformed into story-forms the students knew and were comfortable with. As we can see, their stories reflect the stereotypical family values presented by American media, where, as Taylor notes, problems in the outside world are ignored, or retreated from "into fundamentalist principles of family" (165) and where "genuine argument" is smoothed into "the cozy warmth of domestic affection" (163).

We must also take into account the students' over-acquaintance with images of violence. Through television, the car wreck, the dead soldier, the hurricane disasters—all such images are brought into intimate relationship with the viewer through that piece of living room furniture, the television set. Such a glut of violent images produces a neutralizing effect and their awful immediacy is not felt; they cease to shock. That violence against women is as much a staple of television and film drama as it is of daily life also helps to account for the students' lack of reaction to the crudeness of the operation performed in "Indian Camp." The operation is categorized simply as an errand of mercy.

For the composition students, what Nick "learns," then, is that father knows best. Uncle George's heavily ironic comment, "Oh, you're a great man, all right," goes unremarked by the students, most of whom have written off George as an "unsympathetic" person. They would prefer to have the father play a stereotypical role of wise leader. (Only two women students wondered where Nick's mother was in all of this.) The story was, to many of them, what Jenny said it was: "a typical father and son togetherness" story. That the story also tells of a father who kills himself because of his inability to act during the birth of his son is barely noticed.

What are the implications for teaching in all of this? The criticism students had the advantage of placing "Indian Camp" within the context of the group of Nick Adams stories in *In Our Time*, where babies aren't very welcome and fatherhood is not a condition aspired to ("Cat in the Rain"; "Cross-Country Snow"). The predominantly masculine world of *In Our Time* contains much violence and death, and all relationships with women, whether they be girlfriends, wives, or mothers are problematic. In such a context, "Indian Camp" can be read as Nick's introduction to this violent world. The criticism students, then, were better-informed readers than the composition students, though for the latter group, the addition of the original beginning of the story did at least give them the information that Nick was a relatively small boy with fears of the dark and of death. This information provided some help with their instructor's injunction to identify with a character in the story. Alan wrote, "I can identify with the child's fear of being alone," but "I cannot identify with the two large occurrences [childbirth, death]." Thus he, like almost all the others, reprocessed those two "large occurrences" into digestible gruel. Perhaps in teaching "Indian Camp" one should pose the question, Would the doctor have brought his daugther to be his intern on this occasion? If not, why not? Just whose view of childbirth is being presented here? Men are always only observers of childbirth, and can only describe it from a distanced point of view. They may try to imagine what a woman might be feeling but they can never know, and their presentation of that experience will always have a touch of the alien about it. Another approach would be to begin with Nick's questions and the differences in gender expressed by them and by his father's responses. And the issue of violence must be addressed.

As another way of approaching this story, we might ask, along with Hemingway scholars, why Hemingway wrote "Indian Camp." With a writer who uses autobiographical material as much as Hemingway does, it's a fair question, and one that interests students. In a letter to F. Scott Fitzgerald, Hemingway rates "Indian Camp" as one of the best of the *In Our Time* stories. In the former ending of "Big Two-Hearted River," published as "On Writing" in *The Nick Adams Stories*, an adult, post-war Nick claims:

> Nick in the stories was never himself. He made him up. Of course he'd never seen an Indian woman having a baby. That was what made it good. Nobody knew that. He'd seen a woman have a baby on the road to Karagatch and tried to help her. That was the way it was. (238)

Whether Hemingway actually assisted in this birth, which he witnessed as a young reporter covering the evacuation of Thracians to Macedonia in 1922, is not known. However, as a boy Nick's age, Ernest planned to become a doctor like his father, and later occasionally assisted him with minor cases. But when he finally witnessed his father performing an operation at a hospital where he was chief of obstetrics, though he was interested, according to his older sister Marcelline, "he felt faint and he did not go again" (Sanford 1962, 134). Perhaps this experience of seeing his father cut into someone's flesh was indelibly written in his memory. Perhaps that is the scene that would be transformed in "Indian Camp," where Hemingway's love of going camping with his father would be fused with the horror of what his father actually did to the bodies of others. One might use such a biographical approach in the classroom. But it is equally important to work on the level of events in the story, considering especially the violent yoking together of birth and death. As a binary opposition, birth and death are linked in this story to another binary, women and men. Nick is struggling with these binaries, as his questions to his father indicate. To encourage students to dwell on Nick's "resolution" of oppositions, and thus to ignore the play of gendered oppositions in the story is to invite students to lapse into media-oriented banalities.

Works Cited

Fetterley, Judith. 1978. *The Resisting Reader: A Feminist Approach to American Fiction*. Bloomington: Indiana UP.

Hemingway, Ernest. 1958. *In Our Time*. New York: Scribner's.

———. 1972. *The Nick Adams Stories*. New York: Scribner's.

Sanford, Marcelline Hemingway. 1962. *At the Hemingway's: A Family Portrait*. Boston: Little, Brown.

Taylor, Ella. 1989. *Prime-Time Families*. Berkeley: U of California P.

7

Gender Differences in Response to Literature

Cynthia Ann Bowman

Every year I am faced with the same problem—students who are convinced that there is only one "right" interpretation of a poem, short story, novel, or play. These students want to be told what the work really means and are both baffled and disturbed when I tell them I don't know. They want instant answers that can be taken down as class notes and repeated. Therefore, I have come to use "writing-to-learn" techniques, writing activities which provide students opportunities to focus their thinking and promote enjoyment, understanding, and imagination in their study of literature. As students express their ideas, viewpoints, and questions about their reading, they gradually come to possess their knowledge, eliminating the spoon-fed interpretations memorized for a single exam and then quickly forgotten (Marshall 1988).

For the first few weeks of the year, my students[1] are introduced to a response-based classroom where I encourage them to share their reactions to a piece of literature, discuss the characters as real people, and write about similar experiences they have had. Reactions to my class are initially mixed. Some students quickly adapt to this experience of sharing ideas in a community of learners. Others resist and struggle, finding it difficult to accept the responsibility for their learning and the learning of their peers. For this reason, since 1986 I have been using learning logs which prove invaluable; students who may feel uncomfortable sharing in class discussions tend to write their feelings more openly. Writing becomes a means of promoting cognitive development, a heuristic for understanding, where students discover what they have to say. This discovery, in turn, provides a progressive understanding of the text which promotes the more enthusiastic class discussions and papers.

This enthusiasm doesn't happen overnight. Each nine weeks, I assign a novel or play as outside reading and ask the students to keep a learning log on that work. My only directions are to "talk to me on paper" and tell me what they are thinking as they read—impressions, questions, analyses. During this time, we continue with the regular class curriculum. After the learning logs are turned in, we discuss the work together, and even students who hold back in spontaneous class discussions feel comfortable reflecting on the novel that they wrote about in their learning logs.

In 1988 I began to evaluate the instructional value of this process. My primary research focused only on retention, ability levels, and types of responses in literature learning logs (Bowman 1989). When I was asked by one of the editors of this book if I had observed any differences between learning logs written by the boys and those written by the girls, I could only say generally that my boys' responses were extremely colloquial, even chatty, whereas my girls' logs were more personal. The more I thought about the question, my experience with over five hundred journals from sixteen- and seventeen-year-old boys

Girls' and Boys' Learning Log Statements

Learning Log Statements	*Girls*	*Boys*
Related to females	41	7
Related to males	6	43
Ideological	21	4
Practical	4	22
Compared to life	46	14
Compared to literature	25	11
Compared to television	9	22
Compared to history	7	11
Attempted to answer own questions	26	15
Asked questions but no answer	9	28
Reflective	24	3
Judgmental	6	16
Patient readers	14	2
Less tolerant readers	4	11
Other	2	0
N=120 (60 Boys; 60 Girls)		

and girls led me to believe this would be an interesting area to pursue.

To start, I randomly selected forty learning logs, twenty boys' logs and twenty girls' logs from the past two years on the novels *Crime and Punishment* by Dostoyevsky and *The Stranger* by Camus and Conrad's story "The Lagoon." This test group included juniors and seniors of all ability levels. As I read through the learning logs, I looked for the types of questions the students asked of me, comparisons and specific reflections they made, analyses, and any other interesting comments the students may have made. I kept two charts—one for boys and one for girls—and recorded my observations as well as the students' writing. I became so fascinated that I continued reading eighty additional logs, forty from boys and forty from girls.

Even without a background in gender research, I couldn't miss the significant variations and patterns revealed by these 120 learning logs. Some of these patterns are predictable; most, however, reflect differences I had not noticed until doing this research. Listed in the table are the major categories I derived while reviewing the learning logs. In most of these categories, the boys' tallies are almost the mirror image of the girls' tallies. In the following pages, quotations from the randomly selected learning logs illustrate these differences.

As one would expect, the girls seemed to enjoy taking the part of the female characters and commenting on their situations:[2]

> Will Dounia give in to financial security instead of love? Many women do. I wish I could talk to her.

> Seems to me there weren't many opportunities for women during this time. Makes me feel selfish because I want it all—career, family, home . . .

> What does Marie see in this guy? Well, what did Sonia see in Raskolnikov? I guess every girl falls for a loser once in her life.

> I'd never get along with Meursault. I'd probably slap him for his indifference.

It was also not surprising to see the boys identify with the male characters:

> I am a lot like Raskolnikov because I am harder on myself than others are.

> I understand Meursault because when something goes wrong for me I want to be with a girl I like.

> Sometimes I think of doing things like Meursault and that makes people think I'm weird but I don't do them, I just think about doing them.

Beyond these obvious differences in character identification, the learning logs show other quite interesting differences. For instance, overall, the girls were more reflective about characters than the boys. Typical responses included:

> He is not a soul, just a body walking through life. Maybe something happened to him as a child and he turned off his emotions so as not to be hurt.
>
> Maybe after Meursault dies, he will finally be able to feel.
>
> Just because he didn't cry doesn't mean he didn't care. Sometimes people have to keep something inside to really let it out.
>
> Why does Katherine beat her children? Maybe her anger over giving up a decent life for the one she has now.

The boys were quicker to form opinions and had definite ideas about the characters:

> First I wonder why the story makes a point about how he has his arms crossed. It probably symbolizes that he is either upset or bored.
>
> Usually when I think of a murderer, I envision some derelict man who lives in a trash dumpster.
>
> I wish this guy could come to a decision as to whether he is going to commit the crime or not. I am usually a patient person but this ordeal is killing me. I always thought the actual murder itself would be more difficult but Raskolnikov is proving me wrong.
>
> I don't understand why he went back to the beach with a revolver. If he was hot, he could have gone into the ocean!

The girls tended to look at the individual and search for alternative interpretations:

> Why does he change moods so quickly? Is it that he has something to hide or could he have a split personality?
>
> I wonder if his works are reflective of his personal life because he really seems to know the character.
>
> I think Raskolnikov knew he was not extraordinary but didn't want to admit it because he wanted to give his life some significance.

The boys were quick to look at the character with the power and make judgments:

> Meursault's trial is Camus' way of showing that justice is blind.

> He has two sides—a Mother Theresa type side and the intellectual criminal. This will obviously make him suffer.
>
> I thought it was bad enough he had to contemplate the murder for six long excruciating chapters, but now he has considered confessing. What a wimp.

Besides being more reflective, the girls also seemed to be more ideological:

> Why does Salamano beat his dog when it seems to be his only friend? Maybe it's true we always hurt the ones we love.
>
> It makes me so mad that Raskolnikov, although he loves Sonia, tries to bring down her self-esteem. It doesn't seem right.
>
> Dostoyevsky must have spent many hours observing the poor of his country, examining their triumphs, sorrows with tedious precision.
>
> Marmeladov's death might just save Raskolnikov. Sometimes you can be helped by helping someone else.

The boys were definitely practical:

> It was not a good idea for Meursault to go to the police station with Raymond.
>
> I don't understand how a court can bring someone up on murder charges and question them about their mother's funeral? Meursault should have had a good lawyer, yet nothing meant anything to him.
>
> It's very rare for all eight paddles to hit the water simultaneously.
>
> When Marie asked Meursault if he loved her, his reply, "that kind of question has no meaning to me" makes me think honesty may not always be the best policy.

Probably the strongest characteristics of the girls' learning logs were the comparisons they made to their own lives:

> I was just finishing this book when I got in a car accident. Focusing on Raskolnikov's problems and depression made my situation easier.
>
> "Conflagration of the sunset" reminds me of a time when I was at the beach watching the sunrise with my friends.
>
> Katherine needs to vent her feelings more. When my favorite aunt died, my grandmother cried and screamed, but it seemed to help her get over it.

> Salamano and his dog remind me of my neighbor who lost her husband and the dog is everything to her and she walks it on a schedule just like Salamono.

The girls were also quick to make connections with other literature:

> As I read the part where Raskolnikov talks about what a nuisance the old pawnbroker is, I kept thinking of "The Tell-Tale Heart" and wondering if something similar would occur.

> Raskolnikov's dream about the horse reminded me of the story "The Hunger Artist" and made me remember how scared I was once when I was left alone—loneliness can do strange things to people.

> . . . 'men of the islands' made me think of 'No man is an island.'

> This book shows the wastefulness and uselessness of words in society. Society rarely gets its point across with words, rather society must use actions to communicate. This same idea was brought out in *Rosencrantz and Guildenstern are Dead*.

> Who cares about how much he enjoys washing his hands at noon? Wait a minute, shades of Lady Macbeth and GUILT.

On the other hand, when the boys made comparisons, usually they found the similarities in movies or television shows:

> The whole time I've been reading I've been thinking of the movie *Flatliners*. Have you seen it? It's all about . . .

> I am reminded of Indiana Jones and it sparked my enthusiasm until the narrator switched to third person . . .

> The fog reminds me of Scooby-Doo cartoons . . .

> The part where the white men paddle the canoe reminds me of old movies with boats going down the Mississippi River.

> . . . almost like the Millenium Falcon at the end of the *Return of the Jedi*.

The boys also used current events and history in their comparisons:

> Why has Nikolay confessed to a murder he has not committed? Do we have yet another deranged person, Miss B.? If something like this happened today and that person went to the electric chair—wow, kinda like the case in Tallahassee.

> . . . makes me feel like part of Florida's early history with the Indian tribes and the Everglades . . .

As readers, the girls were open to hope, patient and willing to work through the novel:

> I'm trying to figure out why heat and light are stressed so much. Could Camus be using them to foreshadow Meursault's life and death?
>
> Although the description is extremely detailed, it is funny how even a simple smell can take you back to a place. It almost made Raskolnikov faint at the police station.

As readers, the boys were definitely less tolerant:

> So help me, if Raskolnikov thinks of confessing one more time, I'm going to quit reading.
>
> I understand a story better if I can identify with the characters—these characters are not developed.
>
> This book is ultra-mega boring.

Finally, the girls took a more thematic approach than the boys and often noticed loneliness, isolation, loyalty, and fear:

> . . . how everyone calls out to someone but no one answers is typical of everyday life . . .
>
> It was easier to commit the crime than live with it, so he needs to tell Sonia so she can help him.
>
> Marmeladov represents every family with problems in life.
>
> The only time Meursault might feel any guilt is when he can't tell the warden how old his mother was—how sad.

The boys commented less on theme and more often on the symbolism than the girls—particularly color, temperature, and sound:

> Dostoyevsky presents a typical bar scene—you can almost hear it and feel it—a person comes in, orders a drink, and, bam, someone sits down next to him ready to tell his life story.
>
> The shadows could represent the mysteriousness of the illness.
>
> Did you notice how colors seem to come up a lot?

The more I thought about these apparent differences between the boys' and girls' responses to literature, the more I reflected on our culture and society's expectations of women. Girls are likely to have kept diaries throughout school, at the encouragement of family and/or friends, and are comfortable sharing their personal experiences with others. Boys rarely keep journals for pleasure and are brought up believing they must be tough and keep their problems, thoughts, and concerns to themselves. Girls are allowed to be emotional in our society, but boys cannot. What is interesting in class discussions are the girls' comments that they like a man who can cry, share personal feelings, and break through the "macho" image, while the boys admire women who succeed and demonstrate strength.

Although times may indeed be changing, learning styles are deeply rooted in traditional values. The girls' responses in their learning logs reflect nurturing, patient, sharing individuals, where the boys' logs show very practical, judgmental, and impatient people. In terms of response to literature, it seems that the girls' journals far better illustrate the goals of a response-centered curriculum as espoused by current theorists. All the students who keep the literature learning logs "make their own meaning" of the text (Rosenblatt 1984) through the union of reading and writing (Newkirk 1986). All the students practice being active learners so that the exchange between the reader and text yields meaning and real knowledge (Iser 1978), but it is the girls, particularly, who use the writing to talk to themselves, to work through an understanding, and develop their interpretive strengths (Rosenblatt 1984; Britton 1975; Berthoff 1981). As the teacher of all these students, I am interested in the possibility for change and growth. While the gendered pattern of responses was remarkably consistent throughout the learning logs, I did notice occasional crossovers. More boys, maybe 15–20, gave responses that fell into one or more of the characteristics of the girls' learning logs. On the other hand, fewer girls' logs fell into the categories of the boys' responses, possibly 5–10.

These students, because they do not follow the traditional patterns, might suggest ways to help students move beyond their learning constraints. For example, a boy wrote:

> The scene with Porfiry reminded me of going to the principal's office and trying to B.S. my way out of trouble.

Another boy wrote:

> I liked it when he mentioned we may find ourselves thinking of death as being dead. We imagine ourselves somewhere else alive.

One of the most interesting responses from a boy was his association with the female character:

> Why doesn't Dounia tell Luzhin to get lost? To me, he seems to be a selfish, egotistical dirtball. I have known girls with guy problems, but she takes the cake.

.t another response included:

> Why doesn't Porfiry just haul Raskolnikov off to jail? Maybe he thinks he can help him.

One of my girls in the "crossover" group wrote:

> It says the forest is quiet and dull, but I don't see how because in all the movies you can hear birds and monkeys.

Usually the girls attempted to answer their questions, but the "crossover" girls did not:

> If the white man knew that the slave woman was going to die, why didn't he leave to find his brother?

Another girl asked:

> Why doesn't the white man have a name?

After observing these few logs which varied from the pattern of responses of the group, I considered what I knew about the young men and women who wrote them. The girls who responded with the type of questions and comments typically found in the boys' learning logs were my less academically oriented students, girls who didn't care about school, grades, or learning. They were usually in the bottom percentile of their class in rank. There were also interesting correlations in their personalities. These "crossover" girls tended to be loners; they had a small group of friends with whom they stayed exclusively; and they were from families experiencing problems such as divorce, lack of communication between parent and child, and sibling rivalry.

The "crossover" boys who fell in the pattern of girls' responses were my best students, usually in the top ten percent of their class or extremely hard workers. These boys did well in all their subjects, had high goals, planned to pursue their education, and made academics a priority. What struck me initially was that these boys were my more thoughtful, caring, and perceptive students. Their family situations were stable and, almost always, they had a very positive relationship with their mothers and had many friends of the opposite sex.

The data from my learning logs seem to suggest that what we must do is try to get boys to read literature and write about it more as the girls do, and at the same time encourage even further development in the girls' work. An analysis of the development of the readers and writers in my classes shows that both boys and girls do develop remarkably over the course of the year. But their development is somewhat different. The girls always accepted the learning log assignment much more readily than the boys and usually wrote more. Most were written almost like a diary, in comfortable language with a smooth flow of ideas and comments. On the other hand, the boys had trouble getting started and tended to initially give basic plot summaries. Their journals were often times fragmented and choppy with many personal interjections to me, apparently to deal with their uneasiness about the assignment. As the year progressed, there was a marked difference in the quality of their work, even more pronounced in the boys' responses than in the girls'. The learning logs done near the end of the school year were the ones which reflected this crossover for the boys.

Typically, the first logs of each year are tentative and uncertain. Students are just beginning to develop a sense of confidence in their ability to interpret literature. Each nine weeks the logs become more daring, more analytical, and more exciting. Likewise, class discussions reflect this same growth. The following are excerpts from the first and third learning logs of two students, one boy and one girl.

The junior boy, at the beginning of the year, wrote:

> Nice beginning! God, this guy doesn't seem to care if his mother died or not. Oh, great, now the dork's worried about what his boss thinks and his mom just died.... A nursing home with a warden? Sounds like a prison he sent his mother to, not a home. This guy seems to go through life like a passenger, never making any real decisions, just floating along. The only feelings he has had are those of embarrassment for intruding upon the lives of others. Sounds like a *real* interesting guy to me. ... Gee, he really cared for his mom, too. He thought it was too much trouble going to see her because he had to spend time riding the bus, and it'd be a shame if he actually had to do something for someone else. ... He doesn't even want to see the body! Well, I think I've established the fact that I don't like Meursault. He has no life. What life he does have he spends working, eating at the same restaurant, or staying in his apartment. He sounds extremely boring, like a spectator ...

In the middle of the year, he wrote:

> Dostoyevsky's description of Raskolnikov is deceptive. He is described as being handsome, well-built, dark eyes, and brown hair. This seems to indicate his motive for murder could not have been due to a physical problem. ... Raskolnikov is careful planning his crime. I believe that if he truly wants to murder this lady, he should quit being such a worry wart and just act!. ... I can't believe this dude! He actually has the guts to go see the woman he is planning to kill. What a dork!. ... Now I find out that Raskolnikov had a dual character. One side is a warm and compassionate person who does good for those less fortunate and the other is a cold and intellectual being, much like Ted Bundy. The addition of this split personality to the novel is very beneficial as it stresses he isn't a true hardened criminal. I think this compassionate side is going to be his downfall. I can tell that Raskolnikov has an instant attraction to Sonia—we'll see what

> happens. . . . I love this part in the novel when Raskolnikov is summoned by the police. The stupid idiot thinks they have learned that he is the murderer. I would get over some of my disgust for this freak, then he goes and faints in front of the detective. . . .
> Okay, now who is he trying to fool by wearing new clothes? Symbolically, they represent recovery, but I see no signs of this in Raskolnikov. . . . Raskolnikov is like a lobster about to be put in boiling water. He knows the end is soon and confession is inevitable. He is quaking, fearing for his life. His soft, compassionate side is saying confess, and his cruel side is telling him not to. A return to the scene of the crime prompts once again the confession. In the end, Raskolnikov's theory proves invalid. No man stands above any other—in my eyes, all men are created equal. Miss Bowman, you picked a pretty good book, but next time keep it under 250 pages!

This student's first log was twelve pages and his third was over fifty pages. He had become more reflective and questioning as the year progressed. The junior girl, at the beginning of the year, wrote:

> Now, let's skip to this girl Marie. She seems incredibly naive and insecure. When she asked Meursault if he loved her and he said he wasn't sure but if she wanted to get married it was okay because it didn't matter to him . . . well, I'd have left him! He probably would have said to do whatever, it didn't matter. . . . Celeste's little restaurant reminded me of the story "A Clean, Well-Lighted Place" where the main characters of the respective stories could go and think. It seemed to be a pleasant place, and if there was a similar place in Daytona, I'd like to spend time there, too. . . . This book made me realize how imperfect the world is. Meursault needed something drastic to make him see.

A few months later, she wrote over seventy pages of thoughts, impressions, and questions revealed in the following:

> Why the title *Crime and Punishment*? The crime part is easy to answer, but the punishment part is more difficult. I think the punishment was the waiting and worrying whether anyone would figure out that he was the murderer. I'm not saying he shouldn't have gotten the eight years—I think he should have gotten that and more. Many of my friends think the agony of wanting, needing, to confess was punishment enough, but I disagree. No punishment is hard enough for taking the lives of two innocent people—they'd probably think differently if it was someone in their family. . . . At first I really hated this book, but as I continued reading, I found myself thinking of Edgar Allan Poe, my psychology class, and it made me think that I was really reading, instead of reading *Animal Farm*-type books, I was reading something that made me think. Sometimes I liked it, sometimes I didn't.

In the learning logs, I can observe the processes my students employ in reading and finding meaning. The question of gender differences becomes vital in a subject so inherently personal and emotional. I want to seek out the strength in each student, confirming, not denying, the student's individuality, potential, and knowledge. If this means I need to encourage the boys to respond more like the girls in their learning logs as well as class discussions, perhaps more specific guidelines including personal experience questions would be helpful until the boys become comfortable with this style of learning. One of my strengths as an educator has been the easy rapport I have with my students and the nonthreatening environment I create in class. I do find myself particularly successful eliciting participation and thoughtful responses from the boys. I provide a great deal of positive reinforcement and encouragement as this type of classroom is a risk for adolescents so wrapped up in their images. Thus, I share as much of myself as I ask of them.

Oddly enough, many boys consider English a girls' subject even though the anthologized authors throughout history have been primarily men. When the boys begin improving in English, their scores, for the most part, improve in other subjects as well.

Although not all my girls do well in English, as they begin making the personal connections so apparently characteristic of the girls in my study, they, too, develop more confidence. The type of learning style they employ could be just as easily applied to other subject areas, allowing them to find the relevance to their lives which they must find to succeed academically. Obviously, boys and girls must need this personal connection for learning to truly occur. As an educator who firmly believes in the response-based classroom, I try to encourage all my students to share personal experiences, finding that the boys as well as the girls enjoy the opportunity and become more open as the year goes on. Just a few weeks ago, as I was working on this research, one of my quiet, introverted senior boys wrote:

> Like Raskolnikov, I know all about punishing yourself. The time I wrecked my Mustang was the worst. I couldn't understand how I could have messed up so badly. I planned out what I was going to do all the way home. I took the Jeep and drove down to Bethune Beach. I knew Mom would never suspect me not going back to school. I planned how to avoid seeing anyone and packed a lunch and a shirt, knife, shoes—survival stuff—and drove until there wasn't a soul in sight. It was high tide, so I sat on a dune. The sun and the stress put me in a dilemma much like Raskolnikov's. I felt dizzy and my head was spinning. . . . All of sudden, someone came up behind me. It was my dad and I broke down and cried . . .

Here was a boy who had truly benefitted from making those important personal connections between literature and life.

The girls must also be allowed, in every subject, to make the associations necessary to their understanding and comprehension. Realizing that girls tend to learn best when they apply their knowledge to their own lives and allowing them to utilize their strengths are important keys in making education come alive for each student. We must be open to, and aware of, the differences between genders and create a learning atmosphere which will make our classes meaningful to each unique, individual student.

Notes

1. My students are juniors and seniors at Father Lopez High School, a private regional Catholic school in Daytona Beach, Florida. The students are from diverse socioeconomic and cultural backgrounds ranging from professional families to welfare-assisted families. The grade point averages for the students in this study range from a 1.37 to a 4.13.

2. None of the student excerpts came from the same work and no student's writing appears more than once. All writing is first draft, unedited student work.

Works Cited

Berthoff, A. 1981. *The Making of Meaning: Metaphors, Models, and Maxims for Writing Teachers*. Portsmouth, NH: Boynton/Cook.

Bowman, Cynthia A. 1989. "Effectiveness of the learning log on high school literature achievement." Masters Thesis prepared for Virginia Tech, (August).

Britton, J. 1975. *The Development of Writing Abilities, 11–18*. London: Macmillan Education.

Iser, W. 1978. *The Act of Reading: A Theory of Aesthetic Response*. Baltimore: Johns Hopkins University Press.

Marshall, J. 1988. Classroom discourse and literary response. In B. Nelms, ed., *Literature in the Classroom: Readers, Texts, and Contexts*. Urbana, IL: NCTE.

Newkirk, T. 1986. *Only Connect: Uniting Reading and Writing*. Portsmouth, NH: Boynton/Cook.

Rosenblatt, L. 1984. *Literature as Exploration* (3rd ed.). New York: MLA.

8

Must Boys Be Boys and Girls Be Girls? Exploring Gender Through Reading Young Adult Literature

Lois Stover

Life for young women born in the eighties and nineties and coming of age at the turn of the century differs a great deal from life for their mothers, grandmothers, and great grandmothers. They have more choices. My own mother wanted to be an insurance actuary; since she would not consent to sign papers promising not to marry and have children for at least five years after beginning in such a position, she had to give up her dream. She became, instead, a middle school math teacher. Fortunate young women in school today will select their work because they have made a commitment to a career or profession and receive a sense of identity from pursuing it. They may choose not to marry, may marry and divorce, may remarry. They may choose not to have children; they may have children early in life and then pursue college and careers later on; or they may become established in a profession and delay childbearing until their late thirties. Some will have children as teenagers and will pass their sons and daughters over to their own mothers to raise, waiting for their turn to parent until their children have children. Some will have husbands who stay at home and take over the majority of the responsibility for childraising; some will raise their children singlehandedly. Some will form "traditional" families. All of these changes for women signal increased options for young men as well.

In a society in which traditional roles for men and women continue to be redefined, abandoned, and reexamined, we need to emphasize certain goals of the literature program: a) the exploration of self, including the gendered self and b) the exploration of the relationships between the self and others. The inclusion of young adult novels with characters reflective of various gender-specific traditions and newly developing options should help accomplish these goals. As Donelson and Nilsen (1989) have argued it is through reading good literature that the unique qualities of individuals can be explored along with the similarities of human experience which cross gender boundaries. By discussing young adult novels which explicitly or implicitly deal with sex role stereotyping or the breaking of traditional stereotypes, English teachers can help students reflect upon gender differences and their effects on expectations, communication styles, responses to life's major issues and traumas, and on an individual's planning for the future.

Young adult readers, both male and female, need books to read which validate their own experience as young men or women, but also challenge that experience, perhaps showing them options of which they have been unaware. As Ehle (1982) points out in a review of research about the influence of literature on readers, through reading and vicariously experiencing life from a different perspective, young adults can begin to increase their appreciation for and tolerance of alternate perspectives.

For example, several future English teachers in a methods class I was teaching in London read the adolescent novel *The Turbulent Term of Tyke Tyler* by Gene Kemp (1980) as part of their methods course work. As the author intended, these students were "shocked" to discover, toward the end of the book, that Tyke is a girl. Until the conclusion of the novel, the pronoun usage is non-gender specific, and the language used to describe Tyke is that typically reserved for males. Recognizing that their assumptions were unjustified, these future teachers were made to look inward at their own language use and their expectations for their future students—and for themselves. These students became eager to explore the issue of the impact of language on thought, and several students went on to do research projects about stereotyping in children's and young adult literature. As one "shocked" young man wrote, speaking in many ways for the entire class, "I need to think about how what I say and how I interact with my fellow classmates and my students can set limitations on what we discuss, what we expect from each other, and how we interpret our relationship. I see that women are more like men than I'd ever imagined, though I've been friendly with girls all my life." Similarly, a young, female college student who read Spinelli's *Space Station Seventh Grade* (1982) remarked that she wished she had read the book as a twelve-year-old because "I never realized how unsure of themselves guys could be, how they, too, are concerned about their bodies, about girls as an 'alien' species!"

There are now many young adult novels which provide a catalyst for the kind of insight described above. The Japanese novel *Balloon Top* by Albery (1978) provides a wonderful introduction to the ways in which cultural expectations about men and women come into conflict with an individual's own goals. M. E. Kerr's *I'll Love You When You're More Like Me* (1977), with its alternating first person narratives from male and female perspective, provides a provocative starting point for discussing ways in which gender differences may affect both perception and communication style. Not all young adult novels are equally effective for exploring gender issues, however. The images of reality presented in them are certainly mixed. As we choose books for adolescent boys and girls to read, we need to ask what image of the new world of possible realities they present.

What Mirror of Reality Do Recent Young Adult Novels Present?

After analyzing the 1982 "Books for Young Adults" poll, Stensland (1984) concluded that as of 1984, the books selected by young adults as the best of the young adult field presented "a mixed picture," a reflection of the reality of women's place in the larger society of the mid-eighties. She found that several adolescent female protagonists managed to take charge of their own lives at least to the extent that they refused to become sex objects. Wendy, in Harry Mazer's *I Love You, Stupid* (1981), says, "I don't want to be pawed, Marcus. You don't own me." Tilla, in Ilse Koehn's *Tilla* (1981), tells her boyfriend Rolf that she will not let him endanger her own future as an artist by allowing him to use her sexually. However, Stensland notes that the portraits of the mothers in these books, who represent the future of the young female protagonists, indicate that in society at large women have continued to have difficulty being well-rounded individuals. The mothers in the 1982 books were traditional, stay-at-home mothers. Or, they were professional successes—and personal failures. Or, they may have had professions, but they chose to leave these professions when they had children. For instance, Stensland cites a passage from Karen Ray's *The Proposal* (1981) in which the main character, Sarah, describes her conservative mother; although the mother has always worked alongside the father and has always encouraged Sarah to be whatever she wanted to be, she "was still surprised that the daughter she raised would use that ambition, independence and intelligence to do something as unusual as engineering" (70). The fathers in these books also portrayed traditional patterns of interaction and behavior.

Cooper's analysis of Caldecott and Newbury winners (1989) also indicates that little has changed in the adult role models provided for young women and men. In more recent titles, adult women are

> portrayed as more than mothers. Occupations include teacher, receptionist, nurse, caterer, musician, crazy woman, professor, doctor, storeowner, salesperson, and warrior. However, numbers fail to tell the entire story. For example, when Ramona (*Ramona Quimby, Age 8*, 1982) becomes ill, her mother stays home from work to take care of her. Her father, who is attending college, does not. There is no negotiation on this issue. The mother seems to take it for granted that this is her responsibility. (241)

Cooper points out that motherhood and careers do not seem to mix in award-winning children's literature. In McKinley's *The Blue Sword* (1982), once Harry saves her nation as a warrior, she marries the king, gives up being a warrior, and has five children. Young men, too, have only traditional role models offered to them. Jeff's father in Voight's *A Solitary Blue* (1983) does not want Jeff to cry, and he tells Jeff that boys are more reliable than girls. In describing Speare's *Sign of the Beaver* (1983), Cooper notes, "the father and son are unable to express their feelings. Each is 'locked' in the stereotype of male stoicism" (243).

Cooper concludes her discussion of the Caldecott and Newbury winners by stating that, as of 1990, sexism still exists in books for young people. True, there are more female characters in more recent books, but the roles and characterization of both male and female characters have seen little change. What she says of children as readers applies as well to their older brothers and sisters:

> One of the major socializing forces, particularly for young children, is books. Through books, children become aware of and understand different social roles people play. If stereotyped roles are the primary roles shown, males and females will fail to realize that people, regardless of their sex, can achieve a wide range of roles. (244)

In the September, 1990, issue of *English Journal*, the "Booksearch" column provides teachers' responses to the question, "What young adult novel would you nominate as the best written during the 1980s?" These reviews also indicate that young women still must deal with mixed messages about what constitutes "appropriate" behavior in society. In many of the novels, (e.g., Paterson's *Jacob Have I Loved* (1980), Peck's *Remembering the Good Times* (1986), and Sebestyn's *The Girl in the Box* (1989), females, both adolescent and adult, provide models of strength and integrity; however, the roles they play within the family structure and the careers they pursue still largely reflect traditional options. Also, it continues to be the case that more young adult novels revolve around young men than women. In six of the eight novels recommended in the "Booksearch" column, the main characters are male. A positive change, however, is that several of these books present interesting young women as well. For example Nicki in Kerr's *Night Kites* (1987) continually revels in her own unconventionalism and delights in disturbing others through her untraditional behavior, and readers are convinced that wheelchair bound Wags in Spinelli's *Night of the Whale* (1985) will achieve her professional ambitions. Perhaps if young men are attracted to these titles because they have male main characters, they will, in addition, develop some new insights and appreciation for nontraditional females. Further, in the portrayal of the young men, such as Buck Mendenhall in *Remembering the Good Times* (Peck 1986), or Mouse in *Night of the Whale* (Spinelli 1986) who are learning to express their emotions and accept their need for emotional support, these novels might best encourage both male and female adolescent readers to examine options to traditional visions of "appropriate" male behavior.

Several other studies of male/female roles in young adult fiction also indicate that while in some ways the world of literature is now a more positive place for women, in other ways things have not changed. D'Angelo (1989) did a content analysis of ten award-winning young adult novels from 1945–1985 that had primary female characters. She investigated the efforts of the female protagonists to deal with Havighurst's developmental tasks to see if there were differences in the kinds of tasks attempted and achieved by young women in books published before the beginning of the current women's movement and those attempted by heroines who appear in more recent publications. Her findings are encouraging. The young women from the earlier books dealt with issues at the lower end of Havighurst's spectrum: relationships with peers, developing a feminine social role, and accepting and using one's body effectively. The girls in the earlier books react in stereotypical ways to these issues, reflecting the social realities of their day. Most of their energy is focused on the home, their family, and their physical appearance. If they do think about social concerns, they do so only because an issue directly affects them; for instance, Marjorie from Sattley's *Shadows Across the Campus* (1957) only considers the effects of religious discrimination when she is affected. In contrast, the more contemporary books portray young women, such as Dicey from *Dicey's Song* by Voight (1982), or Vicki Austin in *Ring of Endless Light* by L'Engle (1980), who emerge from the books as "wiser for their efforts" to deal with tasks at the upper end of Havighurst's list: developing intellectual skills, desiring socially responsible behavior, gaining values and ethics. However as D'Angelo (1989) notes,

> Unfortunately, too few of these novels describing identity formation are available to young readers. In a list composed of fifteen years of awards by five prestigious groups only five novels described the female adolescent protagonist in a post World War II setting. (234)

Like Stensland, D'Angelo points out that while females may be more positively portrayed in contemporary fiction as intellectually capable and strong, we still lack books in which female readers are exposed to women working to achieve economic independence or selecting and preparing for varied and challenging occupations. The exceptions seem to occur in the genres of mystery and science fiction/fantasy. Lori, in Peterson's *How Can You Hijack a Cave?* (1990), is the one who pulls Curt into danger and adventure as they rescue a hostage; Karen Prescott, in Nixon's *Silent, Secret Screams* (1990), is a police officer; Kelly Francis, solver of the mystery in Bates's *Final Exam* (1990), spends her spare time fixing cars. Meridith Pierce, Robin McKinley, and Ursula LeGuin write books about intelligent, intrepid heroines in the science fiction/fantasy genres—and they write eloquently about the need for more strong heroines as well.

However, in recent novels for young adults, there are still few examples of mothers who manage to combine profesional expertise with competence at parenting; there are very few examples of fathers who have made untraditional choices about their careers and parenting styles. Ann Fine's *Alias Madame Doubtfire* (1989) is such a pleasant surprise because of its portrayal of a father's response to divorce and subsequent separation from his children—and of his parenting expertise when, in disguise, he manages to spend time with them.

Finding and Selecting Young Adult Novels to Use in Discussing Gender Issues

In searching for books for the library or classroom, teachers have available a wide variety of references and annotated bibliographies such as the older but still useful *Girls Are People Too!* by Newman (1982). She provides annotations about books focusing on young women in the following categories: "classic" young women, young women from American history, "the girl next door," young women representative of cultural minorities within the United States, young women from other lands, and elderly women. Newman even provides information about "non-sexist" books, such as collections of folk tales, compiled specifically to break gender stereotypes. We can turn to chapters such as "Growing up Male" and "Growing Up Female" in NCTE's *Your Reading* (Davis and Davis, eds., 1988) or "Women" and "Sexuality" in NCTE's *Books For You* (Gallo, ed., 1985). We can keep up to date with new publications and critical analyses of issues in the field of young adult literature by reading *The ALAN Review*, or by combing through the "Booksearch" columns of *English Journal* for teachers' recommendations on books, both old and new, which relate to the topic of gender issues.

The British journal *Spare Rib* is a monthly feminist magazine which regularly publishes reviews of children's books. *Hornbook*, *Children's Literature in Education*, *The Wilson Library Bulletin*, and *School Library Journal* also are useful reviewing sources. We can tap other professional resources such as Rudman's *Children's Literature: An Issues Approach* (1985) for additional guidance; her chapter on "The Female" provides selection criteria for teachers to use, as well as suggested titles and annotations. Finally, *The English Curriculum: Gender—Material for Discussion* (1984–85) published by the English Centre in London contains many ideas discussing sexism and gender issues while integrating the use of writing, language study, and the reading of young adult literature in the English classroom.

As teachers select young adult novels for use in addressing gender issues, several criteria should be considered. Most importantly, we need to avoid "tokenism." As Gonzales, writing about the need to include young adult literature reflective of cultural diversity in the literature program notes,

> One piece of literature or one chapter in American history cannot counter the negative social perceptions that children of minority subcultures have of themselves or that society has of them. A significant proportion of the curriculum must be dedicated to positive histories and literature and the many contributions that all groups have made to American life. (18–19)

To the extent that female and nontraditional male perspectives have been limited in the literature curriculum, Gonzales's comments suggest the need to include more works which represent in an honest way the contributions of women and nontraditional men to all aspects of our traditions and our contemporary life.

How can tokenism be avoided? Organizing the literature curriculum by themes representative of issues that cross gender boundaries might better allow for these goals to be met than organizing the literature program through a sequential, chronological order or by genre. If the focus of the unit is on an issue, young men and women can respond to that issue sharing their own experiences, as shaped by their gender, with death, friendship, child/parent relationships, sibling rivalry—as they also respond to the text and its presentation of the issue as shaped by the gender of the author. For instance, it would be interesting to explore whether students think the female S. E. Hinton, who writes primarily about young males, is accurate in her portrayal of their emotional responses and actions in the face of certain situations; or whether Joseph McNair's female main character in *Commander Coat-rack Returns* (1989) is reflective of female thought and feeling.

Teachers and librarians might also do their best to find and stock young adult novels in which characters of both sexes interact realistically, reflecting both the prejudices of our society and the ability of individuals to overcome these, interacting in a more positive way and learning from one another. Obviously, much non-contemporary "classic" literature contains stereotyping reflective of the historical context in which it was written. Also, many contemporary characters in well-written young adult novels do interact with others based on traditional, and even negative, stereotypes. But, as Tway (1981) notes, books which provide "an honest and authentic portrayal of the human condition" (6) will be full of characters who are condescending and even deprecatory. Students need to be exposed to such characters who do reflect current and historic realities, however uncomfortable those realities might be, and then they need to examine why those stereotypes exist and to confront their own stereotyping behaviors as a result.

Using the Novels Once You Find Them: Discussion Topics Related to Gender Issues

The messages about gender roles, both explicit and implied, given to adolescents about their future—and their present—through young adult literature need to be discussed and evaluated with readers. Specifically, teachers and students could explore, both through analysis of young adult literature and through their own responses to this literature, the ways in which young women and men are alike and different in their response to issues of importance to adolescents. The table shown indicates several topics relating to key issues for adolescents, several corresponding sources a teacher might consult, and several young adult novels which present characters (Male and/or Female) responding to these issues.

Books which present two voices, one female and one male, such as Zindel's *The Pigman*, (1968) could be used to initiate discussion of male/female differences in language use and communication style, as could a discussion of contrasting male and female narrators in diary format books, such as Mazer's *I, Trissy* (F) and Townsend's *The Secret Diary of Adrian Mole, Age 13 and 3/4* (M). Tannen's research (1990) suggests that women tend to be more tentative, more questioning, more empathetic in their conversations and relationships, while men, in general, are more assertive, more direct, more focused on external details than on internalized feelings, and more often engage in argu-

Gender Issues and Young Adult Novels

TOPIC: SOURCES	*AUTHOR, TITLE, (GENDER OF MAIN CHARACTER)*
Intimacy/Sexuality: Moffit, Christian, Cunningham	Strasser, *A Very Touchy Subject* (M) Mazer, N.F., *Up in Seth's Room* (F) Chambers, *Breaktime* (M); Koehn, *Tilla* (F) Spinelli, *Jason and Marceline* (M/F) or Blume, *Forever* (M/F)
Communication/ Interaction: Tannen, DeKlerk, Belenky et al.	Oneal, *In Summer Light* (F) versus Paulson, *The Island* (M) or Kerr, *I'll Love You When You're More Like Me* (both alternate M/F narrators)
Puberty/Body Image: Erikson, Carlson	Spinelli, *Space Station Seventh Grade* (M) vs Blume, *Are You There God, It's Me . . .* (F) Smith, *Jelly Belly* (M) Holland, *Dinah and the Green Fat Kingdom* (F)
Crisis/Death: Rofes, Mines, Pierce, Klagsbrun	Wiesel, *Night* (M-holocaust survivor) vs. Klein, *All but My Life* (F-holocaust survivor) Paulson, *Hatchet* (M) vs. George, *Julie of the Wolves* (F) Oneal, *A Formal Feeling* (F) vs Peck, *Close Enough to Touch* (M) Cole, *The Goats* (M/F)
Peers/Friendship: Foreman, Tannen Gilligan	Conrad, *Taking the Ferry Home* (F) Dines, *Best Friends Tell the Best Lies* (F) Myers, *Fallen Angels* (M) Brooks, *The Moves Make the Man* (M) Paterson, *Bridge to Terabithia* (M/F)
Standing Up for Oneself/Dealing with Pressure: Douvan, Gilligan	Cormier, *The Chocolate War* (M) Paterson, *Jacob Have I Loved* (F) Thompson, *Goofbang Value Daze* (M) Albery, *Balloon Top* (F)

mentative exchanges for the joy of doing so—which can be puzzling to women who prefer to compromise.

In Fine's *My War with Goggle Eyes* (1989), a young girl, reminded by something in the class discussion of her angry feelings about her parents' recent separation and her mother's possible remarriage, runs from the classroom and seeks shelter in a closet. The teacher sends the narrator after her; the narrator spends the rest of the book sharing her own story about her "war with Goggle Eyes," who has been dating her mother. She draws the distressed young woman's story from her in exchange. Through the sharing of experience in narrative form, the angry young woman calms down and feels capable of returning to the regular classroom. Also the narrator, through the act of shaping her own experience into story and sharing it, comes to terms with many issues in her own life.

Contrast this pattern of interaction either with that of Jerry in Cormier's *The Chocolate War* (1974) or with the first person narrator in Naughton's *My Brother Stealing Second* (1989). Jerry ultimately faces his crisis in isolation, deciding in *Beyond the Chocolate War* (1984), that he can only be true to himself and his perceptions of the realities of the world by turning his one friend away and by "going it alone." In *My Brother Stealing Second*, the narrator has an urge to *do* something, to take some action against the young man responsible for his brother's death, and he withdraws from his father in anger until his father finally makes a decision to act. These characters do not "share stories" and come to terms with their experiences through empathy as the female characters in *My War with Goggle Eyes* do. The conversations in this novel are argumentative, explosive, confrontational, judgmental.

According to Belenky and her coauthors (1986) female discussion is often characterized by attention to minute detail, intimate feelings, and family and other significant relationships; male discussion and writing tends to be concerned with generalizations and evaluations. These authors contrast E. B. White's effort to portray "grand struggles" in his vignettes and essays with the desire expressed by George Eliot to "listen to a squirrel's heartbeat" in her own writing (199). Ecroyd in "Growing Up Female" (1989) finds, through her own analysis of the writing of women authors and from her reading of others' critical studies of female writers, that this same attention to detail and feeling so often characteristic of women's writing frequently finds form in intimate genres, such as the diary or letter. Heilbrun, in *Writing a Woman's Life* (1989), finds similar traits to be characteristic of much women's writing, and she feels that those biographies of female writers written by males do not fully recognize the power of such a style or its constraints on women seeking to make sense of their universe through writing. Students can examine novels for young adults by men and women themselves to determine whether they share these perceptions, and they can explore how their own gender influences their response to writings by men and women. They might search through the library to find titles written as diaries or in the format of the "personal essay" to see if they can locate such books written by males. (*The Secret Diaries of Adrian Mole, Aged 13 and 3/4* and the "essay" that is *The Outsiders* are both authored by women, though their narrators are young men.)

Students can go on to explore how gender may influence their response to the world in general by reading autobiographies for young adults. For instance, Wiesel describing his experiences as an adolescent male during the Holocaust in *Night* (1960) focuses on issues, on the effect that all he saw and witnessed had on his religious and philosophical beliefs. Klein, describing her experiences as an adolescent girl during the Holocaust in *All But My Life* (1985) focuses on the small kindnesses of others toward her and describes ways in which both conversations and memories of poetry and song sustained her through her ordeal.

In our classrooms we can talk about whether students do and/or should feel constrained by gender stereotypes by explicitly examining gender issues as a significant goal in literature units. We can examine through discussions of young adult books and our responses to them the basis for identity as it is constructed by adolescent men and women, and we can look at how the portrayal of the characters through language choices may reflect the attitudes of the authors. For instance, what does it mean when a novelist says a female character is "spunky"? or a boy is "aggressive"? What would the converse connotations be? *The Chocolate War*'s Jerry would never be described as spunky, and the female characters such as Gilly Hopkins who are "aggressive" frequently find themselves in trouble with peers and adults. It would be interesting to talk about whether *The Chocolate War* could have been written by a female author about an all-female cast of characters; it would be interesting to consider whether Gilly would have acted any differently, made different decisions, if her name was Billy—and if her creator were male.

We must choose books which provide young men and young women with strong, admirable characters who manage to move toward the kind of integration of "male" and "female" morality described by Gilligan (1982). According to Gilligan, the "male morality" is based on *separation*. The individual separates the self from an immediate context and judges the situation based upon what are perceived to be objective rules, moral imperatives, and rights. Each individual is accorded the right to develop as an individual. The "female morality" is grounded in the immediate. Empathy and concern for others grow out of a sense of *connectedness*, and the result of this sense of interconnection is not moral judgment or a hierarchy of absolute values and rules; the effect is to encourage dialogue and networks of care and support. It is important, as Kazemak (1986) states, to note that

> Gilligan takes great care to stress the fact that while male morality is not necessarily a characteristic of the male sex and female morality is not necessarily a characteristic of the female sex, in our society they do indeed tend to be sex-related. .... She also points out that these two moralities are not opposites or sequential; one is not necessarily "better" than the other. Rather, they are complementary. She argues for a psychology of morality and love which combines the two. (265)

In *The Pigman*, published first in 1968, John and Lorraine, the alternating first person narrators, are more reflective of the traditional separation of male and female thinking. For example, after a disastrous party when the young people are taken home by the police, Lorraine's impulse is to share, at least in an abbreviated way, all that happened with her mother—to whom she does not even feel especially close. John, on the other hand, does not even attempt to explain the event to his family. When the Pigman dies, John has the last word, and the book ends with his own judgment about the moral rules he feels he and Lorraine and the Pigman himself had violated:

> I wanted to yell at her, tell her he had no business fooling around with kids. I wanted to tell her he had no right going backward. When you grow up, you're not supposed to go back. Trespassing, that's what he'd done. ... We had trespassed too—been where we didn't belong, and we were being punished for it. Mr. Pignati had paid with his life. But when he died something in us had died as well. (180–81)

In more recent titles, there are characters who reflect an ability to move out of traditional modes of thought. Kate, in Oneal's *In Summer Light* (1986), manages to learn how to make connections with her mother while heeding her own inner compulsion to paint in her own style. She learns forgiveness, a willingness to accept her famous artist of a father, as she wrestles with an essay on Prospero from *The Tempest*, ultimately writing,

> And yet, at the end of the play ... Prospero has become an old man. His magic powers are nearly gone, and then they are gone entirely. In the Epilogue he asks us to set him free. I think Shakespeare means for us to forgive him. I think he means that if we refuse, we will be trapped like Prospero was, in his island. (146)

But Kate also learns to take a stand and to rely on her own judgments even when they conflict with those of others. She asks an art critic "What's this business about 'the mainstream' anyway? ... What's any of that got to do with painting?" He replies, rather smugly,

"Quite a lot, actually." Kate takes him on, stating in no uncertain terms,

> No, it hasn't. ... Painting has to do with knocking yourself out day after day trying to get what you want down on the canvas. Maybe it works and maybe it doesn't, but every day you try. That's what painting is. (149)

Kate has developed what might be considered her own personal value structure on which to build her artistic career, one which is more individualistic than relational in nature.

On the other hand, Walker, from Crutcher's *Stotan!* (1986), provides a model for young men who are learning to see the world in less certain terms. As he looks toward graduation and the end of his high school career, he finds he has fewer and fewer answers and more and more questions—and he decides that this is okay. Walker becomes able to tolerate the ambiguities of day to day life without feeling compelled to know all the "whys." He says,

> I think if I ever make it to adulthood, and if I decide to turn back and help someone grow up, either as a parent or a teacher or a coach, I'm going to spend most of my time dispelling myths, clearing up unreal expectations. For instance, we're brought up to think that the good guys are rewarded and the bad guys are punished; but upon closer scrutiny, that assumption vanishes into thin air. ... Who are the bad guys anyway? (181–82)

This newer generation of young adult characters provides some hope that men and women can learn from one another and help each other toward a more integrated, realistic sense of what it means to be oneself.

Closing Thoughts

The young man in my class who expressed the changes in his perceptions as a result of reading *The Turbulent Term of Tyke Tyler* illustrates that the study of literature can have a positive effect on gender stereotypes. The idea that what adolescents read can affect the way they perceive themselves is based on four assumptions articulated by Purcell and Stewart (1990):

1. Sex roles are learned behaviors and are not solely biologically defined;
2. Sex role definitions can be learned from role models including people presented in media, such as picture books, story books, and films;

3. Role definitions that are narrow or rigid can be harmful to a child's development; and
4. Such narrowly defined sex-role definitions have been found by prior research in children's literature (178)

If, as Reisman stated long ago, "storytellers are the indispensable agents of socialization" (107), and if, as Rosenblatt stated (even longer ago), "through books the reader may explore his [or her] own nature, become aware of potentialities for thought and feeling within himself [or herself], acquire clearer perspective and develop aims and a sense of direction" (1938/1976, v), then those of us who attempt to help young people interact with books must be sensitive to the ways in which young adults and their elders, both male and female, are portrayed in the literature. The role models with which readers are presented should coincide with social realities, not outdated stereotypes, and as D'Anglelo (1989) citing Konopka, notes

> adolescent girls in particular need special understanding because of a new awareness by females of their identities and the rapidly changing expectations made of them in a world of adults who are ambivalent about this change (220).

We will not be able to accomplish significant changes in attitude over night. But we can change our literature programs to indicate that we value and respect diversity and that we appreciate both the similarities and differences between the sexes as one small step toward building a future citizenry that accepts individuals on their own terms rather than imposes roles and unrealistic expectations upon them because of their sex.

Works Cited

Albery, Nobuku. 1978. *Balloon Top*. New York: Pantheon.

Bates, Auline. 1990. *Final Exam*. New York: Scholastic.

Belenky, Mary F., Blyth M. Clinchy, Nancy R. Goldberger and Jill M. Tarule. 1986. *Womens' Ways of Knowing*. New York: Basic Books.

Blume, Judy. 1970. *Are You There, God? It's Me, Margaret*. New York: Bradbury.

———. 1975. *Forever*. New York: Bradbury.

"Booksearch: What Young Adult Novel Would You Nominate as the Best Written During the 1980's?" 1990. *English Journal* 79:5 (September): 94–97.

Brooks, Bruce. 1984. *The Moves Make the Man*. New York: Harper.

Carlson, Dale. 1980. *Boys Have Feelings Too: Growing Up Male for Boys*. New York: Atheneum.

———. 1973. *Girls Are Equal Too: The Women's Movement for Teenagers*. New York: Atheneum.

Chambers, Aiden. 1979. *Breaktime*. New York: Harper.

Christian, L. K. 1984. *Becoming a Woman Through Romance: Adolescent-Novels and the Ideology of Feminism*. Dissertations Abstracts International, 45, 1282 A. University Microfilms 84–13246.

Cole, Brock. 1987. *The Goats*. New York: Farrar, Straus and Giroux.

Conrad, Pam. 1990. *Taking the Ferry Home*. New York: Harper.

Cooper, Pamela J. 1989. "Children's Literature: The Extent of Sexism." In Cynthia M. Lont and Sheryl A. Friedley (Eds.), *Beyond Boundaries: Sex and Gender Diversity in Communications*, 233–49. Fairfax, VA: George Mason University Press.

Cormier, Robert. 1984. *Beyond the Chocolate War*. New York: Knopf.

———. 1974. *The Chocolate War*. New York: Pantheon.

Crutcher, Chris. 1986. *Stotan!* New York: Dell.

Cunningham, John. 1976. "Can Young Gays Find Happiness in Young Adult Books?" *Wilson Library Bulletin*, 50:7 (March): 528–34.

D'Angelo, Dolores A. 1989. "Developmental Tasks in Literature for Adolescents: Has the Adolescent Female Protagonist Changed?" *Child Study Journal*, 19:3. 219–237.

Davis, Jim and Hazel Davis. 1988. (Eds.) *Your Reading*. Urbana, IL: NCTE.

deKlerk, Vivian. 1990. "Slang: A Male Domain?" *Sex Roles* (May) 22: 9–10; 589–606.

Dines, Carol. 1990. *Best Friends Tell the Best Lies*. New York: Dell.

Donelson, Kenneth and Alleen Pace Nilsen. 1989. *Literature for Today's Young Adults*. Glenview, IL: Scott, Foresman.

Douvan, E. 1969. "Sex Differences in Adolescent Character Processes." In D. Rogers (Ed.) *Issues in Adolescent Psychology*. New York: Appleton Century Crofts, 1969. 437–445.

Ecroyd, Catherine Ann. 1989. "Growing Up Female." *Alan Review* 17:1 (Fall): 5–6, 8, 54.

Ehle, Maryann. 1982. "The Velveteen Rabbit, the Little Prince, and Friends: Postacculturation through Literature." Paper presented at the Annual Meeting of the Professional Clinic of Association of Teacher Educators (Phoenix, AZ, February 13–19): ERIC Document ED 221 881.

The English Curriculum: Gender—Material for Discussion. 1984–1985. London: The English Centre.

Erikson, Eric. 1968. *Identity, Youth and Crisis*. New York: W. W. Norton.

Fine, Ann. 1989. *Alias Madam Doubtfire*. New York: Bantam.

———. 1989. *My War With Goggle Eyes*. Boston: Little, Brown.

Gallo, Don. (Ed.) 1985. *Books for You*. Urbana, IL: NCTE.

Gilligan, Carol. 1982. *In a Different Voice: Psychological Theory and Women's*

Development. Cambridge, MA: Harvard University Press.

George, Jean C. 1972. *Julie of the Wolves*. New York: Harper and Row.

Gonzales, Roseann Duenas. 1990. "When Minority Becomes Majority: The Changing Face of the English Classroom." *English Journal* 79:1: 16–23.

Havighurst, Robert J. 1952. *Developmental Tasks and Education*. New York: David McKay.

Heilbrun, Carolyn. 1989. *Writing a Woman's Life*. New York: Ballantine.

Hinton, S. E. 1967. *The Outsiders*. New York: Viking.

Holland, Isabelle. 1986. *Dinah and the Green Fat Kingdom*. New York: Dell.

Kazemek, Francis. 1986. "Literature and Moral Development." *Language Arts* (March).

Kemp, Gene. 1980. *The Turbulent Term of Tyke Tyler*. London: Faber and Faber.

Kerr, M.E. 1977. *I'll Love You When You're More Like Me*. New York: Harper and Row.

———. 1987. *Night Kites*. New York: Harper Keypoint.

Klagsbrun, Francias. 1984. *Too Young to Die: Youth and Suicide*. Boston: Houghton Mifflin.

Klein, Gerda W. 1985. *All But My Life*. New York: Hill and Wang.

Koehn, Ilse. 1981. *Tilla*. New York: Greenwillow.

L'Engle, Madeleine. 1980. *A Ring of Endless Light*. New York: Dell.

LeGuin, Ursula. 1969. *The Left Hand of Darkness*. New York: Walker.

Mazer, Harry. 1981. *I Love You, Stupid*. New York: Avon.

Mazer, Norma Fox. 1971. *I, Trissy*. New York: Dell.

———. 1979. *Up in Seth's Room*. New York: Delacorte.

McKinley, Robin. 1982. *The Blue Sword*. New York: Greenwillow.

———. 1985. "Newberry Medal Acceptance." *Hornbook Magazine*. 61:4. 395–405.

McNair, Joseph. 1989. *Commander Coatrack Returns*. Boston: Houghton Mifflin.

Mines, Jeanette. 1989. "Young Adult Literature Female Heroes Do Exist." *ALAN Review*, 17:1. 12–24.

Moffit, M. A. 1987. "Understanding the Appeal of the Romance Novel for the Adolescent Girl: A Reader-Response Approach." Paper presented at the 37th International Communications Association Conference, Montreal, Canada, May. ERIC Documents ED 284 190.

Myers, Walter Dean. 1988. *Fallen Angels*. New York: Scholastic.

Naughton, Jim. 1989. *My Brother Stealing Second*. New York: Harper Junior.

Newman, Joan. 1982. *Girls are People, Too*. Metuchen, NJ: Scarecrow Press.

Nixon, Joan Lowry. 1990. *Silent, Secret Screams*. New York: Dell.

Oneal, Zibby. 1982. *A Formal Feeling*. New York: Viking.

———. 1986. *In Summer Light*. New York: Bantam.

Paterson, Katherine. 1980. *Bridge to Terabithia*. New York: Avon.

———. 1978. *The Great Gilly Hopkins*. New York: Avon.

———. 1980. *Jacob Have I Loved*. New York: Avon.

Paulson, Gary. 1987. *Hatchet*. New York: Bradbury.

———. 1990. *The Island*. New York: Dell.

Peck, Richard. 1982. *Close Enough to Touch*. New York: Dell.

———. 1986. *Remembering the Good Times*. New York: Dell.

Peterson, P. J. 1990. *How Can you Hijack a Cave?* New York: Dell.

Pierce, Meredith. 1988. "A Lion in the Room." *Hornbook Magazine*. 64 (1 February): 35–41.

———. 1982. *The Dark Angel*. Boston: Little, Brown.

Purcell, Piper, and Lara Stewart. 1990. "Dick and Jane in 1989." *Sex Roles*, 22.3–4: 177–84.

Ray, Karen. 1981. *The Proposal*. New York: Delacorte.

Reisman, D. 1950. *The Lonely Crowd*. New Haven, CT: Yale University Press.

Rudman, Marsha Kabakow. 1985. *Children's Literature: An Issues Approach*. Lexington, MA: D.C. Heath.

Rofes, Eric. (Ed.) 1985. *The Kids Book about Death and Dying: By and For Kids*. Boston: Little, Brown.

Rosenblatt, Louise. 1938/1976. *Literature as Exploration*. New York: Noble and Noble.

Sattley, H. 1957. *Shadows Across the Campus*. New York: Dodd, Mead.

Sebestyn, Ouida. 1989. *The Girl in the Box*. New York: Bantam.

Smith, Robert Kimmel. 1982. *Jelly Belly*. New York: Dell.

Speare, Elizabeth. 1983. *Sign of the Beaver*. Boston: Houghton Mifflin.

Spinelli, Jerry. 1986. *Jason and Marceline*. Boston: Little, Brown.

———. 1985. *Night of the Whale*. Boston: Little, Brown, 1985.

———. 1982. *Space Station Seventh Grade*. New York: Dell.

Stensland, Anna Lee. 1984. "Images of Women in Recent Adolescent Literature." *English Journal*. 73:7 (November). 66–72.

Strasser, Todd. 1985. *A Very Touchy Subject*. New York: Delacorte.

Tannen, Deborah. 1990. *You Just Don't Understand: Talk Between the Sexes*. New York: Morrow.

Thomas, Joyce Carol. 1982. *Marked by Fire*. New York: Avon.

Thompson, Julian. 1989. *Goofbang Value Daze*. New York: Scholastic.

Townsend, Sue. 1986. *The Secret Diary of Adrian Mole, Age 13 3/4*. New York: Grove Press.

Tway, Eileen. 1981. Ed. *Reading Ladders for Human Relations*. 6th ed. Urbana, NCTE.

Voight, Cynthia. 1982. *Dicey's Song*. New York: Atheneum.

———. 1989. *Seventeen Against the Dealer*. New York: Fawcett.

———. 1983. *A Solitary Blue*. New York: Atheneum.

Wiesel, Eli. 1960. *Night*. New York: Farrar, Straus and Giroux.

Zindel, Paul. 1968. *The Pigman*. New York: Harper and Row.

CONTINUING THE CONVERSATION: GENDER AND LITERATURE

Gilligan, reading *The Tempest*, notes that Miranda's central questions on hearing her father's version of her life history are "in short, why all the suffering? and where are all the women?" Think of a literary work you teach almost every year because it is a "classic," vital to the development of the students' cultural literacy. Who are the women characters? How do you know about them? What is not said about them? Try, for a moment, speaking in one of the women's voices. Notice if you had to do anything to your own voice to make yourself sound like her: Did you have to whisper? To shout? To laugh?

If, as Nancy Comley's and Nancy McCracken's essays report, students tend not to hear the voices of certain characters in the literature they read—even when those voices are screams—how can we help students regain their hearing? Why is this tricky? Is it the fault of the readers? the texts? the teachers?

What literature could you add to your curriculum to increase the gender perspectives available to your students? How could you plan your teaching of the "classics" so that all of the young men and women in your classes might find some way into them?

Look at the table of contents of the literature anthologies and texts you are using. Is there an imbalance between male and female writers? Ask your students to reflect on how they see this imbalance and ask them to reflect on how they feel themselves reacting to this question.

Cynthia Bowman's excellent ideas for the use of literature learning logs might be a good place to start (or continue) your use of journals in your teaching of literature. Consider using a split-entry journal, where students put what is happening down the left side of a page (to record their comprehension and understanding), then put down the right side their feelings about what is going on in the story. Ask the students to consider how they respond to the gendered aspects of the characters in the stories they read. Consider even a triple-entry journal, where the students share journals and react to each others' responses in the third column.

Poll your students on their favorite young adult novels. Do they select books to read that reinforce gender stereotypes? Lois Stover's essay includes a number of alternatives you might suggest as well as several ideas for units you can teach in your classes to help students look for more complex characters in the literature they read independently.

Part III
Gender and the Teaching of Composition

In this section we include essays on the teaching of writing from a variety of perspectives. McCracken opens the section with an overview of gender issues and the teaching of writing in schools and colleges. Roen's research on how teachers use the real or assumed gender of the writer in reading students' essays will probably surprise you and challenge you to read and respond to students' writing much more aware of ways your own rhetorical assumptions are stereotypically gendered. Finally, Sanborn's essay, including the voices of her college students, challenges the efficacy of the narrowly prescribed academic essay and illustrates more promising approaches.

9

Gender Issues and the Teaching of Writing

Nancy Mellin McCracken

The 1970s and early 1980s were decades when Americans were making every effort to erase gender role differences in the academy. Gender virtually disappeared as a research variable in landmark studies of writing in academic settings e.g. Emig, 1971; Britton *et al.*, 1975; Flower & Hayes, 1977; Shaughnessy, 1977; Perl, 1978; and Sommers, 1980. In Hillocks' 1986 *Research in Written Composition*, gender is not even listed in the index. Graves (1975) noted gender-related differences in the topics selected by his seven-year-old male and female subjects, but for the most part, research on adolescents and adults was what Jane Roland Martin, in another context, has called "gender-blind." This gender blindness in composition research in recent decades is not difficult to understand. In an era of newly established graduate school quotas based on gender and mandated affirmative action in higher education, most academics had seen all that they wanted to of discrimination based on claims of gender-based differences. Just as efforts to eliminate sexist language often resulted in the elimination of gender markers in language usage (e.g., not waiter or waitress, but server; not chairman or chairwoman, but chairperson), efforts to eliminate sex discrimination against students and faculty is reflected in the absence of reference to gender as a variable in research in the teaching of composition (e.g., not male or female writers, but "Twelfth Graders," "Basic Writers," "College Students"). As Elizabeth Flynn has noted, we were working hard in those times to "erase difference in a desire to universalize" (1988, 425). While it is not difficult to understand the historical lack of attention to gender as a research variable in the teaching of composition, it is no longer reasonable to continue such research without reference to the growing body of knowledge from philosophy, psychology, and communication studies concerning gender-role differences in the ways men and women learn to use language. Beginning in the latter half of the 1980s theorists began to turn their attention to gender issues in the teaching of writing (e.g., Annas, "Style as Politics," 1985). With the publication in 1986 of *Women's Way of Knowing* by Belenky, Clinchy, Goldberger, and Tarule, and the collection of essays titled *Teaching Writing: Pedagogy, Gender, and Equity* in 1987 by Caywood and Overing, gender became a significant issue for many composition teachers and theorists.

There are still those who would prefer to leave gender out of composition studies: A rose is a rose, and good writing, it is argued, is good writing without regard to the gender of the writer. It is important to ask if there is sufficient evidence to justify revising the traditional goals and approaches for composition teaching and research, when one might argue that the traditional approach has done quite nicely. Martin has argued that we must pay attention to gender in education wherever gender makes a difference, just as we must ignore it where it does not: "In acknowledging gender without making us its prisoners, a gender-sensitive ideal allows us to continue . . . building into the education of females traits genderized in favor of males without victimizing women" (1988, 12). Gender makes a difference in a composition course perhaps more than in any other course because it is in writing classes that women and men learn to extend their voices beyond the private sphere, and voice is an aspect of our culture in which sexism is so deeply ingrained we hardly even notice it.

Why Both Men and Women Might Profit from a Gender Balanced Approach to Composition Teaching and Research

Women and girls come into high school and college writing classes with different discourse experiences than men and boys. Myra and David Sadker provide important research on gender in pre-collegiate education that strongly suggests that our women students arrive with a prior educational experience that has not encouraged the development of their voices. In over a hundred fourth, sixth, and eighth grade classrooms in rural, urban, and suburban schools in four states and the District of Columbia, in which black and white, male and female teachers and students worked on math, science, and English language arts, the Sadkers and their associates found that

> at all grade levels, in all communities and in all subject areas, boys dominated classroom communication. They participated in more inter-

actions than girls did and their participation became greater as the year went on. (1985, 57)

Perhaps even more relevant for this discussion is the Sadkers' three-year study of teachers' perceptions of male-female student participation in class discussion. When shown a film of a classroom discussion in which boys clearly dominated ("a ratio of three to one"), most teachers said the girls were talking more than the boys:

> Even educators who are active in feminist issues were unable to spot the sex bias until they counted and coded who was talking and who was just watching. Stereotypes of garrulous and gossipy women are so strong that teachers fail to see this communications gender gap even when it is right before their eyes. (57)

The discovery of male dominance in the discourse in classrooms is echoed in sociolinguistic research on cross-gender conversations of adults. West and Zimmerman (1975, 1983), for example reported that men accounted for 96 percent of the interruptions in recorded conversations between male and female acquaintances. Deborah Tannen's book, *You Just Don't Understand* (1990) traces this pattern of difference in the ways males and females converse from early childhood through adulthood.

Besides the fact that girls don't get as many opportunities as boys to use their voices either in school or outside it in cross-gender conversation, there are strong cultural pressures against women using their voices too freely. Those who risk speaking out at length publicly often suffer the experience French feminist philosopher Helene Cixous described so well in "The Laugh of the Medusa":

> Every woman has known the torment of getting up to speak. Her heart racing, at times entirely lost for words, ground and language slipping away—that's how daring a feat, how great a transgression it is for a woman to speak—even just open her mouth—in public. A double distress, for even if she transgresses, her words fall almost always upon the deaf male ear, which hears in language only that which speaks in the masculine. (1976, 251)

It is not "ladylike" even in contemporary American culture for a woman to be too outspoken. Belenky and her colleagues review the terms many of the women in their study used to indicate their own beliefs that silence is a desirable trait in women, that punishment is warranted for a woman who "mouths off" (24, ff). Xaviere Gauthier expresses the views of many women toward the language they are expected to write in school:

> The frightful masculine fashion of speaking always surprises me. Speaking in order to be right!—how ridiculous! In fact, to put someone

> else in the wrong. Speaking to nail the listener's trap shut. Speaking to put her in her place. ... this machine-gun language ... this war machine. ... Let's leave the practice of every-one-out-of-my-way-or-else to the football players. (199–200)

Learning to speak what is perceived as "machine-gun language" creates a real conflict in many women, and many men as well. The acquisition of public, academic language is particularly difficult for those socialized as women, however. In her essay, "The Contradiction and the Challenge of the Educated Woman," Martin (1988) describes the common fate of many academically talented women who master the dominant discourse, get A's in their writing courses, graduate, and then turn sharply away from graduate study and career achievement. They discover that their educations have left them disabled in important ways. As Shaw's Eliza Doolittle explains to her Professor Higgins:

> You told me, you know, that when a child is brought to a foreign country, it picks up the language in a few weeks, and forgets its own. Well, I am a child in your country. I have forgotten my own language, and can speak nothing but yours. That's the real break-off ... (1951, 100)

Martin believes this phenomenon is the result of the unbearable "contradiction of the educated woman." Carol Gilligan, in her book, *In a Different Voice* (1982) explains this contradiction in terms of developmental psychology:

> Woman's place in man's life cycle has been that of nurturer, caretaker, and helpmate, the weaver of those networks of relationships on which she in turn relies. .... When the focus on individuation and individual achievement extends into adulthood, and maturity is equated with personal autonomy, concern with relationships appears as a weakness of women rather than as a human strength.

Martin, however, sees a way to turn this contradiction into a challenge by tapping the qualities that psychologists such as Gilligan and Belenky, *et al.* have found characteristic of women's ways of knowing in our society. Unless, says Martin, we find ways to help our students wed their central ways of knowing—care, concern, connection—to our academic goals of rationality, critical thinking and autonomy ultimately our efforts will have failed. If these researchers are right and most women create their knowledge in a context of care, concern, and connection, then those who would help their women students achieve success with writing in school and *beyond* school would do well to revise their approaches to teaching to allow for this kind of learning.

The healthy trend at the elementary school level to encourage children of both sexes to develop a repertoire of voices in a whole language environment has met with greater resistance in the upper grades. When children reach secondary school, opportunities to develop personal knowledge and personal voice are replaced with the requirement to master theme writing. Young men and women are discouraged from writing about topics that do not fit into the fixed form of the five-paragraph essay with its certain thesis and predicted conclusion. The collaboration fostered in the primary grades is cut off in favor of competition in the higher grades.

The traditional college composition course pits individual students against one another in competition for grades which, it is assumed, students acquire like consumer goods (c.f. Friere). In efforts to train their students to enter the academic community, instructors teach their students to write with a voice characterized by distance and disinterest, and thereby, unwittingly, they cut them off from a needed sense of community. It seems clear that the teaching of composition should be reviewed in the light of gender sensitivity if all our students, males and females, are to fully develop the potential to use their own voices strongly and to hear the voices of others clearly.

Kenneth Burke once compared education to joining a conversation. Imagine, he said, walking into a room in which a conversation has already been going on for quite some time. One listens quietly for a period of time, and then, puts one's oar in to join the conversation. If learning to write in the academy is as Burke describes it, then insights gained from sociolinguists who study men and women in conversation will be important for those of us who teach composition to men and women. Tannen observed that when men talk together, they limit their topics to simple, relatively safe, public topics. Their conversations proceed by one-up-manship, a series of assertions and evidence, one man's contribution not necessarily connected to the other's. When women talk together they open complex, difficult, and often private topics. Their converasations proceed collaboratively, questioning and embellishing each other's statements. Each speaker's contribution is interwoven with the prior speakers'.

Tannen's book has achieved popular attention because her research offers explanations for cross-gender linguistic battles men and women have been fighting for years outside as well as within the academy. Tannen explains, for example, that when women express a problem or concern they are likely seeking a listener who will share the concern, embellish it, and offer solace and, perhaps descriptions of similar problems. This is the way women—but not men—usually respond to each other. When men express a problem or concern they are more likely seeking a solution to their problem. When their feminine conversation mates, instead, offer sympathy, embellishment of the problem, and anecdotes of similar problems, they become impatient.

What does this research suggest about the ways we might best help women join the academic conversation? If we imagine a man and a woman walking into the parlor in which a conversation of men has been going on for a long time, we must imagine significant differences. The man will speak almost immediately. He will offer his knowledge on the given topic and then feel free to change the topic as he wishes. The woman will likely remain silent until she gets a sense of the direction of the conversation and a sense of the speakers' attitudes and purposes. Then she will offer some related experience of her own or otherwise express support for the speaker and the topic in progress.

The implications for those who would prepare women—and men socialized in similar ways—to enter the academic master discourse are clear.

What Would a Composition Class That Incorporated Recent Gender Research Look Like?

First, the students would be helped to discover a way to make their contribution to the academic conversation *useful beyond the classroom*. If, as developmental psychologists are learning, most girls and women and many boys and men as well, are primarily motivated by care, concern, and connection, then it makes sense to provide writing projects that will engage students' sense of care and concern, projects that have the potential to alleviate suffering, to provide needed care, and projects that invite connection to the life of the writer. The opportunity to engage in sustained discourse about topics to which the writer is personally connected through care and concern will likely be helpful to males, but not so comfortable for them because, as research indicates, there is really no place else in their lives where they can acceptably talk and write in this way. For females this opportunity will likely be both helpful and comfortable because it allows them to take a mode of learning that is central to their lives outside of school and apply it to their learning in school.

Second, the students would be given the *opportunity to read* a variety of writers and genres on a given issue before being asked to contribute to the "conversation." Women conversants are used to participating in collaborative conversations, and their contributions are often the very skillful "weaving" of prior contributions. They should be very good at writing "synthesis" papers, and these papers should provide a firm base for later analytic ones. Providing opportunities to write about topics on which the students are already authorities would ease the students' entry into the academic conversation.

Third, the students would be given the *time to listen* long before they are asked to put in their oar and join the conversation. Many women writers will profit from assignments where they have time to develop deep knowledge of their topic. This goal could be met by the sequential writing assignments advocated by Bartholomae and Petrosky (1987), and others. Instead of asking students to write nine (or however many) papers on a series of unrelated topics, students would gain more command of their writing if they wrote nine parts of one longer paper on a single broader topic.

Fourth, writers would likely profit by an opportunity to engage in *dialogue with texts* they are reading, to keep a dialogue journal in which they ask and answer questions, embellish the text with their own experiences, and offer affective responses. Writers also would have ample oportunity to talk in groups in which they could play both Elbow's (1973) "doubting and believing games" before writing. Without awareness of the characteristics of "women's ways of knowing," teachers might view these kinds of responses as inappropriate digressions from the academic task at hand. One of the teachers in Gilligan's study at the Emma Willard School explains, "Had I not had this approach validated by the Gilligan research, I would have enjoyed these stories yet harbored an uneasy feeling that these were diversions" (1990, 304).

Fifth, *social context* is important to the conversant. Advice to students to develop an uninterrupted discourse is misguided unless those students who are unused to delivering such monologues outside of school have been given the opportunity to explore the rhetorical context for their writing. Ong (1975), in "The Writer's Audience Is Always a Fiction," imagines a teacher's assignment to write about your summer vacation. His hypothetical student's response, "Who wants to know?" is likely to be raised by a woman, along with a host of other questions: "Does it have to be true?" "How long can it be?" These questions which may suggest insecurity or, worse, a kind of negotiating for a minimal commitment, may instead signal the quite sophisticated recognition of the writer that writing is entering a social context. To cut these questions off is to miss the opportunity to build on a strength of many writers to see invention in writing as a social act (LeFevre 1987).

Sixth, both men and women should be given the *opportunity to collaborate* in same-gender and mixed gender writing groups. As Ede and Lunsford (1990) have shown, collaboration is the norm in the world of work, and male and female students need to learn to write together. Women's likely practice with collaborative discourse can be used as a strength in the writing class. Unless males and females are given opportunities to learn to communicate effectively with one another there is little chance they will avoid the cross-gender communication gap described by Tannen and others.

Seventh, if response to student writing is to be helpful to students it makes sense for *teachers to practice women's ways of listening* that are known to facilitate discourse, especially when they mark papers or conference with students about drafts. Fishman (1983) found that providing frequent "supportive utterances" and questions enabled women's conversation mates to initiate and develop conversation topics, whereas withholding such comments and questions had the opposite effect. McCracken, Green, and Greenwood (in press) show a number of examples of men and women instructors responding in gender-stereotypical ways and suggest that the women in their studies responded more positively to teacher comments that were like Fishman's women's responses. Research reported in the essays in this volume by Sanborn and Greenwood suggests that when authoritarian teachers respond to students' writing they appropriate the students' texts and silence their developing voices.

Finally, a writing course based on what is known about gender and language would give all students *the opportunity to hear other voices like theirs*, not confine their assigned reading to a limited sampling of linear argument or exposition. Students who have an opportunity to read a rich variety of essay types beyond the syllogistic or expository essay will discover models on which to develop their own written discourse. Essayists from Alice Walker to Annie Dillard to Virginia Woolf need to be read by students who have spent their time outside of school finely tuning a collaborative, exploratory, personal mode of discourse in their speech and letters and diaries. It would be both unhelpful and unfair to pretend to such students that the most effective, most memorable, most informative, and clearest kind of writing is the linear academic essay.

Linear, Aristotelian rationality is one mode of thinking and writing. But it has been privileged so as to exclude from serious consideration any other mode. Students are required to practice it constantly in defending their positions in class and in writing their exposition and arguments. Feminist theorists such as Adrienne Rich, Helene Cixous, and Catherine Clemont, have taught that gender has entered into the very core of our thinking, our logic, and how hard it is to see that the ways women think cannot be dismissed as irrational, intuitive, purely emotional expression, but are powerful alternative ways of thinking. These theorists point out that the academically privileged mode of thinking and writing is hierarchical and adversarial: *either* this *or* that proposition is true, not both *and*; either this statement supports or refutes a single proposition, or it is irrelevant. There are other modes, women's modes and non-western modes, of writing and thinking which are effectively used by both men and women. These modes are less linear and less hierarchical, but no less truth bearing.

Gender studies have important implications for us as writing teachers because they suggest that we must, ourselves, learn additional forms and logics and listen for them in our students' writing. We must help students try to discover how to write about what they know that goes beyond where the linear, hierarchical, completely certain mode of thinking and writing can take them. Where we once listened only for major and minor premise, we must now listen also for truth statements shaped in different patterns such as metaphors and parallel narratives. In addition to the modes of narration, description, exposition, and persuasion, after all, there are—and there have long been—the non-academic, but central, modes of celebration, lament, and puzzlement. These writing purposes don't often fit well into the canonized patterns of organization—comparison-contrast, cause-effect, problem-solution, process-analysis—so we will also need to learn and teach a greater variety of forms. Fortunately we can find those forms almost everywhere we read outside the academy, and more and more even within it. Although it will take some work at change, it appears that a gender-balanced composition course would be the best for all students, and perhaps for their teachers as well.

Works Cited

Annas, Pamela. 1985. "Style As Politics: A Feminist Approach to the Teaching of Writing." *College English* 47.4: 360–71.

Bartholomea, David and Anthony Petrosky. 1987. *Facts, Artifacts, Counterfacts*. Portsmouth NH: Heinemann.

Belenky, Mary Field, Blythe McVicker Clinchy, Nancy Rule Goldberger, and Jill Mattuck Tarule. 1986. *Women's Ways of Knowing: The Development of Self, Voice, and Mind*. NY: Basic.

Britton, James, *et al.* 1975. *Development of Writing Abilities (11–18)*. London: Macmillan Education.

Caywood, Cynthia L., and Gillian R. Overing. 1987. *Teaching Writing: Pedagogy, Gender, and Equity*. Albany: State U of New York P.

Cixous, Helene. 1981. "The Laugh of the Medusa." *New French Feminisms*. Ed. Elaine Marks and Isabelle de Courtivron, 245–264. New York: Schocken.

Cixous, Helene and Catherine Clement. 1975. *The Newly Born Woman*. Trans. Betsy Wing. Minneapolis: University of Minnesota P.

Ede, Lisa and Andrea Lunsford. 1990. *Singular Texts/Plural Authors: Perspectives on Collaborative Writing*. Carbondale: Southern Illinois UP.

Elbow, Peter. 1973. *Writing without Teachers*. New York: Oxford UP.

Emig, Janet. 1971. *The Composing Processes of Twelfth Graders*. Urbana: NCTE.

Fishman, Pamela M. 1983. "Interaction: The Work Women Do." In *Language*

Gender and Society. Eds. Barrie Thorne and Nancy Henley, 89–101. Rowley, Mass: Newbury.

Flower, Linda and John R. Hayes. 1977. "Problem-Solving Strategies and the Writing Process." *College English* 49: 19–37.

Flynn, Elizabeth. 1988. "Composing as a Woman." *College Composition and Communication* 39: 423–435.

Friere, Paolo. 1970. *Pedagogy of the Oppressed*. New York: Seabury.

Gauthier, Xaviere. 1981. "Why Witches?" In Marks and de Courtivron, Eds. *New French Feminisms*. New York: Schocken. 199–203.

Gilligan, Carol. 1982. *In a Different Voice*. Cambridge: Harvard UP.

Gilligan, Carol, Nona P. Lyons, and Trudy J. Hanmer, Eds. 1990. *Making Connections: The Relational Worlds of Adolescent Girls at the Emma Willard School*. Cambridge: Harvard UP.

Graves, Donald. 1975. "An Examination of the Writing Processes of Seven Year Old Children." *Research in the Teaching of English*. 9: 227–41.

Hillocks, George. 1986. *Research on Written Composition: New Directions for Teaching*. Urbana, IL.: NCRE/ERIC.

LeFevre, Karen Burke. 1987. *Invention As a Social Act*. Carbondale: Southern Illinois UP.

Martin, Jane Roland. 1985. *Reclaiming a Conversation: The Ideal of the Educated Woman*. New Haven: Yale UP.

———. 1988. "The Contradiction and the Challenge of the Educated Woman." Address to the Gender and Education Conference, Kent State University.

McCracken, Nancy, Lois Green, and Claudia Greenwood. In press. "Resisting Gender in Composition Research: A Strange Silence." In Susan Hunter and Sheryl Fontayne, Eds. *Unheard Voices*. Carbondale: Southern Illinois UP.

Ong, J. Walter. 1975. "The Writer's Audience Is Always a Fiction." *Publication of the Modern Language Association*. 90: 9–21.

Perl, Sandra. 1978. "The Composing Processes of Unskilled College Writers." *Research in the Teaching of English*. 13: 317–36.

Rich, Adrienne. 1979. *On Lies, Secrets, and Silence: Selected Prose 1966–1978*. New York: Norton, 1979.

Sadker, Myra, and David Sadker. 1985. "Sexism in the Schoolroom of the '80s." *Psychology Today*. March, 54–57.

Shaughnessy, Mina. 1977. *Errors and Expectations*. New York: Oxford UP.

Shaw, Bernard. 1951. *Pygmalion*. Baltimore: Penguin.

Sommers, Nancy. 1982. "Responding to Student Writing." *College Composition and Communication* 33: 148–56.

Tannen, Deborah. 1990. *You Just Don't Understand: Women and Men in Conversation*. NY: William Morrow.

West, Candace, and Don H. Zimmerman. 1983. "Small Insults: A Study of

Interruptions in Cross-Sex Conversations between Unacquainted Persons." Thorne, Barrie, Cheris Kramarae, and Nancy Henley, eds., 103–17. *Language, Gender and Society*. Rowley, MA: Newbury.

Zimmerman, D. H., and C. West. 1975. "Sex Roles, Interruptions, and Silences in Conversation. In *Language and Sex: Difference and Dominance*. Ed. Barrie Thorne and Nancy Henley. Rowley, MA: Newbury, 105–130.

10

Gender and Teacher Response to Student Writing

Duane H. Roen

Interest in gender differences in writing is not new.[1] More than forty years ago, Stalnaker (1941) reported gender differences on essays written by high school students for the 1940 English examination of the College Entrance Examination Board. With a sample consisting of 3,879 boys and 2,178 girls, the mean score for girls was 527 while that for boys was 485. This difference of 42 points, said Stalnaker, was "large and significant" (533). His concluding sentence summarizes his discussion: "Girls in the type of culture from which these groups are drawn seem to show a superior ability in writing English" (535).

Britton, Burgess, Martin, McLeod, and Rosen (1975) considered the gender of writers and found that adolescent boys and girls preferred different audiences and different functions in their writing. While girls preferred "trusted adults" as audience, boys preferred "teachers." While girls preferred expressive writing, boys preferred pseudo-informative (111).

Diederich (1974) briefly reports on a study conducted by Rosner (no citation) in which labels such as "grade 9" or "grade 10," "regular" or "honors," and "girl" or "boy" were attached to papers evaluated in the context of a larger study. In Rosner's study the labels "regular" or "honors" did affect grades that secondary teachers assigned to papers, but no other labels, including "girl" or "boy" did.

Published results from the National Assessment of Educational Progress (1980) point to gender differences in the writing of nine-, thirteen-, and seventeen-year-old students. Results pertaining to the oldest group, the group closest in age to students in the present study, are interesting and perhaps revealing. NAEP results have suggested that girls at this age generally wrote better papers than boys.

More specifically, among seventeen-year-old girls' narrative papers, 73.8 percent were judged to be competent or better in 1969, 67.9 percent in 1974, and 82.8 percent in 1979. Percentages of "competent or better" narrative papers for boys, on the other hand, were 64.5 percent, 59.4 percent, and 74.8 percent, respectively, for those three years (1980, 16).

In both 1974 and 1979 seventeen-year-old girls did better than boys in persuasive writing. In 1974, 28.2 percent of the girls wrote competent or better papers, but only 20.3 percent did so in 1979. While only 14.4 percent of the boys wrote competent or better persuasive papers in 1974, and even smaller percentage (8.9 percent) performed that well in 1979 (1980, 27).

In 1974, 49.2 percent of seventeen-year-old girls wrote competent or better explanatory papers; 53.0 percent did so in 1979. The percentages for boys for those two years were 43.6 percent and 39.1 percent, respectively (1980, 33).

In the report of the 1984 National Assessment of Educational Progress (Applebee, Langer and Mullis 1986), female students in grades 4, 8, and 11 again had significantly higher achievement in writing than males.

The aforementioned responses to students' papers point to yet another set of problems that seem to stem from teachers' stereotypes of male and female students. Sears and Feldman (1974) have reviewed a number of studies investigating the ways in which teachers interact with their elementary and secondary students. Many of these studies suggest that teachers dole out differential rewards (expressions of approval or disapproval, praise or blame, attention, and even grades) depending on complex interactions of factors such as gender of the student, students' personalities, the types of behavior exhibited, and conformity to school norms of behavior. For example, Spaulding (1963) reported that teachers' criticisms of boys tend to be harsh or angry in tone while their criticisms of girls tend to be "normal" in tone. While no one is certain how such differential treatment may affect boys, Sears and Feldman hypothesize that defiance and independence may result, which in turn may be detrimental to effective thinking (Maccoby 1966). Given our field's prevalent belief that effective writing requires effective thinking (indeed, it may even be synonymous with effective thinking), we need to consider carefully the tone of our comments on students' papers.

Research spanning several decades suggests that teachers—because we all suffer from the frailty that comes with being human—can bring a wide array of gender-related stereotypes—some founded, others not—to the task of reading students' papers. For example, our grading, especially at the secondary level, has tended to favor females over males (Baker 1954; Donelson 1963, 1967; Martin 1970, 1972; National Assessment of Educational Progress 1980; Stalnaker 1941; Woodward and Phillips 1967). However, this documented preference needs to be qualified. For instance, Daly and Miller (1975) and Dickson (1978), in examining levels of writing apprehension, have found that women are less apprehensive than men and that apprehension is inversely related to perceptions of previous success in writing. Further, Daly (1979) found that teachers have differential expectations of students' achievement based on gender and level of apprehension. Specifically, teachers most positively regarded high apprehensive males and low apprehensive females. That is, teachers most highly regarded students who most fully approximated their stereotypes.

First Part of the Study

Studies such as those that I have cited here have for a long time made me wonder about the ways and extent that gender influences teachers' responses to students' writing. I have also been curious about the ways in which we can reveal those influences. Several years ago these and other curiosities led me to conduct a study to test gender differences in teachers' responses to students' papers (Roen 1989). In both parts of that study, I asked teachers to read four persuasive letters written by high school juniors: two written by males and two written by females. Students wrote these letters as part of an earlier study (Piche and Roen 1987). In that study, students read a letter from a fictitious school nurse, who argued that schools should not establish smoking lounges for students because the creation of such lounges could easily be construed as schools' condoning an activity that is clearly hazardous to health. In response to the nurse's letter, each student, adopting the persona of a student council member at the fictitious high school at which the nurse worked, wrote a persuasive letter to the nurse. I present the four letters below and invite readers to speculate on the gender of each writer. Later, I will reveal the gender of each writer.

> Dear Mrs. Anderson:
> #1 In regard to your letter condemning the proposal of a school smoking lounge for students, I must disagree.
>
> I feel that banning smokers to hide in cars and bathrooms is much more of a health and education risk.
>
> The health risk being obvious, non-smokers will suffer by the fact that they too must use the smoke-filled restrooms. Providing a area for smokers to indulge their habit without being offensive to non-smokers was a major reason for the proposal.
>
> Both students' rights are now being neglected—the smoker to smoke and the non-smoker to avoid the smoke.

The education risk is the fact that students who smoke are missing three days of school because of their habit, therefore contributing to the downfall of the educational process and ultimately their grade point average. Do adults suffer pay losses from indulging this habit at work? No, I think not.

#2 As a non-smoker, I understand how you feel; however, I do not agree with your argument.

I feel a smoking lounge for students would be a good idea, for the simple reason that if the faculty tells the students that they can't smoke on school grounds, the students will take rebellious action.

Those who smoke will smoke, even if it does break the rules. Students will begin to "sneak" cigarettes, smoking them in the bathrooms and such. This would then expose non-smokers to cigarette smoke whereas a smoking lounge would be only smokers and the non-smokers could go in the bathrooms being able to breathe fresh air.

I feel that it is only fair that if the faculty can have a smoking lounge, the students should be allowed a smoking lounge.

Sure, smoking is definitely injurious to one's health, but think about what I have said. Wouldn't it be better to let the smokers smoke in one room rather than pollute the bathrooms?

Thank you for taking time to listen to my point of view.

#3 In regard to your letter you wrote to the student council, I personally disagree strongly on your stance to abolish the proposed student smoking lounge.

You mention the safety and well-being of the people in this school. Let me state that if someone chooses to smoke, it is their own choice. The smoke from their cigarettes won't kill anyone that doesn't smoke. People that don't smoke won't have to even set foot in the lounge.

If we had a lounge, people wouldn't have to go and sneak around just to have a smoke. The teachers have their own lounge. They can smoke anytime. Why not hit them with you anti-smoking campaign? See what kind of response you get. And because kids are sneaking around, many are getting suspended. What good is this? It won't stop them from smoking.

I'm not saying that everyone should smoke. You have your opinion and that's fine, but let others have theirs, too! Let people make up their own minds. If they don't want to smoke, they won't have to use the lounge.

#4 Thank you for your response; I know this is a touchy subject because either way the vote goes, someone is offended.

We, the Student Council, are trying to work out a plan where no one is offended. If fifty percent of juniors and seniors smoke, most of them will probably not quit, so we have to live with the fact that fifty

> percent of the students in the Senior High smoke. We (the Student Council) have proposed a plan that would put the smokers in a smoking area away from the other non-smoking students.
>
> This resolution would:
>
> a) keep the smokers happy on their free time,
> b) keep the nonsmokers happy by keeping the smokers secluded in their own area,
> c) keep smoking out of the bathrooms,
> d) no smokers would be punished for smoking if they stayed in their area.
>
> We feel this is the strongest proposal yet because we know it pleases both groups of people. I myself feel smoking is bad and I hope that you can help people from not smoking, but this proposal keeps both groups satisfied for the meantime.

In preparing the papers for this part of study, I typed each paper, correcting spelling and punctuation errors. I created eight fictitious names of student writers—one male name and one female name for each of the four papers. The names were all intended to sound Anglo-Saxon: Patricia Dunn, Gary Hopkins, Jane Cooper, Edward Davis, Thomas Brown, Linda Rogers, Jeffery Hunt, Gloria Winthrop. The two letters written by females in the earlier study were assigned two female names (Patricia Dunn, Linda Rogers) and two male names (Gary Hopkins, Thomas Brown). Likewise, the two letters written by males were assigned two male names (Edward Davis, Jeffery Hunt) and two female names (Jane Cooper, Gloria Winthrop). As teachers for the present study read the letters, they wrote the student writer's name at the top of each scoring sheet. This procedure ensured that teachers attended to those names. The names on two of the letters that each teacher read correctly identified the gender of the writer while the other two names incorrectly identified the gender. I arranged the two sets of papers so that a paper with a correct label in one set had an incorrect label in the other set. As each teacher read a paper, he or she wrote the student writer's name at the top of a scoring sheet to ensure that he or she attended to those names—that is, to the gender label. My assumption was that the names—gender labels—would influence teachers' evaluations of the papers in such a way that papers with female labels would receive higher ratings than papers with male labels, regardless of the real gender of the writers.

I randomly assigned each of 28 high school English teachers (14 males, 14 females) to read one of two sets of four papers. Each teacher read the two letters written by males and the two written by females. The names on two of the letters correctly identified the gender of the writer while the other two names incorrectly identified the gender. The order in which teachers read the four letters was counterbalanced to avoid order effects.

Each teacher was given the following instructions:

> Attached are four essays written by ninth-grade students. Their assignment was to write a letter designed to persuade the school nurse, Vanessa Anderson, to reconsider her stand against a smoking lounge for students. Her main objection to establishing such a lounge was that it constituted tacit approval of an unhealthy activity. Please read the papers, and using the criteria you normally use for evaluating student essays, assign a numerical value (1–5) and complete the remainder of the attached evaluation scale. Please include your name and the name of the student writer on the evaluation form. Thank you.

After reading the instructions, each teacher read the first of the four persuasive letters. After reading the first paper, the teacher completed a scoring sheet (see figure, page 132). The first item on the scoring sheet was a holistic scale, with 1 as the lowest possible score and 5 as the highest. The teacher then completed nine Lykert-type items designed to measure teachers' assessments of writers' personal qualities. Scores of 1 to 4 were possible for each of these items. Each teacher then followed this procedure for the remaining three persuasive letters.

On the holistic measure, as well as most of the analytic measures, the gender of the teacher and the labeled gender of the writer made no significant difference in scores. There was, however, a strong, consistent interaction between gender of reader and real gender of writer. That is, male readers assigned significantly higher scores to persuasive letters written by male students, and female readers assigned significantly higher scores to persuasive letters written by female students, regardless of the gender label. This trend showed up in holistic scores, as well as scores for six of the nine analytic measures. The six significant interactions involved the following readers' judgments of writers: respect for the writers' opinions, their intelligence, the confidence they inspire, their experience with the topic, their qualifications to write about the subject, and their truthfulness. The nonsignificant interactions were as follows: the writers as sources of information on the topic, their informedness, and their honesty. The consistency of the interaction across the measures suggests that gender-specific linguistic and rhetorical discourse features, rather than gender stereotypes evoked by the gender labels attached to the texts, had differential effects on male and female readers.

I have tried to find features of these four papers that might account for the results. For example, the males' papers have roughly 50 percent

Figure 1

Teachers' Response Form

(Please print)

Your Name ________

Writer's Name______

I. Please rate the overall quality of this paper by circling one of the five numbers that follow.

LOW QUALITY				HIGH QUALITY
1	2	3	4	5

II. Please indicate your response to each of the following items by circling one of the five possible responses: 1 = Strongly Disagree, 2 = Disagree, 3 = Agree, 4 = Strongly Agree.

1 2 3 4 I respect this writer's opinion on the topic.
1 2 3 4 This writer is very intelligent.
1 2 3 4 This writer is a reliable source of information on the topic.
1 2 3 4 I have confidence in this writer.
1 2 3 4 The writer is well informed on this subject.
1 2 3 4 The writer has had much experience with this subject.
1 2 3 4 This writer is well qualified to write on this subject.
1 2 3 4 This writer is basically an honest person.
1 2 3 4 I trust this writer to tell the truth about the topic.

III. Personally, I find this writer:

Unreliable				Reliable
1	2	3	4	5
Unintelligent				Intelligent
1	2	3	4	5
Inexpert				Expert
1	2	3	4	5
Dishonest				Honest
1	2	3	4	5

more T-units[2], but I can find no evidence that this difference should make a difference for male and female readers. A second difference—that the males focused on their own needs more than twice as many times as the females—may make a difference, though. Tannen (1990) cites a study by Goodwin (in press) in which "boys typically did not give reasons for their demands, other than their wishes" (Tannen 156–57). Not giving reasons for demands or assertions, as in a persuasive letter of the type under consideration here, reinforces hierarchical social structures, to which males tend to subscribe (Gilligan 1982, 163; Tannen 1990, 156–58). The female writers engaged in slightly more refutation than males, but I'm not certain that that difference matters. In a third difference, the males directly addressed the school nurse, the person whose own letter served as part of the prompt for the students' writing, approximately 2.5 times as often as the females. Directly addressing the school nurse, who happened to be portrayed as a woman, may have been the males' way of establishing their separation from the nurse—something that Gilligan says is common for adolescent males, who are struggling to achieve personal masculine identity by separating themselves from their mothers (8). In the letters, when *I* as a writer explicitly address *you* as a reader, especially in an argument, I may be marking our separateness or even the antagonism that exists between us in this dispute. That is, I may be saying, "*I* know; *you* don't."

Second Part of the Study

In the second part of the study, I asked twelve graduate students in rhetoric and composition at a major university in a Rocky Mountain state to look at the same four papers. This time, though, I removed the fictitious names from the papers before asking the graduate students, all teachers of writing, to guess the gender of each paper's writer. I also asked them to explain the reasons for their guesses.

While two of these readers guessed the gender of the writer with 0 percent accuracy, two others were accurate on 25 percent of their guesses, and the remaining eight readers were accurate on 50 percent of their guesses. No one was accurate 75 percent or 100 percent of the time.

I repeated this part of the study with readers from a major university in the Southwest. The results were similar. While no one guessed with 0 percent accuracy, twelve readers guessed with 50 percent accuracy. Three readers were accurate 75 percent of the time; one guessed with 100 percent accuracy.

When I compared the accuracy of the male and female readers at both universities, I found some interesting patterns, which are evident in the table shown on page 134.

Although both males and females were accurate just over 52 percent of the time, which is approximately at the level of chance, the individual papers yielded widely differing rates of accuracy. Readers were not very successful at guessing the gender of the writers of papers 1 and 4; they were moderately successful with paper 2 and very successful with paper 3.

Table 1
Rates for Accurately Guessing Gender of Writer

	Paper 1 (female)	Paper 2 (female)	Paper 3 (male)	Paper 4 (male)	All Papers
Females					
School 1	3/8 (37.5%)	4/8 (50.0%)	6/8 (75.0%)	1/8 (12.5%)	14/32 (43.75%)
School 2	3/9 (33.3%)	8/9 (88.9%)	9/9 (100.0%)	2/9 (22.2%)	22/36 (61.1%)
Subtotal	6/17 (35.3%)	12/17 (70.1%)	15/17 (88.2%)	3/17 (17.6%)	36/68 (52.9%)
Males					
School 1	2/4 (50.0%)	1/4 (25.0%)	4/4 (100.0%)	1/4 (25.0%)	8/16 (50.0%)
School 2	2/7 (28.6%)	6/7 (85.75%)	5/7 (71.4%)	2/7 (28.6%)	15/28 (53.7%)
Subtotal	4/11 (36.4%)	7/11 (63.6%)	9/11 (81.8%)	3/11 (27.3%)	23/44 (52.3%)
Total	10/28 (35.7%)	19/28 (67.9%)	24/28 (85.7%)	6/28 (21.4%)	59/112 (52.7%)

I won't repeat here all of the reader's reasons for their guesses but I do wish to offer some of the more interesting ones from readers who guessed incorrectly.

Paper #1, which was written by a female:

> Male. The writer's sense that (he) is writing to a kind of crazy old bat—I guess I feel that (his) willingness to make her seem stupid is "male." (female reader)

> Male. No emotional appeal; objections are structured, and closing sentence is *overly* formal. (female reader)

> Male. It sounds like the statement a male would make. (male reader)

> Male. I see the writing as forceful and direct, usually considered a male trait, but more than that I see some male-type choppiness. (male reader)

Paper #2, which was written by a female:

> Male. The last paragraph hints that a man wrote this. He asks the questions back at the reader and Mrs. Anderson. I can't picture a girl

> saying "Think about what I have said." It doesn't fit a girl's image in my opinion. (male reader)

> Male. Some of the word choice was like a male. That he was very sure about himself. (female reader)

Paper #3, which was written by a male:

> Female. This sounds like a woman because she is more concerned about the student than most men would. (female reader)

> Female. "Let me state" is a strident young female mind hitting its stride. (male reader)

> Female. I can hear one of my female students saying this. (male reader)

Paper #4, which was written by a male:

> Female. The conciliatory tone—the willingness to humor the reader in the beginning—the willingness to identify with the reader at the end. (female reader)

> Definitely female. A gentle approach, yet fair. "I know this is a touchy subject" sounds like a feminine introduction to me. (female reader)

> Female. Tries to see others' opinions—cares.
> Empathetic. Not very assertive ("We feel"). (female reader)

> Female. Starts out politely. The writer says "happy." A male would probably say "satisfied." (male reader)

> Female. Wants to please everyone. Uses a variety of persuasive strategies; my experience suggests that women seem more open to a variety of prose strategies. (male reader)

The reasons offered by these readers reveal some stereotypes that they hold *or* that they perceive others to hold about males and females and their written discourse. Of course, the stereotypes seem incongruous, given that the guesses were wrong. However, the reasons offered by readers who accurately guessed the gender of writers revealed some equally strong stereotypes:

Paper #1, which was written by a female:

> Female. Presents disagreement in less aggressive language. (female reader)

> Female. Possibly because of the nature of the argument, i.e., talking in general terms. (male reader)

Paper #2, which was written by a female:

> Female—placing such a significance on "bathrooms" seems typically female to me. (female reader)
>
> Female. It's empathetic and takes others into account in a more concerned voice. (male reader)

Paper #3, which was written by a male:

> Male. Aggressive voice. (female reader)
>
> Male. I feel this is more aggressive male rhetoric. It's the typical male argument that if I can vote and go to war then I should be able to do X. (male reader)

Paper #4, which was written by a male:

> Male. The way the letter has been broken down into certain areas is somewhat characteristic of a man. (female reader)
>
> Male. Wimpy final sentence betrays a well-groomed and mannered young Jim Kolbe sort. (male reader)
> (Note: Jim Kolbe is an Arizona Republican serving in the U.S. House of Representatives.)

The rates of guessing accurately and the comments that readers offered suggest an explanation: Papers 1 and 4 have features that violate readers' stereotypes quite often while paper 2 and especially paper 3 conform to their stereotypes.

Paper #2, for instance, exhibits some of the features that Tannen (1990) says are common in women's discourse. For example, the writer begins with "I understand how you feel," the kind of statement that, according to Tannen, women tend to use and like to hear. Such a statement is "the gift of understanding" (50). The first sentence also contains "I do not agree," which may mute the argument more than "I disagree." The final sentence in the paper is both a sign of politeness, as well as gratitude for the nurse's listening, the first step toward the kind of understanding that Tannen describes.

Paper #3 also contains some of the features that both Tannen and Gilligan (1982) attribute to males' discourse. The first sentence, for example, includes "I personally disagree strongly," which conforms to Tannen's observation that men tend to be more combative, as well as Gilligan's observation that men strive for individuation and separateness ("personally"). There is little indication in this letter that the male writer is willing to understand the nurse's position or that he wants to be personally *connected* with her—in Gilligan's sense of the word—as they discourse on this matter.

I note these features of these two letters while remaining cautious, for as Coates (1986) demonstrates, we have many unsubstantiated stereotypes about men's and women's language use (103). The results that I report, like results of studies that Coates surveys, indicate that what we believe to be true of men's and women's language—both written and oral—sometimes lacks empirical support.

Some Reflections

The two parts of the study that I have thus far described, when taken separately and together, suggest that reading and evaluating students' writing may be more hazardous than we usually consider it to be. The first part of the study suggests that male and female secondary English teachers respond differently to features of the discourse, at least some persuasive discourse, that male and female students write. I have suggested several possible discourse features that may account for these differences, but it will take much additional investigation with all sorts of discourse types before we will know how males and females *may* differentially use—both as writers and readers—particular discourse strategies.

The second part of the study is in some ways both more interesting and potentially more disturbing than the first part. The comments offered by the readers in this part of the study reveal what powerful stereotypes we can bring to the task of reading students' papers.

Of course, many social institutions besides school contribute to the learning and socialization of boys and girls, men and women. We teachers should not consider ourselves responsible for the gender-specific roles that males and females assume in life, but we do need to consider carefully our contributions to stereotypical behavior. When we teach English, we must be critically conscious of the ways in which we interact with our male and female students—as they write, read, speak, listen, think, and cooperate in our classrooms. Our interactions with them, even in the margins of their papers can greatly influence their work in our classrooms and their lives outside our classrooms.

If we consider our composition classrooms as academic discourse communities, we may need to be attuned to special needs that may differ for some of our male and female students. I believe this because I believe that Cayton (1990) may be right when she says,

> while men entering academic discourse communities may be more likely to see themselves as apprentices mastering a process that will allow them to contribute to a generalized body of knowledge, women are—for good reason—more likely to see themselves as outsiders with misgivings about entering the circle of the elect. (333)

In the past I have urged writing teachers to use strategies that coaches use to help athletes learn to play more effectively (Roen 1987), and I still feel that the best coaches can offer us many insights into effective teaching (e.g., principles of modeling, cooperative collaboration, and practice). However, there is another metaphor for effective writing instruction, offered by Socrates (Plato, ca. 394–369 B.C./1928) in *Theaetetus* nearly 2400 years ago. This concept, that of the midwife teacher (490–494), has recently been renewed by Belenky, Clinchy, Goldberger, and Tarule (1986): "The midwife-teacher's first concern is to preserve the student's fragile newborn thoughts, to see that they are born with their truth intact . . ." (218). Further, the midwife-teacher follows Vygotskian (1934/1962; 1978) and Bakhtinian (1975/1981) principles of dialogic thinking and learning: "Midwife-teachers help students deliver words to the world, and they use their own knowledge to put the students into conversation with other voices—past and present—in the culture (Belenky et al. 1986, 219). And, as Socrates suggests, if the midwife-teacher is working effectively, students "all make astonishing progress" (Plato, 492).

By assuming the role of midwife-teachers, we can more easily foster not only the writing but also the thinking and learning of students who put words on paper in our classrooms. As we respond to students' writing, we must more often play Elbow's (1973) "believing game" than we play his "doubting game," keeping in mind that "most students appreciate a less rather than more confrontational rhetoric of response" (Kraemer 1990, 312). As much as possible, we need to be attuned to each student's—male or female—individual cognitive and affective needs. I believe that if we act in these ways, ways that are human and humane, we will encourage our students to become what Freire (1970) would consider fully empowered language users.

Author Note

I thank Bruce Appleby, Nancy McCracken, and Margaret Fleming for their comments on earlier versions of this chapter. I am indebted to my colleagues Donna Johnson and Gerri McNenny for helping me to think critically about gender differences. I wish to thank Michael Gessner, Susan Miller, Jan Rowe, and their colleagues for their help in gathering data for the studies that I report here. I also thank my students for their assistance and support.

Notes

1. In an earlier version of this paper, I discussed gender as a cultural construct. Since the editors discuss that construct in detail in the introduction

to this collection, it is unnecessary for me to cover the same ground in this chapter.

2. A T-unit, "minimal terminable unit," consists of an independent clause and any dependent or reduced clauses attached to it or embedded in it. See Hunt (1977) for a more detailed discussion of T-units.

Works Cited

Applebee, A. N., J. A. Langer, I. V. S. Mullis. 1986. *The writing report card: Writing achievement in American Schools*. Princeton, NJ: Educational Testing Service.

Bakhtin, M. M. 1981. *The dialogic imagination*. (M. Holquist, Ed. and Trans.). Austin: University of Texas Press. (Original work published in 1975.)

Baker, W. D. 1954. In investigation of characteristics of poor writers. *College Composition and Communication*, *5*, 23–27.

Belenky, M. F., B. M. Clinchy, N. R. Goldberger, and J. M. Tarule. 1986. *Women's ways of knowing*. New York: Basic Books.

Britton, J., T. Burgess, N. Martin, A. McLeod, and H. Rosen. 1975. *The Development of Writing Abilities (11–18)*. London: Schools Council Publications.

Cayton, M. K. 1990. What happens when things go wrong: Women and writing blocks. *Journal of Advanced Composition*, *10*, 322–37.

Coates, Jennifer. 1986. *Women, men, and language: A sociolinguistic account of sex differences in language*. New York: Longman.

Daly, J. A. 1979. Writing apprehension in the classroom: Teacher expectancies of the apprehensive writer. *Research in the Teaching of English*, *13*, 37–44.

Daly, J. A., and M. D. Miller. 1975. Further studies in writing apprehension: SAT scores, success expectations, willingness to take advanced courses, and sex differences. *Research in the Teaching of English*, *9*, 250–56.

Dickson, F. C. 1978. *Writing apprehension and text anxiety as predictors of ACT scores*. Unpublished master's thesis, West Virginia University, Morgantown.

Diederich, Paul B. 1974. *Measuring growth in English*. Urbana, IL: National Council of Teachers of English.

Donelson, K. L. 1963. Variables distinguishing between effective and ineffective writers at the tenth grade level. *Dissertation Abstracts International*, *24*, 2734A. (University Microfilms No. 63-07998)

Donelson, K. L. 1967. Variables distinguishing between effective and ineffective writers in the tenth grade. *Journal of Experimental Education*, *35* (4), 37–41.

Elbow, P. 1973. *Writing without teachers*. New York: Oxford University Press.

Farrell, T. J. 1979. The female and male modes of rhetoric. *College English*, *40*, 909–921.

Freire, P. 1970. *Pedagogy of the oppressed*. New York: Seabury Press.

Gilligan, C. 1982. *In a different voice: Psychological theory and women's development*. Cambridge: Harvard University Press.

Goodwin, M. H. In press. *He-said-she-said: Talk as social organization among black children*. Bloomington: Indiana University Press.

Hunt, K. W. 1977. Early blooming and late blooming syntactic structures. In C. R. Cooper and L. Odell (Eds.), *Evaluating writing: Describing, measuring, judging*. Urbana, IL: National Council of Teachers of English.

Kraemer, D. 1990. No exit: A play of literacy and gender. *Journal of Advanced Composition*, *10*, 305–319.

Maccoby, E. 1966. *The development of sex differences*. Stanford, CA: Stanford University Press.

Martin, W. B. 1970. Applying and exploring the Diederich method for measuring growth in writing ability in a high school. *Dissertation Abstracts International*, *31*, 2616A. (University Microfilms No. 70-23921)

———. 1972. The sex factor in grading composition. *Research in the Teaching of English*, *6*, 36–47.

National Assessment of Educational Progress 1980. *Writing achievement, 1969–79: Results from the third National Writing Assessment; Volume 1–17-year-olds*. Denver: Education Commission of the States.

Piche, G. L., and D. H. Roen. 1987. Social cognition and writing: Interpersonal cognitive complexity and abstractness and the quality of students' persuasive writing. *Written Communication*, *4*, 68–89.

Plato. 1928. *Theaetetus* (B. Jowett, Trans.). In I. Edman (Ed.), *The Works of Plato* (481–577). New York: The Modern Library. (Original work published circa 394–69 B.C.)

Roen, D. H. 1987. Learning to bunt/learning to write. *Journal of Business Communication*, *24* (1), 65–72.

———. 1989, March. *The effects of gender of writer, labeled gender of writer, and gender of grader on the judged quality of students' writing*. Paper presented at the meeting of the Conference on College Composition and Communication, Seattle.

Sears, P. S., and D. H. Feldman. 1974. Teacher interactions with boys and with girls. In J. Stacey, S. Bereaud, and J. Daniels (Eds.), *And Jill came tumbling after: Sexism in American Education* (147–58). New York: Dell.

Spaulding, R. L. 1963. *Achievement, creativitiy, and self-concept correlates of teacher-pupil transactions in elementary schools*. (Cooperative Research Project No. 1352). Washington: U.S. Department of Health, Education, and Welfare, Office of Education.

Stalnaker, J. M. 1941. Sex differences in the ability of writers. *School and Society*, *54*, 532–35.

Tannen, D. 1990. *You just don't understand: Women and men in conversation*. New York: William Morrow and Company.

Vygotsky, L. S. 1962. *Thought and language*. (E. Hanfmann & G. Vakar, Trans.). Cambridge, MA: M.I.T. Press. (Original work published in 1934)

———. 1978. *Mind in society*. (M. Cole, V. John Steiner, S. Schribner, & E. Souberman, Eds.). Cambridge, MA: Harvard University Press.

Woodward J. C., and A. G. Phillips. 1967. Profile of the poor writer—the relationship of selected characteristics of poor writing in college. *Research in the Teaching of English*, *1*, 41–53.

11

The Academic Essay: A Feminist View in Student Voices

Jean Sanborn

Jill is a student who struggles with a conflict between her ways of knowing and the demands of the academic essay.[1] When she says, "I think that this course is taught in a certain way and I don't work that way so I, I don't know, I don't expect to have my papers taken seriously," she is illustrating what Adrienne Rich said years ago: "Listen to a woman groping for language in which to express what is on her mind, sensing that the terms of academic discourse are not her language, trying to cut down her thought to the dimensions of a discourse not intended for her" (1978, 243–44). Jill clearly connects her writing frustration with a required essay form:

> form means, to me, a paper has to be academic, which to me seems there has to be some kind of style involved that is stuffy and it maybe shouldn't seem that way to me, and the idea that you have to come up with a little grain of an idea and prove it, leave no questions unanswered is difficult to do. ... I always have to leave questions unanswered. I really just start to feel dumb. I feel dumb.

Linda has similar perceptions:

> I sometimes wonder how really strongly students feel about their work because I almost feel like you have to separate yourself from your emotions if you want to write these papers that are so controlled. ... The student has kind of had to kind of block themself from that uncertain feeling that maybe they can't explain something. I mean why lead people into thinking that's not a good way to feel?

Indeed, that "uncertain feeling" is the moment of disequilibrium when learning can occur. The tightly controlled academic essay denies uncertainty and limits thought to a little grain of an idea. Historically, the essay has been a very open genre. Annie Dillard has said: "The essay is, and has been, all over the map. There's nothing you cannot do with it, no subject matter is forbidden, no structure is proscribed. You get to make up your own structure every time, a structure that arises from the materials and best contains them" (1988, xxii). William Carlos Williams, who explored the boundaries of form in both prose and poetry, says, "an essay is multiplicity, infinite fracture, the inter-crossing of opposed forces establishing any number of opposed centres of stillness" (1970, 321).

This malleable, fertile form originating in Montaigne is not what we mean when we say "essay" to students. We mean not "put your ideas to the trial"; we mean rather "choose a point, a thesis, a 'grain of an idea' as Jill puts it, and line up support for it." The academic essay is not a vehicle for exploring ideas and making knowledge; it is a vehicle for presenting formed ideas, a didactic, authoritative model rather than an interactive form.

The academic essay as we know it fell firmly into place late in the nineteenth century when it was assumed that the hierarchical essay represented the "natural" way of thinking of the human mind, all human minds. Representative of the voices of composition text writers of that era is Henry Pearson of MIT: "The planning of the simplest theme, if done intelligently, is an exercise in ordering thought, and properly shaping a series of ideas. . . . Even more necessary is it for the learner to perceive that this same literary form is an absolute essential of all clear thinking, and that thought, to be adequate, must be orderly" (1898, xii). Sixty years later, in 1958, Cleanth Brooks and Robert Penn Warren claim: "The division into introduction, body, conclusion, or, if you like, into beginning, middle and end, is the natural sequential division of a piece of writing. It is the mode of organizing that naturally occurs to anyone who is getting down to the actual business of writing, whatever the topic" (213). Carol, a student in college now, learned this essay in high school as "TAB CocaCola = Thesis-A-B-C-Conclusion." Unity, singleness, is one hallmark of the academic essay. Of unity Williams has this to say: "Unity is the shallowest, the cheapest deception of all composition. In nothing is the banality of the intelligence more clearly manifested" (1970, 321).

Students also object to the limiting linearity of the academic essay. Says Sam, "My problem with papers is that I see them as linear processes – one sentence and then another sentence and then paragraph and then page. . . . I think writing should be a spherical process. . . . I've just been expanding ideas linearly and all it gives me is a chain of sentences." And Matt: "I'm not very good at making a single line, logical argument. . . . I often know when I'm doing something that is not logical but I'll believe that it is true—in contradiction to its being illogical." These students are thinking in what Carol Gilligan (1982) calls a web rather than a hierarchy. Rose has another image:

> I guess the papers that kind of go like a hydra are ones where the ideas, one idea will spin off of another idea and then another will spin off and another idea—and they all are intertwined and seem to back each other up and so I don't know how to get them all in without the paper sort of exploding under it. But I want to get them all in because I think they are so important.

Rochelle's description is close to Gilligan's imagery: "My outlines often look more like something with little radii coming out than a ladder or whatever. They are not very linear." My own metaphor for this kind of writing is woven.

Thinking in different ways from the academic norm has serious consequences for these students. Not all good literature follows the Aristotelian unities, an understanding we share with our students. Neither does all good expository writing follow the dictates of the thesis-driven, hierarchical essay. This understanding we too often keep a secret from our students, though if they read published essays they must guess. When they fail to find many examples of the academic essay in print, they quite reasonably make a separation between "school" writing and "real" writing. Nothing of themselves is invested in school writing, so it becomes an impotent exercise, at best boring, at worst paralyzing. We can empower our students by letting them in on the secret that thinking and writing are not monolithic, that they come in many forms, thus freeing these students from the suspicion that they are just dumb. Recent research, especially in feminist studies, suggests that the variety of forms found in essays is not just a matter of style but is connected with ways of thinking, ways of making knowledge.

I want to give a hearing to the voices of students, so I will refer only briefly to some of the research which illuminates intellectually the struggle that these students experience, often painfully and physically. Psychologist Carol Gilligan illustrates in the field of moral development how women tend to make ethical decisions based on relationships while men take stands based on principle; women think in webs, men in hierarchies. In previous studies women who stood inside the problem in this way were considered less developed ethically than men who achieved an autonomous, separated stance, a conclusion which Gilligan challenges. Mary Belenkey, Blythe Clinchy, Nancy Goldberger, and Jill Tarule (1986) extend Gilligan's work into women's ways of knowing. Among their categories, the most useful here are separate knowing and connected knowing. Elizabeth Flynn (1988) has elaborated the connections between these psychological theories and some of the problems of women composing. I want to add to the theories what women students themselves say about composing in academic formats.

The Gilligan and Belenkey, *et al.*, theories also create some problems. Early theoretical breakthroughs often set up dichotomies, as these do. Both are also stage theories, which establish a hierarchy of development. Dichotomies help to elucidate a problem in the beginning, but ultimately they are both false and destructive. Hierarchies undercut the values of connection which feminist theorists espouse. Despite disclaimers that results are not gender specific but gender related, gender studies tend to polarize people because they challenge ways of thinking that have long been assumed to be "natural." In fact, of course, not all women think in webs, and some men do. The "natural" way is the way of those in power, and "other" ways are considered inferior.

A more productive way to look at cognitive differences is through multiplicity, which also extends the possibilities to the problems of ethnic, cultural, and socioeconomic groups which were not included in the early studies. Howard Gardner (1983) identifies seven different ways of thinking. Vera John-Steiner (1991, 69) goes a step further in her concept of "cognitive pluralism," claiming not only that different people think differently, but that a single individual can access different modes of thinking in given situations: "While an individual may have a dominant mode of representation (or internal code), there is no single universal language of thought. As human beings, we each embody a subset of human possibilities" (17).

If the mind has multiple possible forms for thought, then the single form imposed by the academic essay does violence to the perfectly legitimate and potentially valuable thinking of some students. Their own words indicate best what this limitation does to their attitudes, to their learning, to their academic lives.

Every year I have encountered in my first-year writing classes at least one student, usually but not always a woman, who could write beautifully when she or he perceived the subject to be experiential, but whose writing fell apart totally, even at the syntax level, if the topic seemed academic. A particularly vivid example is Polly. Here is a selection from an essay she wrote about her "Gahmie":

> Her blue eyes were faded, the color of an old jean jacket, and her rims were slightly bloodshot. Her skin remained a dark brown due to trimonthly trips to Arizona or Florida. I remember watching her wrinkly arm as her hand delicately held on to her coffee cup. She held a balled up napkin in the left fist and rubbed her right forefinger and thumb together until she reached toward the cup handle. She would

> slightly wince as the hot liquid touched her tongue. I used to sit closely to her as she drank her coffee so that I could smell her herbal hand lotion rubbed into her cuticles. She sat straight, properly, of course, and gazed across the landscape as she watched the children's games and recalled memories. . . .
>
> Gahmie went into the hospital shortly after Christmas. . . . The smell of the room didn't contain the slightest hint of her hand lotion and the decorations on the wall didn't have the familiarity of her white wickered porch.
>
> I had difficulty recalling conversations with Gahmie because her disintegration was so foreign to my young mind. I sat next to her bed and drew pictures while she reminisced. My sister cried in the corner; my mother helped the nurse with bedpans, needles, and sheets; my father remained in the hallway most of the time. I explored the room and bathroom for signs of the "real" Gahmie.

In the same first month of the semester, this observant student who wrote with such precision and rhythm about her grandmother was asked to respond to two essays about education in light of her own educational experience. She began:

> As Chisholm states in her essay "Needed Equal Educational Opportunity for All," higher education brings about the purpose of upward mobility. Education involves the training of minds and intellectual training. The skills mastered in higher education become important for society's intelligence basis in a democratic hierarchy. Opportunity for higher education leases fulfillment of individual intellectual goals and voluntary contribution to society's achievements. . . .
>
> Fulfillment of intellectual goals is a common motivation for many higher education students. As one interested in the field of law, a search for challenge and satisfaction prevails in my endeavor pursuit. Employment in a professional field seems to exist as a challenging goal and satisfying position.

I began this study because I wondered how the woman who wrote "My sister cried in the corner; my mother helped the nurse with bedpans, needles, and sheets; my father remained in the hallway most of the time" could write a sentence so meaningless as, "As one interested in the field of law, a search for challenge and satisfaction prevails in my endeavor pursuit." The gap is so great that it seemed there must be more at work than the distinction between personal writing and "school writing," between what Janet Emig (1971) calls reflexive writing and extensive writing, what James Britton (1975) calls expressive writing and transactional writing, what we now often call exploratory writing and analytical writing. Whatever the terminology, crossing this great divide is the central struggle for composition classes. The issue also marks a division among composition theorists. Should the focus in writing courses be on developing the students' voices or on initiating the students into academic discourse? We want students to be able to use their experience informed by theory, to be able to analyze without resorting to empty jargon, to be able to write with strength and voice whatever the rhetorical situation. Yet when students who have demonstrated their ability to write well in some contexts perceive the rhetorical situation to be an academic essay, they often revert to language and form like Polly's, though her distress is so extreme that her writing seems to be a parody.

Jill and Linda, who opened this chapter, are among fifteen subjects in a study I have been conducting for the past five years, a study involving interviews and writing samples with upperclass college students in an attempt to discover what they think about their writing and about the academic essay. Twelve of the fifteen are women, three men; eight are successful writers, seven distressed writers. At first I selected students whom I knew from my experience with them or from their records were serious and intelligent but were having major problems with writing. Later I added students who had been especially successful in academic writing because after a presentation I gave at an on-campus colloquium about how cramped and frustrated some students felt when confronting the academic essay, a woman came up to me to say, "That's exactly how I feel." Yet she was an extremely successful student, a psychology major, who had never seemed to have any trouble at all with academic writing.

In order to gather data that might be useful, I set up a format: an interview covering their writing autobiographies plus a series of three fifteen-minute writing protocols. The first writing sample is the student's open choice, the second is in response to a poster of a chimpanzee, the third is an assigned topic (Do Animals Have Language?) following a ten-page reading about animal communication. When Polly was a senior, she agreed to take part in the study. Although I anticipated that the free writing would give Polly the best opportunity to use her own forms of expression, it was the chimpanzee poster that elicited her most interesting writing:

> I see a hunger that cannot be satisfied with food. She looks female. I guess that assumption comes from my experiences of the depths of sadness women have potential for.
>
> I'm reading Anna Akhmatova's poetry. She speaks of her country, its constraints and its madness. I wonder what Akhmatova would say about Ethiopia and the starvation that descended to its soil.
>
> Depths of sadness is what fascinates me in women. I've been writing lately fantasizing that I am Ophelia and I leave Hamlet for Heathcliff. Heathcliff is one fired by passion, he sets her free while Hamlet constrained her love.

> I feel an obligation to fulfill some sort of writing rule and make one string of connection with all the subjects I've mentioned. Maybe if I let go of that intellectual constraint, I would be more free to explore original possibilities of thought.
>
> I don't know why I always turn to my father when I become introspective.

Although Polly believes she has failed to make connections in this passage, I see it as an example of what Belenkey, *et al.*, call "connected knowing," a deep involvement in her reading. In fact, it is also a coherent piece of writing despite its many subjects. Polly weaves the threads of sadness and constraint, even repeating the key words so that her reader can follow the path of her thinking. The reference to her father becomes clearer in her interview: "My father has a great influence over me. He is an extremely intelligent man who is constantly challenging me intellectually. And it's a very healthy challenge. . . . But when I think of an intellectual challenge I think of him and that's how I see academic writing. I see it as somebody giving me a problem or saying 'prove it otherwise' and the . . . content of your writing is valued, the quality of intellectualism that you've used. . . ." Later she talks about a friend who is successful in academic writing:

> We have a real intellectual relationship and she sees writing as a challenge. And it's funny because her relationship with her father is quite parallel to the relationship with my father and that is very high expectations. Her father expects her to go into law school and a lot of challenges posed there so she sees this academic writing as something in like a law court, where she's out to prove a point and she's going to win the case. It's effective for her, it really is because she pumps out good quality stuff.

Both of these women equate academic writing with male authority and success, even with adversarial combat.

In Polly's assigned topic writing sample the tone is distinctly different from that of the previous sample—less "fired by passion," more held by "intellectual constraint":

> I'm tempted to answer affirmatively to this question ["Do Animals Have Language?"] because I'd like to believe that animals communicate within their societies in a recognizable human form.
>
> Although science has not yet been able to determine whether animals have a language, their ability to communicate certainly has been established.
>
> I think a lot of the controversy in science's dilemma concerning whether animals have the capability to learn language stems from science's own self importance and pride in its commitment to objective testing and conclusions that are beyond a reasonable doubt. Science mirrors Swift's attitude towards science in Part III of *Gulliver's Travels*.

> Then again, the human race owes much to science for its advances in technology. Where would we be in medicine without their diligence in pursuing cures or preventions? What about in agriculture to hasten farmer's productivity? Or opening up new worlds to us through space travel, telescopes, and satellites?
>
> We can't always consider animals in relation to humans. It is helpful in science to have relations in order to maintain objectivity, but wouldn't it be refreshing (and idealistic) to consider the animal race in its own context?

Polly changes not only tone but form in this sample. She presents a tentative answer, a critique of science, a concession, a possible new approach. Curiously, she even changes her paragraph style. The reference to Swift seems gratuitous and unconnected here, but in her oral protocol Polly did elaborate the connection with human arrogance, the assumption that "everything revolves around us." Only the brief allusion reached the paper. Despite the skeleton of academic form, the answer rather than the exploration, this piece of writing is internally less coherent than the response elicited by the chimpanzee poster.

In the interview with Polly, I never asked her specifically about the academic essay, but in the course of her autobiography, she mentioned it frequently, in strong language:

> When I sit down to write an academic paper I feel already in my cage because I'm being forced to write about a subject, the subject is given to me and so I feel like I'm in a zoo, a zoo animal. . . . When I sit down to do something creative, I feel like I'm skydiving, that I can go in any direction I want. . . .
>
> I just couldn't jam into a form like that, it was something that was too constricting for me; my thoughts made me feel constricted.

In the following comment Polly feels the "dumbness" that Jill expressed:

> I felt as though somebody was trying to cram a square peg into a round hole. And, I had feelings that had to be expressed in a certain form and all of a sudden people were telling me that my form was not acceptable.

Most of the students I interviewed used similar language to express their discomfort with the academic essay. Although I never asked them explicitly about the form, every one of them talked about it. Linda says:

> I felt violated . . . I think it's because I put a lot of time into finding things that I wanted to say and I just could not find the right way to say it . . . the paper was just not taking the right form that I had in my mind. And it got to the point where I could not form paragraphs.

Violated . . . crammed . . . jammed . . . constricted . . . caged—

these were typical of the vocabulary of students who were distressed in their writing. Among the students who were successful academic writers, the language applied to the academic essay included "boring" and "grunt work." Siobhan, an honors graduate in English, adds: "I feel somehow I cheated myself out of doing anything creative. . . . I can write pieces like the essays, you know, in my sleep." Martha, a highly successful psychology major who also graduated Phi Beta Kappa, says of her academic work:

> There was really nowhere for my own feelings or projections even though it was just my paper, it was my research, and the only freedom that was really allowed was to make very tentative conjectures and I understand that, I mean it's supposed to be professional style, that's important. . . . But I felt very cramped.

These frustrations, these blocks created by the academic essay, interfere with the learning of these students, men as well as women. Sam was never able to finish a paper because he knew he had more to say. Siobhan once wanted to write a paper on *Paradise Lost* through Eve's voice, but because she got no support from her instructor and because she worried about her GPA, she "scrapped it and wrote a straight analysis of something." Rochelle expresses a sophisticated concern for audience but with some ambivalence about her learning:

> I think that often times I come to an anti-conclusion rather than a conclusion, which is also a little bit frightening. I think it can be good for me just as a learning exercise to explore different avenues and to arrive somewhere that I didn't really plan on arriving—at the same time I think it can make life for a reader a little more difficult than it should be. I think I have to think about communicating with other people more than just exercising my own ideas.

Later she adds:

> Maybe I like wading through ambiguities rather than actually trying to find anything, or maybe I'm incapable of actually finding any conclusions. I don't know why it is.

It may be because Rochelle's ways of thinking are not fully compatible with the essay form which she understands so well.

Peter Elbow's analysis of the "doubting game" and the "believing game" helps to illuminate the gender connections in the learning environment of these students. The doubting game is "hard," accepting as truth only what can be proved beyond challenge; the believing game is "soft," inhabiting a variety of positions in a search for truth. "The doubting game emphasizes a model of knowing as an act of discrimination: putting something on trial to see whether it is wanting or not. . . . The believing game emphasizes a model of knowing as an act of constructing, an act of investment, an act of involvement" (173). Elbow makes the gender connection explicitly, but he remains within a dichotomy rather than multiplicity (180).

For many women and some men the model of knowing as an act of investment is more "natural." Even Polly has one course where it all comes together for her. In a poetry course she is able to combine what she calls her "passion" and her "intellect," and in this connected state her learning flourishes:

> I could connect to the poetry and it made me feel good and I felt as though it got my intellectual juices going so I also had the language, my language is conducive to the issues of the course. For some reason that semester my language was just very powerful and I wrote some good papers.

Students who are not at home in the model of knowing that prevails in the schools cope in a variety of ways. Some, like Linda and Sam and Rose, are paralyzed. Rose explains, "I'm supposed to be writing a paper right now and if I'm not writing a paper I shouldn't be doing anything at which point I sit there in a catatonic state and the next thing I've gone to sleep." Adrienne Rich describes a similar state: "I was writing very little, partly from fatigue, that female fatigue of suppressed anger and loss of contact with my own being" (1971, 43). Rarely do students have the understanding of Rich's perspective. Usually they are like Matt: "I was really bogged down and I really couldn't see out, see in the linear way."

Short of paralysis, students procrastinate, as Pamela Annas points out, "in a dazzling and creative variety of ways, leaving themselves so little time that they can't possibly write something that satisfies them, thus self-fulfilling their expectations of failure" (1985, 366). Polly developed a pattern of withdrawing from courses whenever she blocked on a paper. Her transcript is sprinkled with "W's." Her expectation of failure once drove her to plagiarism after she had earned an "A" on a paper, fearing she could not live up to expectations. She actually called it "fear of success."

Some students function by drawing a rigid barrier between school writing and their own writing, either by enrolling in creative writing courses as Rose and Rochelle and Matt did, or by trying to silence their creativity, as Polly and Siobhan did. They acquiesce by writing what Polly calls "crud": "I choose something that is very obvious, that's almost embarrassing to write a paper about." Martha found her outlet in a minor in Women's Studies where she could bring herself into her writing. Linda and Jill each designed an independent study where they could explore from more freely. Linda made the comment that even the designation of "adviser" rather than "teacher" in this situation was more conducive to her learning. Matt and, to some extent, Linda challenged the system and insisted on handing in papers in their own forms. Jessica, the most recent student to take part in this study, chose confrontation. Her sense of compromise comes not from form but from what she perceives as an inability of some instructors to accept her ideas. Once, when a paper was returned marked "I don't agree. B−," Jessica marched into the instructor's office saying, "Wait a minute. You can't do this." After a discussion of her ideas, she was allowed to rewrite the paper. She claims she made few changes but incorporated some of the instructor's ideas and received an A− on the revision. Her narration of this experience reflects a certain cynicism about the learning process which many students feel. Psyching-out the teacher is, however, one way to cope with an uncongenial system.

Sam's breakthrough is instructive. He went away as an exchange student and during that semester took a course on eastern religions. He blocked on a paper about Confucianism so totally that he went for psychological counseling and ultimately refused to write the paper. Luckily, he had an instructor who accepted his refusal. Then came Taoism, and Sam wrote what he calls the best paper of his life. From that experience he gained an insight into the writing process that provides us with a useful metaphor, using the eastern philosophies. Confucianism, like the academic essay, is the form, the mold, into which one pours thoughts and actions. Taoism, like writing to discover, seeks meaning from within, allows meaning to grow. Once Sam had this larger framework of understanding, he was even able to write a "confucian" paper when it was called for.

At this point it is important to remember Jane Roland Martin's analysis of gender in education:

> When the educational realm embodies only male norms, it is inevitable that any women participating in it will be forced into a masculine mold. The question of whether such a role is desirable for females needs to be asked, but it cannot be asked so long as philosophers of education assume that gender is a difference that makes no difference. The question of whether the mold is desirable for males also needs to be asked; yet when our educational concepts and ideals are defined in male terms, we do not think to inquire into their validity for males themselves. (1982, 147)

It may indeed be that the mold of the academic essay is educationally unsound, for both women and men, and that the pedagogical methods that I will consider next would enhance the learning of both women and men.

How can we help students like those whose voices are raised here to learn, even to function, in the present academic world? Gender issues arise not only in the way students write but in the way we teach. The academic essay thrives in a learning atmosphere that is authoritative and competitive. "Rhetoric," says Walter Ong, "developed in the past as a major expression of the rational level of the ceremonial combat which is found among males and typically only among males at the physical level throughout the entire animal kingdom" (1979, 615). There is much talk these days about the "feminization" of rhetoric, a term which, however positive the intentions are, has pejorative connotations of softening. Yet as Janice Moulton points out:

> The Adversary Paradigm accepts only the kind of reasoning whose goal is to convince an opponent, and ignores reasoning that might be used in other circumstances: to figure something out for oneself, to discuss something with like-minded thinkers, to convince the indifferent or the uncommmitted. The relations of ideas used to arrive at a conclusion might very well be different from the relations of ideas needed to defend it to an adversary. (1983, 159)

Talking about classroom climate, Jessica makes a startlingly direct connection between gender and essay form: "The ones who aren't sympathetic to women's issues are going to want you to stay in the text, they're going to want you to have a very tight paper with the thesis at the top—very linear." She has also noticed that teachers who use "non-mainstream" materials, such as Native American literature, are more open to varieties of essay forms. It would appear that once we have opened the canon of literature we can begin to open the canon of student writing.

The classroom that can help the students who are paralyzed or bored by the academic essay needs to be collaborative rather than authoritative. We need dialogues and conversations more than assignments and grades. I believe that we must work in two directions. First, we must reassure students whose modes of thinking are not primarily linear that they are not dumb. To begin with, we can let them in on the secret of cognitive pluralism by introducing them to the views of Gilligan and Rich and John-Steiner, larger frameworks that will increase their self-confidence, as Sam's experience did. Then we can give them examples of woven essays to read or, better yet, paired essays on similar topics, one linear and one woven. Working with peers on their writing rather than with authority figures can help students to concentrate on conveying meaning rather than replicating form. A technique that I have found successful with many students is to ask them to draw their writing, to make a graphic representation of their draft. By changing the mode of thinking from verbal to graphic, the students gain distance from the words they often are drowning in, and they also see that their thinking does have a shape. Then they can decide whether the shape is appropriate to their thoughts. This process can also give them experience in accessing their own plural cognitive possibilities.

Having found a shape of their own, however, is not enough. Because teachers have the academic essay imprinted in our heads like a template, we may unconsciously reject any less straight-line forms as disorganized. If we are trying to help students such as those I have been talking about, we need to take a second step to enable them to convince readers of the appropriateness of whatever non-standard forms they have chosen to write. This is an extraordinarily difficult task and can only be undertaken when students have gained confidence in themselves. Linda is a good example.

Linda's crisis began in a Shakespeare course in the first semester of her junior year. She had never been easy with writing because, like Sam, she felt that she could never get in all she wanted to say. Moreover, she perceives herself as a visual thinker. She also clearly expresses her frustration about having to separate herself from her reading and writing: "I had to program my mind this way so that I would not get so emotionally involved in the reading." In a Shakespeare paper she hit the wall and scrawled a despairing cry at the bottom: "I am ashamed to hand this in, but it's done. I must meet with you—something is wrong—this must change." The instructor was sympathetic, told her she had perceptions which required a three-step argument, and proceeded to write a three-page outline for her. But the grade was "D," and Linda never rewrote the paper.

I first met Linda the following year when she came to the Writers' Center in tears with a paper on *Wuthering Heights*. She had allowed herself to become emotionally involved in this reading, and she could not find a way to write her perceptions. Several weeks and many drafts later she handed in a paper that still did not satisfy her but to which her instructor responded: "Though perhaps not a wholly consecutive argument, this is much more coherent than I'd realized. In concentrating on the 'process of understanding' and *mis*understanding instead of on narrative technique, you've given the paper some unity."

A truncated look at these two papers may illustrate one way to recognize and to help students who are not predominantly linear thinkers to survive in the current school atmosphere. A segment from the middle of Linda's Shakespeare paper illustrates her struggle:

> In *Titus Andronicus*, the dominating force is embodied in a single character. Throughout the play, we can trace incidents of Aaron's regulation of the action [examples from the text]. . . . In other words, the fate of the characters has been determined by one individual.
>
> The controlling force in *Romeo and Juliet* transcends human form. The Friar admitted that "A greater power than we can contradict/ Hath thwarted out intents." (*Romeo* V, III, 153–43) His statement

> implies that man's effort to determine his destiny can be intercepted by an element outside of his domain. Romeo killed himself after discovering what he thought was Juliet's dead body. But if he had been aware of the circumstances—if he had arrived ten minutes later—he would have realized that Juliet had just been in a deep sleep.
>
> After having established the main distinction between the two plays, we can begin to account for the variation in the effectiveness of each of the final scenes.

The language of this paper indicates that Linda is trying mightily to write an academic paper. When we make a skeleton by looking at only the first and last sentences of these body paragraphs a startling dissonance in language becomes evident. Paragraph two begins, "In *Titus Andronicus*, the dominating force is embodied in a single character" and ends, "In other words, the fate of the characters has been determined by one individual," which is a direct translation of the first sentence into another language. In the opening sentence of the next paragraph Linda pulls herself back to "The controlling force in *Romeo and Juliet* transcends human form," a detached, critical level of language. By the end of the paragraph she has worked herself into the play and concludes, "But if he had been aware of the circumstances—if he had arrived ten minutes later—he would have realized that Juliet had just been in a deep sleep." Then she yanks herself out of connection with the play to start the next paragraph with academic language, "After having established the main distinction between the two plays, we can begin to account for the variation in the effectiveness of each of the final scenes." It seems to me that Linda is in terrible conflict between what she wants to say about these plays and the way she believes she has to say it, though we never talked about this paper since she sent it to me after she had participated in the interview study and had graduated.

Linda is not incapable of writing linear prose. For a summer job she wrote a report that gave her no difficulty at all. As she says, "I had no problem sitting down and writing that because I had an audience in front of me ... I was communicating something. It wasn't like there was this person above me that was judging what I was writing." For the Shakespeare paper she was fighting her personal connections with the texts in order to write in the forms of separate knowing.

Because she was already engaged in *Wuthering Heights*, Linda was willing to struggle for a form that would express her ideas. Here is a skeleton of her final draft, with the road signs that she developed to allow her readers to perceive the structure of her essay emphasized:

1. The "passionate love" between Catherine and Heathcliff would seem to be the focal point of *Wuthering Heights*. However, Emily Bronte's narrative technique often places the reader at quite a

distance from the actual plot. What we are in fact reading is Lockwood's documentation of a series of events from the past that are recalled by Nelly—an account which is often based upon second- and even third-hand information. However, the complex network of voices can in fact direct our understanding of the conflict which erupted between Catherine and Heathcliff. By working our way through the chain of characters, we can recognize Bronte's comprehensive presentation of the cause and resolution of the conflict that was set into motion by Catherine and Heathcliff and concluded by young Catherine and Hareton.

2. The scene where Catherine revealed her feelings about Heathcliff to Nelly triggered the chain reaction of conflict. . . .

3. The conflict between Catherine and Heathcliff spread to the other characters and introduced a motif of relationships which portrayed examples of interdependence and inequality—one character's obedience to another. . . . [the rest of this paragraph is about Nelly as director of the action]

4.–7. [These paragraphs are all about Nelly. 7. concludes:] The motif is continued as the next example presents a more basic case of dependence and implied obedience—the subservient child and the guardian.

8. When Linton first appeared in the story, he was under the care of his Uncle, Edgar. . . .

9. Young Catherine also admitted to her naivete as she underwent a similar process of questioning [by Heathcliff] which revealed her ignorance of the circumstances. . . .

10. The quarrel between adults—traceable to the confrontation that had been induced by Nelly—was ultimately fought through the children.

11. Whereas Nelly directed the action from the sidelines, the extent of control seems stronger in this relationship. . . . The adults had exploited the children's ignorance in order to suit their own needs.

12. The motif is carried through the example of young Catherine and Hareton, as the issue of ignorance and the possession of knowledge was a key point that established the initial inequality between the two characters. . . . However, young Catherine's ultimate treatment of Hareton's lack of knowledge became the device through which the conflict was resolved.

13. The tension between young Catherine and Hareton was alleviated once the two confronted the issues at hand, worked out their differences, and were able to come to an understanding of each other. . . .

14. A comparison can be drawn between this scene and the previous one with Catherine, Nelly, and Heathcliff. . . . The older Catherine

had also intended to provide Heathcliff with her assistance, but she never allowed him his part in establishing the guidelines for some kind of an agreement.

15. The other two examples that have been discussed—servant and master, and parent and child—both exemplify relationships which are classically understood to involve one party's obedience to the other. . . . [with Catherine and Hareton] One was dependent upon the other, but each strove to achieve love together.

16. We were provided with the image of Catherine and Heathcliff's union as two who were one in the same—sharing one soul. However, their relationship was encircled by various examples which emphasized the distinction between individuals, and the rift that can occur because of one's possession of knowledge and the other's lack there of, and the resulting conflict. The relationship between young Catherine and Hareton began in conflict, but they soon resolved their differences through a kind of learning process of sharing of knowledge; they learned about each other. Through give and take, they fit together like a puzzle piece, reflecting the ideal image of unity, but through realistic terms.

Not only is the language free of academic abstractions, but the voice is strong and clear. Linda is engaging both her interest in human relationships and her longstanding interest in learning. In the tutorial process that arrived at the final draft of the *Wuthering Heights* paper, Linda drew pictures and trees, diagrams and clusters, cut and pasted. She was already conscious of form and through her interest in visual arts ready to manipulate it. As a sophomore she had appeared for a conference with an instructor with a draft composed of pasted-together strips of yellow legal paper. She was a little uncomfortable with this process, however: "I don't know if that's a very good system because if your ideas flow in a certain way what I would do is cut apart that flow and try to rearrange it into something, like I said I'd put it into a format that I thought was the right way to make an argument and I don't think that's the natural way to do it. . . ." Her comment clearly reflects the conflict between her way of thinking and the demands of the essay.

My contribution to Linda's revision process was to help her develop road signs for the reader, terminology that would bring the underlying structure of the paper to the surface. Her instructor underlined the two "howevers" in the opening paragraph, presumably suggesting that it was illogical to take two turns. The turns do, however, prepare the reader for the circles of narration which the paper will take, circles that to some extent mirror the narrative patterns of the novel. Linda could help her readers by bringing this circular movement to the surface of the paper whenever she could. For example, in paragraph two the "chain of characters" of the opening paragraph becomes "chain reaction of conflict." The "complex network of voices" becomes in paragraph three "a motif of relationships" ending in the final paragraph with the phrase "their relationship was encircled." In paragraph four "The motif is continued" and in paragraph twelve the terminology comes back with "The motif is carried through." This terminology enables a reader to grasp a thread and circle with it as Linda weaves her picture. As Shirley Brice Heath points out: "It is the case not that essays under the pen of good writers are written according to a formula, but that they are written so that the structure is built within the essay. Put another way, the reader must know how to anticipate what is coming—anticipation must precede comprehension" (1987, 102).

A paper without a recognizable thesis and with several circles of development, like Linda's, is not a paper without a point, but it may be difficult to follow for readers who subconsciously expect the thesis-driven essay. It requires a suspension of closure. I have used these papers in workshops and found faculty, usually women, who read the *Wuthering Heights* paper easily and found it an example of good academic writing. On the other hand, a male student who read Linda's paper wrote: "I don't care if writing is linear, non-linear, or blue with pink polkadots. If it doesn't have a thesis sentence in the first page, I'm not going to wade through the rest of it." A faculty member might not make such a ruthless, impatient statement but might feel the same way. Even recognizing cognitive pluralism, we cannot expect a form that has been entrenched for a century to relinquish its hold on the subconscious expectations of readers of student essays, but we can validate other forms, can help our students to write in forms that are congenial to their thinking and still be heard. To do so, we must recognize that gender plays a role in thinking and thus necessarily in writing. If we stop at the male/female dichotomy, though, we are likely to do further damage. The more we recognize difference as multiplicity rather than dominant/other, the more students we can empower.

Note

1. I want to thank all the students who have participated in this study for their generosity and honesty and for their permission to use their words publicly. The names are not their own; in some cases they have chosen their research names themselves. I also thank the colleagues and students who have read drafts of this manuscript and given valuable suggestions, especially Mary Bartosenski and Erika Sayewich.

Works Cited

Annas, Pamela J. 1985. "Style as Politics: A Feminist Approach to the Teaching of Writing." *College English* 47.4 (April): 360–71.

Belenkey, Mary Field, Blythe McVicker Clinchy, Nancy Rule Goldberger, and Jill Mattuck Tarule. 1986. *Women's Ways of Knowing: The Development of Self, Voice, and Mind*. NY: Basic.

Britton, James, Tony Burgess, Nancy Martin, Alex McLeod, and Harold Rosen. 1975. *The Development of Writing Abilities (11–18)*. London: Macmillan Education.

Brooks, Cleanth, and Robert Penn Warren. 1958. *Modern Rhetoric*. 2nd ed. NY: Harcourt, Brace & World, Inc.

Dillard, Annie, ed. 1988. *The Best American Essays, 1988*. NY: Tichnor and Fields.

Elbow, Peer. 1973. *Writing Without Teachers*, 147–91. NY: Oxford University Press.

Emig, Janet. 1971. *The Composing Process of Twelfth Graders*. Urbana: National Council of Teachers of English.

Flynn, Elizabeth A. 1988. "Composing As a Woman." *College Composition and Communication* 39.4 (December): 423–35.

Gardner, Howard. 1983. *Frames of Mind: The Theory of Multiple Intelligences*. NY: Basic.

Gilligan, Carol. 1982. *In a Different Voice: Psychological Theory and Women's Development*. Cambridge: Harvard University Press.

Heath, Shirley Brice. 1987. "The Literate Essay: Using Ethnography to Explode Myths." In *Language, Literacy, and Culture: Issues of Society and Schooling*, Edited by Judith A. Langer, 89–107. Norwood, NJ: Ablex Publishing Corporation.

John-Steiner, Vera. 1991. Cognitive Pluralism: A Whorfian Analysis." *The Influence of Language on Culture and Thought*. Mouton 61–74. Ed. B. Spolsky and R. Cooper. See also John-Steiner's *Notebooks of the Mind: Explorations of Thinking*. NY: Harper and Row.

Martin, Jane Roland. 1982. "Excluding Women from the Educational Realm." *Harvard Educational Review* 52: 133–48.

Moulton, Janice. 1983. "A Paradigm of Philosophy: The Adversary Method." In *Discovering Reality*. Edited by Sandra Harding and Merill B. Hinlikka, 149–163. Holland: D. Reidel.

Ong, Walter. 1972. "Review of Brian Vickers' *Classical Rhetoric in English Poetry*." *College English* 33.5 (February): 612–16. Quoted in Rich, "Toward a Woman-Centered University," in *Lies, Secrets and Silences*. NY: W. W. Norton, 1979: 128.

Pearson, Henry G. 1898. *The Principles of Composition*. Boston: D. C. Heath and Co.

Rich, Adrienne. 1978. "Taking Women Students Seriously." In *Lies, Secrets, and Silence*: 237–245.

———. 1971. "When We Dead Awaken: Writing as Re-Vision." In *Lies, Secrets, and Silence*: 33–49.

Williams, William Carlos. 1970. "An Essay on Virginia." in *Imaginations*, 319–322. NY: New Directions. [first published, 1921].

CONTINUING THE CONVERSATI[illegible]
GENDER AND WRITING

Write, or dig up and re-read, your own writing hist[illegible] you learn to write? Who taught you? What are the ear[illegible] your writing you can remember? What kinds of purpo[illegible] early memorable pieces of writing serve? Who have been the most frequent audiences for your writing? Who have been your most valued audiences for your writing? What is the hardest writing you have ever done? Why was it so hard? What is one of your favorite pieces of writing? What makes it so special to you? How did you go about writing it? Who was the audience? Was it difficult to write? As you look over your writing history, notice at what points gender roles enter into it. How, if at all, might you have developed differently as a writer if gender roles had been less clearly divided during your life history?

Find a piece of writing you've published (turned in, mailed, seen in print, or just saved for posterity). Read it again to see how it might be said to be gendered. How, if at all, would you revise it in the light of your awareness of the ways gender roles influence writing?

List several of the writing assignments you give regularly to your students. Label each one according to the following scales which reflect some of the writing traits said to be gendered: open—closed, certain thesis—uncertain thesis, factual approach—speculative approach, local focus—universal focus, unknown/distant audience—intimate audience, purpose to explain, describe, narrate, persuade—purpose to connect with others or perform action. See how you might change your assignments, just slightly, to tip the scales in the opposite direction some of the time and to offer students more choice.

Try assigning your students numbers or have them use pseudonyms after putting their real name and the number or pseudonym on cards. Read and respond to the set of papers without knowing who really wrote them. Look, then, at the cards to see if there are any papers that surprise you. Ask if you may not be honoring the gender of the writers by assumptions about how males and females write, as Duane Roen has found in his research.

Try the same with your students. Have them read an essay without knowing the gender of the author and ask them to guess at whether it was written by a male or female, giving the reasons why they think it was by a male or female. Consider with your students how much the topic of the article may bear on their ideas about the gender of the author. Are there topics that are commonly acceptable or exclusive to one gender or the other?

Part IV
Gender and the Profession

In this section we include essays that reveal the ways gender roles shape our behavior as developing teachers and researchers. Greenwood describes the complex interaction between her gender role as graduate student and as college professor, and illustrates from her own research the ways even obvious interpretations may be masked from researchers and their mentors. Miller reviews literature on gender and curriculum theory and reflects on ways her own professional development, and by implication, ours, as teacher and as researcher has been affected by gender stereotypes and roles.

12

Voiced and Voiceless Findings: The Gender Gap in Composition Research

Claudia M. Greenwood

Not many of our colleagues return to the pages of the dissertations that afford them legitimacy in our profession. I am told that I am among a very few who have returned not only to the printed pages, but also to the notes that preceded the text reporting my study (*Factors That Influence Re-entry Women in College Composition Classes: A Descriptive Study* 1987). I have done so because I have been haunted by a cacophony of voices seeking a hearing—not the least among them my own.

Current interest in feminist issues in the profession that has encouraged open discussion within journals and at conferences has, for me, encouraged the retrospection necessary to close the gap between my knowing—and my telling. Such retrospection has revealed missed opportunities for understanding, for celebrating, and for influencing.

In 1985, as I was nearing completion of my doctoral studies, the number of students identifiable as re-entry women (Wheaton & Robinson 1982, 44) was steadily increasing on my campus and in my classes. These women, who had interrupted their formal education to marry, begin or, in some cases, complete—a family, represented an opportunity for me. Exactly what the opportunity was remained unclear for a period of time as I sought research that would help me focus a study of this population. Extensive reading yielded no research that examined, specifically, re-entry women in composition classes. Research by Kasworm (1980, 40–47) and other adult educators offered a generalized description of adult learners as active and self-directive, demonstrating in the classroom a developed self-confidence, various strategies for learning, and effective time management skills. My classroom experience with re-entry women students, however, did not then, nor has it yet, supported these assumptions. This extended experience suggests, in contrast, that re-entry women do not enjoy a well-defined sense of direction or an established identity; they have conflicting self-expectations and demonstrate a low tolerance for uncertainty. They seem not to value their experience and lack confidence in their ability to learn. Most apparent, they lack the ability to manage academics and other responsibilities to their satisfaction. My study was motivated, in part, by my desire to identify factors that distinguish re-entry women students from the general adult student population.

Aware of the numbers of nontraditional students in my workplace, a two-year commuter campus, my committee didn't question the appropriateness of the population. They never challenged my intention to study only women. I would suspect that their interest at this point was similar to mine: the population represented unturned ground for analysis. Their concern focused, primarily, on methodology. I foresaw qualitative research as the only possible way to get in touch with the answers to the questions that had begun to form regarding factors that influence re-entry women students in college composition classes. Although the committee's prior experience had been primarily quantitative, once again, they did not object, suggesting combined qualitative and quantitative approaches to secure certain pre- and post-instruction data. Their primary concern—and mine—was that I complete a study that would inform the teaching of the population. Pedagogy became a controlling focus, not only in the shaping of research questions, but also in the selecting of appropriate intersecting research methods and data sources, and in my reporting the findings.

Although the sample population was limited to twelve women, it yielded a wealth of data, enabling me to delineate a number of influencing factors, both internal and external, which affect re-entry women as writers. Curiously, however, I never identified *gender* among them. Further examination suggests that omission of the gender factor may explain some of the interpretative gaps remaining in the study; however, at the time of the writing, the oversight forced me to look beyond what might have been a more facile explanation, pushing me toward triangulation, toward proof, and away from conjecture. I do not regret that fact because I am a product of socio-political constructs that have made it difficult for me to believe sufficiently in *my* knowledge to have the courage to test my ideas in the public forum. Clean research, research unmuddied by implications of gender was safe then. Today it would be supported by the additional work of women such as Belenky and her colleagues (1986), Caywood & Overing (1987), and Hayes (1989). Like the subjects of my research, I had accepted a challenge at considerable risk and was eager to stay within the pedagogical template I had negotiated with my committee.

Findings Re-considered

To accomplish a meaningful discussion of the gender gap as I perceive it in my research I will examine several *voiced*, or stated, findings closely in an attempt to articulate the *voiceless*, or unstated, findings eclipsed by the pedagogical focus.

The research question was: taking into consideration the internal and external factors that affect the way re-entry women learn and write, are there certain modes and focuses more appropriate than others in their writing instruction? (Hillocks defines mode of instruction as the role assumed by the instructor, the types and order of activities involved, and the specificity of learning tasks; he defines focus as the dominant content of the course [1984, 141–150]).

Following data collection from a variety of sources including several surveys, interviews, videotaped writing sessions and retrospective protocols, portfolios, and teaching evaluations, I was able to enumerate many influencing factors, including the following:

- fear of failure
- doubt about the ability to learn
- low self-esteem
- diminished value of life experience
- guilt about neglect of family/home
- concern about not fitting in
- intimidation by instructors
- spousal non-support

Of course none of these factors would surprise feminist writer-researchers Adrienne Rich (1979), Carol Gilligan (1982), or Mary Belenky and her colleagues. They had observed the lack of confidence in meaning-making and meaning-sharing and had reported, "Feeling cut off from all internal and external sources of intelligence, women fail to develop their minds and see themselves as remarkably powerless and dependent . . . since they cannot trust their ability to understand and to remember what was said, they rely on the continued presence of authorities to guide their actions" (Belenky 1986, 28).

As my research pushed beyond the point of entry, beyond the fear, the doubt, and the guilt to examine the development of the women, observing the extent to which, as Belenky remarks, "the development of a sense of voice, mind, and self were intricately intertwined" (18), it became clear that the intricate web of internal and external factors that affects the attitude and performance of the re-entry woman in her many roles is not at all distinct from that which impinges on her role as writer.

The first blatant example of the exclusion of gender-based explanation is found in my reporting of the Writing History Survey data. This survey asked the subjects to explore their experience with writing prior to college, including personal as well as school-sponsored writing. I reported such rich responses to questions about the value of writing as "Writing is very important! I only wish I could" (Greenwood 1987, 78). And I found value in responses to questions about perceived strengths and weaknesses in the use of language which confirmed the re-entry student's preoccupation with correctness and sensitivity to audience: "I choose my words carefully. I care about people and would never intentionally hurt someone," (76); "I wrote in a journal because that was the only place I could say what I thought without being sent to the principal's office." Responses about instruction seemed important as well: "He was prejudiced against girls," or "I always seemed to get good grades, but felt I didn't deserve them because I never liked my content" (82). Yet *my* text reads simply:

> The portrait of the re-entry woman writer, with the addition of the historical data, now includes external factors relating specifically to the act of composing. The extent to which its value, its conception, and for most, its implicit risk created constructs upon which college instructors and instruction had to build will be revealed in other data. This writing history data reveals that the students had received traditional instruction. (82)

This *voiced* interpretation, quite clearly, was controlled by the pedagogical focus.

The *voiceless* interpretation would have posed the question: "How can we teach women to move beyond the desire for male approval and getting 'good grades' and seek and write their own truths that the culture has distorted or made taboo?" (Rich 1979, 240). Or, as Belenky et al. observed, it would have noted that

> Women typically approach adulthood with the understanding that the care and empowerment of others is central to their life's work .... Authorities hold considerable leverage and can be in particularly strategic positions to help these women find the power that can reside in their own minds, as well as in the minds of others. (48–49)

It is appropriate at this point to mention the four instructors of the composition classes from which data were collected. Two were male, two female, a gender split resulting from staffing and scheduling. While I surveyed and reported the instructors' attitudes toward the re-entry students, I did not elaborate on the now-obvious differences between the male and female instructors. Rather, I summarized their observations, identifying them, *collectively*, as strongly supportive of the students. I failed to note, for instance, that it was one of the male instructors who observed: "Though few in number, regularly [note the contradiction] problems interfere with their studies—children, current or ex- or future spouses, illness, work schedules, emotional crises"; also, "I probably expect more of the women because they've worked harder in the past. I expect them to be more fluent, too." He concluded his reply with the statement, "Since as a group over the years women have delivered more valuable goods, I have come to look for superior products. They seem to sense this condition and, as a result, try harder." (Greenwood 1987, 56–57). The *voiced* interpretation of the data cited the positive difference the women made in the ambience of the classrooms as well as in the instructors' attitudes toward the classes. The observation that the male instructors had dangerously high and unjustifiably certain expectations of these students remained unexpressed. Yet, as Belenky et al. observe, "In accepting the authorities' standards, the separate knowers make themselves vulnerable to their criticism" (107). As *vulnerability* was not isolated for study, neither was the possibility of its gender-role explanation.

High expectations, of course, influence the mode and focus of instruction in subtle ways, ways consistent both with the anticipation of superior performance by this group of students, and consistent with the misapprehension of the students' constructs, including the lack of confidence and diminished sense of creativity. Once again, in my original examination of data, the pedagogical focus eclipsed any other explanation for the conflicts that arose in the classes of one of the male instructors. Carefully I delineated his philosophy of teaching; carefully I assigned the clearly problematic features of his instruction to old-paradigm English education. That was easy to do. He believed in formal instruction of grammar; he believed that he was responsible for correcting the students' oral language; he believed that class time should not be devoted to peer activities of any kind, but rather to lecture; he believed that successful writing could be achieved only if all writing was carefully marked by the instructor; he believed that an instructor should mark every detected error on a student's paper, and used red ink to do so; he demanded perfect copy without giving students the benefit of instruction in the writing process.

Even as the data accumulated and I noted that comments on his papers differed considerably from those of the female instructors, I did not attribute either those comments or the students' reactions to gender. I saw them as the effects of unfortunate, uninformed pedagogy. And yet, as I review my data and my reporting of it, I see missed opportunities for understanding; especially when I note that the female instructors were responding to the students' voice and tone, "Your voice is clear. I feel your pain" and "Very clear and strong. What a fine paper. What a good point" (Greenwood 60), while his comments were generally limited to mechanics—as they were, for instance, on the very first essay submitted by one of the students, "See the mechanics closely. Work to prepare nearly perfect copy" (60), or on a paper of 435 words, "No more shortees" (101). Reviewing my data, I have discovered the distressing exclusion of additional commentary such as: "Essay by essay we can expect, I believe, a hardening of thought and control."

I did not seek an explanation other than pedagogical when I noted the apprehension of the group in this instructor's class as they faced their first in-class writing assignment: "I'm afraid of the subject he might pick. I won't have time to refine my work. He'll get it raw" (Greenwood 103), or when I spoke with them in a mid-term interview and heard them remark about their inability to estimate their chance for success and one of them said, "Why did I get a 91 on this paper and a 75 on this one? I didn't do anything different. How am I ever going to get through this" (111). Or even after a final interview when one of the students stated, "He gave us a lot of proofing symbols and when he put them on my paper I had to go back and figure out what he meant, then I had to run to a dictionary or his little handbook to figure out what it was I did wrong. I am still not sure what I ever did right." Following this observation the student showed me a paper peppered with bold red marks and one final comment: "There is no vitality, no energy in your writing" (101). In this instance I made no connection between her attempt to satisfy what she believed he had identified as a goal in composition—an average of eighteen words per sentence—and his perception of lifelessness in her text. By semester's end, this student as well as her writing lacked energy. One of her classmates dealt with the expectations somewhat differently, yet the results were similar: "He made me feel the need to challenge him, to show him I could do those things right that he showed me I was doing wrong, but the harder I tried, the more I did wrong. I had to learn from my mistakes—that's how he taught" (111).

In my reporting and interpreting of this data I did mention that the common factors of little initial confidence and strong goal orientation led to the students' indefatigable pursuit of their instructors' composition goals; I did not, however, apprehend the gender-specific explanation of their behavior: "The women see blind obedience to authorities as being of utmost importance for keeping out of trouble and insuring their own survival, because trying to know 'why' is not thought to be particularly possible or important" (Belenky 28). Reviewing raw data,

I find it distressing that I didn't even report the following comment by one of the students: "Now, after this class, every time I write it's like he's sitting on my shoulder with his red pen poised. . . . I can hardly write a word without thinking it must be wrong."

Voiced in my discussion of the reported data was the achievement of an acceptable solution by a third student: "Her solution to lack of encouragement or advice was simple: 'I just felt no matter what I did it wasn't going to please him, and I thought that that is too bad, so I just kept writing to please me, and I didn't care if it pleased him or not'" (Greenwood 1987, 111). *Unvoiced* was the rich interpretation possible, acknowledgment of the students' struggles for independence, for empowerment; their tough-mindedness—heretofore the privilege only of their critic—in an environment that represented not only traditional instruction, but traditional obstacles to the women's development.

Thinking about the education of women, Adrienne Rich wrote, "A woman, like any other human being needs to know that the mind makes mistakes . . . that she is capable of intelligent thought, and she needs to know it right away . . ." (240). *I* knew that. But these students of my study knew only that their thinking and its expression were both inadequate; their instructor reminded them of that fact regularly in his marginal comments. Unvoiced also was the observation by one of the women in the Belenky et al. study, "You need a little bit of praise to keep you going" (197), and the researchers' conviction that intellectual development can be impeded rather than promoted by unrelenting academic pressure.

Although I did make the statement in the dissertation that none of the students of the professor in question had requested a conference, I did not follow through with that information, either, leaving *unexpressed* the gender-related explanation: the women were afraid of confrontation. They hesitated to challenge the instructor's authority, believing that what he taught must be what was most important in the teaching of writing.

Conclusion

Even though only a cursory review of the data has been possible here, I believe that it is necessary to reflect on the broader scope of gender-related implications for feminist research and its communication. Having reconsidered both my project and its process, I have come to understand that my failure to identify and pursue the understanding of gender as a factor in my research is itself gender-based.

In earlier discussions of my data and in subsequent recommendations for instruction based on the findings, I did not move beyond the limits of the template I had negotiated at the outset of my research: pedagogy. I suggested that the re-entry student responded and grew in certain classroom environments—that mode and focus were significant, contributing factors. My own voice failed, however, when I took the carefully considered position: "What I can recommend after observing this group of women enter and complete a semester of collegiate work is neither special treatment nor separate treatment, but rather considerate treatment not unlike that which ought to be given to all of our students all of the time" (Greenwood 148).

The written conclusion, in its entirety, voiced my endorsement of the process methodology of writing instruction, but not, it seems, for all of the right reasons. It was not, of course, grounded in the rather recently formulated rationale of *feminist pedagogy*, a mode and focus of instruction recognized for "its potential to better meet the particular needs of women," (Hayes 1989, 59). Nor did it appropriately reflect the sense of celebration or respect for the tough growing the women had accomplished:

> I think I have grown mainly because having not gone to school for so long it is almost as if my mind had stopped. You can go to work every day and you can deal with your family, your children every day, but that's different. There's something—a third type of thing you can do—and that's *real thinking*. I was amazed at some of the things I was able to come up with or think, because I hadn't thought like that before I went to school. But now that I've been forced into thinking, I can see that the possibilities are unlimited. (Greenwood 1987, 116–17).

It was a conclusion that reflected, most of all, the extent to which I, the researcher, listened to an internal voice that warned against risk and tempered my message, allowing neither the public celebration of the women's accomplishments nor the unrestricted criticism of instruction that perpetuates the myth of the all-powerful male authority figure in the composition classroom. Like the women of my study, I had allowed personal goals to be subsumed by the dictates of the academy, dictates which prevented the development of a strong, clear, authentic voice.

The extent to which my voice appeared restrained was, indeed, noted by one reviewer (male) of my work who observed, "Seems unsure ... some parts have a clear voice, others lack an authorial voice ..." I suspect that the lack of authorial voice also caused a journal editor to respond that the readership of his journal "already sense the special needs of the group," and guess that research specialists would "have questions about the extent and design of the project." Like other women in our profession, I have, as a result of these responses, been hesitant to seek public confirmation of the importance of my findings, stifling my own voice, however clear and authentic.

As authority figures that stifle voices exist not only within the classroom, but beyond it as well, both factors have implications for our profession. Instruction that frustrates the attempts of non-traditional women students to develop their voices must be replaced with a pedagogy that encourages them to realize their full academic potential. Research that examines the process of empowerment of this growing student population must not, itself, be stifled by outmoded attitudes in university research communities or on editorial boards.

Works Cited

Belenky, Mary, et al. 1986. *Women's Ways of Knowing: The Development of Self, Voice, and Mind*. New York: Basic Books.

Caywood, Cynthia L., and Gillian R. Overing. 1987. *Teaching Writing: Pedagogy, Gender, and Equity*. New York: State U of New York P.

Gilligan, Carol. 1982. *In a Different Voice: Psychological Theory and Women's Development*. Cambridge: Harvard UP.

Greenwood, Claudia M. 1987. "Factors which Influence Re-entry Women in College Composition Classes." Diss. Indiana U of PA.

Hayes, Elizabeth. 1989. "Insights from Women's Experiences for Teaching and Learning." *Effective Teaching Styles*. Ed. Elizabeth Hayes. San Francisco: Jossey-Bass. 55–66.

Hillocks, George Jr. 1984. "What Works in Teaching Composition: A Meta-analysis of Experimental Treatment Studies." *American Journal of Education* 93.1 (Nov.): 133–70.

Kasworm, Carol. 1980. "The Older Student as an Undergraduate," *Adult Education* 31:1, 30–47.

Rich, Adrienne. 1979. *On Lies, Secrets, and Silence*. New York: W. W. Norton.

Wheaton, Janilee, and Daniel Robinson. 1983. "Responding to the Needs of Re-entry Women: A Comprehensive Campus Model." *NASPA Journal* 21 (Fall): 44–51.

13

Gender and Teachers

Janet L. Miller

The early morning sessions at this annual conference of English teachers were adjourning, and the conference center hallway swelled abruptly with the movement and chatter of eager session-goers. Teachers paused only momentarily to discuss and critique the latest presentations, and then surged toward the next scheduled events. This rather frenetic scene has invariably been repeated during every professional conference that I have attended. And I always feel, in that rush from one session to the next, that we all are somehow trying to juggle both the ideas gleaned from each session and those inevitable plastic shopping bags that we lug around, filled with books, handouts, and splashy posters designed to capture our students' often wavering attention.

As I watched this ritual yet once again, I was waiting this time not for jugglers of theory and practice to emerge from these countless sessions, but rather for a reunion with a friend. And, staring at the parade of teachers flowing past me in order to find Donna, I thought of the ways in which I once believed that a plastic bag filled with materials could bring me pedagogical bliss. I smiled as I began to remember how much I thought I knew about teaching and my discipline when I greeted my very first classes of high school juniors and seniors.

I had spent the week before school opened working in my new homeroom, decorating with some plants and posters as well as with photographs which I had carefully cut from magazines and mounted on brightly colored paper. I had filled the back wall, a giant corkboard that went from floor to ceiling, with book jackets and hand-made letters, announcing the various novels that we were going to read together. And, as I introduced myself on that first day of school to my students, who gazed at me with mild curiosity, I was armed with my bag of nifty activities and lesson plans and an introduction that emphasized how much I wanted them to *love* literature. That introduction, of course, set me back months.

Now, I was pressed against the hallway wall of the conference center cavern, scanning this predominantly female crowd, and wondering if I would recognize my friend Donna, with whom I had attended both high school and college. And as I waited and watched, I continued to think about my teaching of high school juniors and seniors, and I began to ponder all that Donna and I had needed and didn't get in our teacher preparation classes and in our ensuing professional teaching careers. In the years since college, I had learned that those needs went far beyond those plastic shopping bags filled with the pedagogical conceptions and packagings of others. But, in our undergraduate education program, we had only been presented with courses that emphasized the sequencing and end-product aspects of particular "methods and materials" in the teaching of English. And so, of course, we thought that those plastic shopping bags, if filled with just the right activities and books and motivating posters, could guarantee smooth teaching and learning in our classrooms.

Eager as I was then to see pictures of Donna's two children and to hear about her life since our college years together, I also was hoping that we could talk about ourselves as teachers. I wanted to know if Donna had been met with the same blank stares and the same resistances that I periodically had experienced in my high school teaching career. I wanted to share with her how I had frantically dug to the bottom of my shopping bag in search of just the right approach to entice that group of seniors in my after-lunch sixth-period class who seemed so bored with Modern Literature. I wanted to know what she thought and did once she too realized that those shopping bags of methods and materials were not sufficient in dealing with the multiple needs, desires, interests, and positions of students, of colleagues, of parents, of administrators. And I wanted to know how she had changed, as a woman who teaches, and who now also administers her high school English department as chairperson. I knew that I wanted to share the changes that I had experienced as a woman who had moved from high school to university teaching. In particular, I wanted to ask Donna about her present perceptions of what we had *not* received or constructed for ourselves in our undergraduate program and in our early years of teaching. As well, I wanted to share ideas about what we now knew we needed and wanted as experienced teachers.

And I knew that we would have to do this kind of talking away from the bustle and segmented sessions of this huge annual conference. For I wanted to talk in depth about our teaching lives, just as we had been able to do so long ago in our dorm room. And the shopping bags and the two-hour sessions at this conference, in which we usually sat passively as others imparted wisdom from their own particular shopping bags, did not encourage the kind of conversations that could enable us to make connections between our past and present roles as women who teach, or to examine the similarities and the differences that might characterize our professional lives.

Just days before this conference began, Donna had announced herself back into my life on my answering machine, suggesting that we meet here after twenty-plus years of exchanging holiday notes. As I searched the faces of the women ebbing through the halls and into the next session rooms, I also remembered those countless dorm conversations with my friend, especially as we were completing our college years together and preparing to become teachers. Yes, we agreed, we wanted to teach; the school schedule would easily accommodate our plans for marriage and eventual families and summer travels and study. No, we agreed, we did not want to become administrators in schools; we didn't want to relinquish the flexibility of time and approach that we were sure our own classrooms would afford us. And besides, most administrators were men. Yes, we agreed, we were excited about sharing our love of literature and language with our future high school students.

Twenty-five years later, as we finally found each other near the coat racks, Donna and I embraced, surrounded by umbrellas and rain hats and other people's smiles. And, amidst the clatter of breakfast dishes being set and then cleared, we picked up the threads of those college conversations in our morning-long reunion in the hotel coffee shop. And even as we were able to talk as if few years had intervened in our conversations, our discussions during that easy yet intensely emotional morning-long reunion were markedly different from those dorm-room sessions during our senior year.

It wasn't just that we were older now, and thus could talk about our lives and our teaching from experienced stances. What was striking to us both during that morning reunion, and what I want to describe in this essay, were ways in which our conversation now emanated from very different perspectives than those that we shared in our constant dorm-room discussions. For our morning reunion talk focused on ways in which our early teaching expectations and assumptions and ensuing experiences reflected socially constructed, and therefore gendered versions of our work and of our roles as teachers. Analyses of the ways in which teaching, both as a profession and as a process, and curriculum, both as content and process, are filled with gender-biased assumptions and expectations had been absent from our teacher preparation as well as early inservice programs. These were the analyses that we had needed but had never received or constructed for ourselves during our early years in the profession. And so, in this essay too, I discuss reasons why both Donna and I have had to reconstruct versions of teaching and curriculum for ourselves and our students that incorporate analyses of gender as well as of race, class, and other positions and identities that influence what and how and why we teach and learn.

Gender-Neutral Versions of Teaching and Curriculum

Our talk that morning was interspersed with cups of coffee and stories of the twists and turns of our individual lives in those years following our college classes together. And yet most of our talk centered on our still-present preoccupation with the difficulties and joys of being teachers. We moved back and forth between the spaces of our initial preparation for teaching and the spaces that we now occupied as professional educators. But especially in the initial stages of our conversation, we reminisced about our college experiences together as English majors and future teachers.

We giggled as we remembered the audio-visual class that we were required to take as part of our education minor; the professor was particularly known for his insistence on colorful bulletin boards, and Donna and I recalled sitting in our dorm quad for hours with five or six other young women, cutting out over-sized tag-board letters for the mandatory weekly bulletin board display in his classroom. We hadn't questioned the dubious value of this activity in his classroom, only in our paper-cutting sessions in our dorm. And we hadn't wondered why all of our education courses were filled with women, even in our secondary education component; the few men enrolled talked, even then, of moving quickly into administrative lines.

And as we continued to review our college courses together, we laughed as we remembered our favorite Shakespeare professor's tendency to relax once in a while and allow us to deviate from the text a bit in order to wonder about the life and times in which such literature was created. We loved those deviations, but now Donna and I marveled that we had not wondered, too much anyway, about the constant focus on our professor's interpretations, rather than on our own. We had carried our conjectures back to the dorm and had spent many hours constructing our versions of Shakespeare's friends and lovers and the economic and political atmosphere in which he might have been working. But we did not offer those conjectures in our classes. We listened to our professor, and exchanged delighted smiles when one of his interpretations coincided with our own.

Now we also wondered how we could not have wondered then about the dearth of women writers in the literature canons that we had studied. Nor had we questioned, initially anyway, that lack in the textbooks from which we began teaching. Nor had we puzzled then about who got to say what counted as literature "classics," or what constituted "serious" writing, or whose worlds and perspectives those canons represented.

Nor had we even wondered about ways in which we might acknowledge the diversities and differences among our future students' needs and interests, because, of course, as Donna wryly noted, we had not ever acknowledged our own. We recalled that instead, we wanted to share with those students the great pieces of literature and language that we had studied, and in the ways that we had studied, in order that they too might come to love what we loved.

As we recalled those college experiences, then, we could see ways in which conceptions of teaching, learning, and curriculum, as we had experienced them in our undergraduate studies especially, were presented as gender-neutral processes and contents. We never were encouraged to question our professors' positions behind the lecterns as representing and dispensing knowledge that most often portrayed men's perceptions and ideas and constructions of the world. And we never were encouraged to identify the ways in which the women characters in the literature that we were studying, or the professors who were interpreting their literary lives, were like, or different from, ourselves. For the most part, we had accepted our roles as students who received information and authoritative interpretations of the canons that constituted our studies as English majors. And, although we now were appalled at our passivity during those college years, we agreed that we had been wonderful representations of the "good girl/good student" syndrome. We had learned early on to nod agreeably, to read conscientiously, and to keep most of our questions confined to those of classroom procedures and requirements.

Teaching as "Women's Work"

And, as we sat at the breakfast table, we were well aware that twenty-five years ago we also had unquestionly accepted teaching as appropriate "women's work." As we discussed the possibilities of my niece becoming a veterinarian, one of many careers about which she daily changes her mind, we agreed, with a shared glance filled with our sixties existential irony, that neither of us had considered a profession other than teaching. Neither of us had wanted to be a nurse or a secretary (although we both had taken typing in high school, "just in case.") These were the two other major professions for women that were socially sanctioned as we were growing up in the 1950s and 1960s. As an English major, I had thought briefly about a career in publishing or in journalism, but had quickly dismissed those possibilities as not fitting in with my marriage and family plans.

When Donna and I graduated from college in 1966, we were among many of our classmates who immediately married, some to evade the Vietnam war draft, and who began careers in a time of political upheaval in the United States. But we both moved to small communities, settling where our new husbands' positions took us. Our teaching was less informed by the political strife surrounding the war, or the civil rights movement, or the women's movement, for example, than by the immediate concerns of simultaneous marriage, family, and professional responsibilities.

And now, years later, with both of us working in careers that we have honed and crafted by choice at this point, we discussed ways in which those initial understandings of ourselves as supplemental to our husbands' careers and in some ways as isolated from the ferment that surged through colleges and universities in response to the war and to the various political movements of the times, are understandings that we still are attempting to deconstruct.

Only in the ensuing years since college graduation, for example, have I become aware of analyses that have enabled me to see ways in which I had internalized the socially sanctioned role of woman as teacher/nurturer/responder to others' needs and as conveyer/transmitter of other's ideas and interests. Just as I had learned to respond to my professors' remarks with smiles, and to craft written exams that reinforced their interpretations of particular pieces of literature, for example, I too assumed that I should nurture my students, my male chairperson, and my male principal by attempting to please them. And I also assumed that the ways in which my professors had transmitted knowledge, as if it were fixed and agreed upon by everyone, and the ways in which I returned that knowledge to them, in exams and papers that replicated their versions, were the ways in which my students and I should engage in these processes called teaching and learning.

I only began to examine the underlying assumptions around which such constructions of myself as teacher were based when the supposed securities of marriage and one life-long teaching position were no longer my choices. As I pursued my doctoral degree, especially, I started to hear remarks such as "Well, does this mean you will never get married again?" And, "Now you will really get to play the expert!" Such remarks contained not only assumptions about women who teach beyond the accepted boundaries of elementary and secondary education, but also about the hierarchical relationships between university and classroom teachers. And those various assumptions reflected some of the contradictory aspects that frame academic women's lives.

As I began my academic career in the university, then, I began to experience conflict between the role of professor as "expert" and my simultaneous role as woman teacher. It was at this point that I began to more fully investigate those assumptions as aspects around which I had constructed my personal and professional life.

> Women have been led to feel that they can integrate and use all their attributes if they use them for others, but not for themselves. They have developed the sense that their lives should be guided by the constant need to attune themselves to the wishes, desires, and needs of others. The others are the important ones and the guides to action. (Miller 1986: 61–62)

And so, I began to consider ways in which, without thinking and without questioning, I had transferred an expectation of myself as a woman to my professional role, especially during the time that I taught high school English. Now that I was experiencing expectations within university structures that I teach and research as "expert" rather than as "nurturer," I began to struggle with ways in which I could engage in those activities in reciprocal and collaborative ways that could acknowledge both the supportive and the inquiring aspects of my role as female academic.

Thus, I began to investigate social, economic, political, and historical junctures that had led to the "feminization of teaching" in the United States. I read Nancy Hoffman's historical accounts (1981) of the development of teaching into "women's 'true' profession"; her accounts emphasize the voices of women as they struggled, within the confines of social expectations and schooling structures that relied on women's accustomed roles as subservient, genteel, and docile replicators of the status quo, to create and choose teaching as their vocation. And I read Madeleine Grumet's gender history of American common school teachers during the nineteenth and early twentieth centuries (1988), where she argues, like Hoffman, that some women were interested in escaping the compulsory domesticity of nineteenth-century rural family life. But Grumet notes that, ironically, in their desire to create for themselves careers as teachers, these women had to work for men who functioned not only as administrators but also as the ones who determined the content and processes of the classroom as well as the functions of schooling. Thus, in having to support patriarchal school authority in order to keep their positions as teachers, these women ensured and enacted a "pedagogy for patriarchy."

And I noted that Michael Apple's analyses (1986) emphasize the political economy of schooling, in which de-skilling, depowering, and de-personalization of teaching are related to the devaluing of a profession which is comprised mainly of females.

Within these analyses which consider the deleterious effects of the feminization of teaching, Susan Laird's work (1988) identifies five distinct sets of interpretations to the slogan of teaching as "women's true profession":

1. The Descriptive Thesis: That the vast majority of American schoolteachers are women.
2. The Normative Thesis: That schoolteaching, on account of its nature and women's nature, should be women's work.
3. The Problematic Thesis: That intelligent women somehow become devalued by schoolteaching.
4. The Negative Thesis: That schoolteaching somehow becomes devalued through its identification with women.
5. The Critical Thesis: That schoolteachers' own public, collaborative, self-definitive responses to the other four theses are crucial to a reconception of teaching that can address our current teaching crisis.

The Negative Thesis is what Apple (1986) and Grumet (1988), in particular, are pointing to in their analyses, and the Normative Thesis is the one that probably most dramatically framed my initial understandings of how I "should" be as a teacher. Both of these theses assume "woman" to be an essential category; that is, all women supposedly share an essential nature, and that nature is often conceptualized as caring, nurturing, and compliant, rather than as independent, visionary, and authoritative. These theses set up an "either/or" construct that situates women's "nature" in opposition to men's supposedly inherent "nature" as aggressive, autonomous, and often stoic. So, for example, in the teaching profession, men, because of their supposedly more developed leadership and authoritative "nature," still assume the majority of administrative positions, while women remain in the classroom to enact the dictates of curriculum and pedagogy that have been forged by those in authority. And both are supposedly enacting those roles that biology and society have deemed appropriate for them.

Daniel Liston and Kenneth Zeichner (1990) utilize Susan Laird's theses and their implications not only to explore the social contexts of schooling with their students who are prospective teachers, but also to examine their own positions within teacher education:

> As male elementary teachers and now as male teachers of predominantly female prospective teachers, we have observed subtle and overt reactions to men's participation in "women's work." Many of our prospective women teachers express surprise that a man would want to be an elementary teacher. Many of our male college mentors thought we should choose more appropriate careers. And, more

> recently, many of our colleagues have advised us to focus on matters other than teacher education. . . . Committed as we are to a nondiscriminatory and non-repressive educational agenda, the strong possibility that gender dynamics in schools and society may contribute to antidemocratic biases seems good enough reason to examine these relations. (630–31)

These scholars, and many others, have heightened my awareness of the ways in which I had internalized expectations for myself as woman/teacher/nurturer; further, they have provided critiques that enable me to understand more fully the ways in which such essentialized notions of women and our work effectively guarantee our marginalization and devalued status not only in the workplace but also in our relational lives. And, as Daniel Liston and Kenneth Zeichner note, such gendered constructions of teaching influence both women and men in their conceptualizations and enactments of teaching and teacher education. For we all are fighting deeply internalized notions, constantly reinforced by historical and social arrangements and expectations, and by media and print representations, of how we "should" be as women and men in the world. And those internalized notions, then, often reinforce unequal power relations within school classrooms, corridors, and in the central administration offices.

Thus, realizing the limited career options that were socially sanctioned during the 1960s was an important initial aspect of my evolving understandings of the myriad implications of teaching as women's work. However, as I continue to explore those implications, I also am influenced by feminists who argue that although expanded career options or equal compensation for equal work are necessary, they are not sufficient in attempts to address and to change the unequal power relations that characterize myriad aspects of people's lives. And so to move into analyses that question the hierarchical structures that reflect power relations inherent in every aspect of teaching requires that we question the social structures and representations that school reflect and maintain. We can ask, for example, why males still continue to dominate the field of educational administration, or why most of the teachers at the annual English teachers' conference are women, or why that conference program still contains little if any discussion of these kinds of gender issues, or why the organization of the conference still reflects the authoritative and hierarchical structures in which those "in charge" or who are deemed as "experts" impart their wisdom to teachers in lectures and other monological formats. These structures and arrangements reflect subtle and not so subtle gender-biased roles and assumptions within a profession that claims as a priority the acknowledgment of individuals' cultural and social diversities.

Further, then, we also must acknowledge that the very structures of the disciplines that we teach, the ways in which we teach them, and the ways in which we research and write and represent ourselves among our professional colleagues and others in our educational communities constantly create new disciplinary and pedagogical knowledges that are filled with issues of power. Who gets to decide what and how we teach? Who gets to say what is "good" teaching? Who gets to say what counts as "knowledge" in my classroom? And on standardized tests? In my professional organizations, publications, and relationships? And in whose interests are these decisions made? Mine? My students? The school's public image? The administrators? And how do those decisions reflect unequal relationships of power, based on gendered, raced, and classed constructions of teaching, research, and curriculum?

Curriculum as Gender Text

As Donna and I continued to recall the linear and sequential conceptions of curriculum with which we were presented as part of our secondary English education program, we also remembered that we had connected such conceptions, even then, with the ways in which our literature courses were organized and presented.

We had marched our way through the Norton Anthologies of American and English literature. We remembered the time-lines that we constructed in our dorm rooms, in order to maintain the chronology of those whose biographies and works we were studying. And we recalled one long night of studying "Childe Roland to the Dark Tower Came." We had agonized through every verse of Robert Browning's Victorian age version of "Star Wars," knowing that we would be required to cite specific lines from this work in our essay exam the next day. Now, we recalled tearing the pages of this work from our text, throwing the crumpled pages at one another, and shrieking "Why is it always the guys who get to face the dragons?"

We talked at length about curriculum as we had experienced the concept in our undergraduate English and education courses. In our exasperation with "Childe Roland," we agreed that we were finally expressing, in our junior year, not only our frustration with the linear "marching through the curriculum" in which we had been engaged, but also our dismay in the constant masculine views of the world which this "official" English major curriculum had presented us. There was no Norton Anthology of Literature by women, as there is now, and so we read Tennyson and Whitman and Eliot and Dickens and Hemingway and Lewis and Fitzgerald and Malamud and Camus and Sartre, among many others. We read these men, usually in chronological order and by genres, all neatly categorized and sequentially ordered for our consumption.

Our education courses had only reinforced the notion of curriculum as discipline-specific content areas that are bound by testable, measurable, and deliverable categories. Nowhere in this definition of curriculum could Donna or I acknowledge the multiple interpretations and understandings of the particular contents and processes and contexts that emerged in our dorm dialogues and study sessions. Nowhere did that official definition of curriculum allow for our feelings of exclusion or distortion that emerged as we read, once again, of a young male's attempts to meet the challenges of life's battles. Nowhere did that official definition of curriculum as unitary and objective representation of the world, of reality, of life, allow for the divergent experiences that Donna and I brought to those official readings.

We had been presented with an "official" English major curriculum that presented stable, unified canons that supposedly represented consensus on singular and universal traditions and knowledges. And we had been presented with "official" versions of teaching that portrayed that activity as means by which to convey or transmit a particular and predetermined body of knowledge to others. These official definitions seem to refer to knowledges constructed most often through male-centered frames of inquiry and experience, and translated, pedagogically, through metaphors such as assembly line production or factory models. Those metaphors reinforce notions of curriculum as knowledge that can be created only by those "in charge" of a discipline's content and modes of inquiry, and that can then be transmitted to others in the forms of products or outcomes.

Only as we have been teaching and grappling with the discrepancies between these "official" definitions and our relational and always changing experiences with students and colleagues have Donna and I both been able to question these "official" conceptions of curriculum and pedagogy. And so as breakfast turned into lunch, we began to share our frustrations and puzzlements about curriculum that still excludes or trivializes or stereotypes the contributions of women and others who have not been a part of the construction of "school knowledge." We worried further about those constructions of curriculum that replicated social orders and forms that would have us think of those exclusions and marginalizations as the norm. We questioned the ways in which curriculum conceived as product or course of study denied the particular perspectives and interactions of teachers and students as aspects of classroom curriculum. And we shared the ways in which our present positions, Donna's as chairperson of her high school English department, and mine as university professor in a school of education, are filled with examples of gendered constructions of teaching in which we, as women, often still are posited as caretakers, as nurturers, as conveyers of others' knowledges rather than as creators of our own.

For example, Donna talked of her current frustration with an administrator who was insisting that Donna, as chairperson of the English department, must supply standardized scores to justify continuation of the writing-across-the-curriculum program that she had instituted. Donna of course was arguing that such processes could inform students' learning on multiple levels, and that such learnings might not be reflected through "objective" measures. We discussed ways in which the high school curriculum, as traditionally organized, still reinforces notions of that "official" curriculum definition which posits knowledge as fixed and therefore measurable. Such a definition would allow her administrator to insist on such separations of students' learning processes from the "end products" of knowledge conceived as a series of facts or skills to be mastered.

As we discussed ways in which writing had become a way for both of us to reflect on as well as to create multiple versions of ourselves as teachers, Donna and I also talked about possible ways in which she might continue her writing program in the face of these standardized testing constraints. Interwoven in our conversation were issues of students' and teachers' voices, linear conceptions not only of curriculum but also of the processes that inform teaching and learning, and the ways in which gender considerations frame these particular issues.

Embedded in these issues, of course, are discrepancies. Donna saw this particular situation in terms of separations between what counts as official school knowledges and what students and teachers construct daily as knowledges lodged in their interactions as well as in the spaces between and among those interactions. Who gets to say what counts here? The administrator, a male, was deciding how and why Donna, as chairperson, must account for *his* versions of teaching and learning. And those versions replicated standard conceptions that were initially developed and administered by males in the field of education. These spaces in which we teach and learn, we agreed, always contain multiple social positionings and power relations.

For me, these discrepancies have emerged too in the spaces created between my understanding and experiencing of curriculum and teaching as interwoven and as situated in the multiple interpretive frames that my students and I bring into the classroom. We create the curriculum of the classroom as we interpret and re-frame the "content" or "material" of our coursework through our own understandings and biographical experiences. These understandings and experiences reflect and yet often contradict the social, historical, and political frames that constitute "official" school knowledges. And so thus, as part of our work together, my students and I might investigate the manifestations of these frames as part of the "hidden" curriculum of our classroom and of our various "methods and materials."

As the discrepancies between what is presented as "official school knowledges" and our own experiences become more pronounced, I share with students the various work of teacher-researchers who are attempting to address such discrepancies from frameworks that enabled them to challenge the unequal power relations that exist within linear and transmission-like curricular and pedagogical conceptions.

Ann Berlak, for example, addresses such issues by examining her own teaching (1989; 1991). Via reflective journal writing, including detailed journal entries on her current teaching practices, and via examination of notes on her teaching over the course of her teaching career, Berlak attempts to uncover traces of unconscious and unintended imposition of her beliefs on her students. By focusing on inequalities perpetuated by social structures, including those of race, class, and gender, Ann Berlak autobiographically traces examples of inequalities in her own teaching practice.

> What will matter is that I remain an experiencing teacher, that I encourage questions and contradictions to emerge, that I and the students recognize them when they appear, that we take the time to engage in edifying conversations about them, that I encourage students to continue to examine what they are doing as teachers, in order to increase the likelihood that after they leave our classroom, they continue to converse. (1991, 39)

Like Berlak, Elizabeth Ellsworth (1989) acknowledges the contradictions that emerge in attempts to enact reciprocal and non-impositional forms of curriculum, pedagogy, and research. Such forms encourage the dialogue and the constant questioning to which Berlak refers. However, Ellsworth notes the difficulties of such attempts within hierarchical and often authoritarian settings such as universities as well as even within forms of pedagogy that claim to be emancipatory and critical:

> While I had the institutional power and authority in the classroom to enforce "reflective examination" of the plurality of moral and political positions before us in a way that supposedly gave my own assessments equal weight with those of students, in fact my institutional role would always weight my statements differently from those of students. (1989, 308)

Deborah Britzman (1991) also highlights the processes of intersubjective critique among herself and her students; she focuses on ways in which she works with students as well as on ways in which students work with her to reproduce and challenge traditional relations of power and authority. Britzman conceptualizes curriculum as relational and thus as necessarily infused with a diversity of cultural expressions and productions that enable students and herself as teacher to construct their educational and lived worlds:

> When student teachers encounter a curriculum, they are always encountering more than a body of traditions. They have the difficult work of helping their students make sense within a context that stifles interpretive risks and creative thought, and of constructing relevancies and common ground necessary for the creation of effective pedagogies. Simultaneously, student teachers must also confront their own subjective experience with school knowledge, how their deep convictions, investments, and desires have been structured by it. (1991, 46)

In researching issues of pedagogy and curriculum, Patti Lather (1991) also questions concepts that are basic to those "official" definitions, those positivist ways of knowing—concepts such as neutrality, objectivity, and "observable facts." Lather especially questions the impositional tendencies inherent within positivist versions of research and curriculum that separate the researchers or "experts" from those who are the subjects of their inquiry:

> [There is] the need for intellectuals with liberatory intentions to take responsibility for transforming our own practices so that our empirical and pedagogical work can be less toward positioning ourselves as masters of truth and justice and more toward creating a space where those directly involved can act and speak on their own behalf. (1991, 164–65)

My own work in recent years has focused on such relational issues in both teaching and research. I continue to examine assumptions regarding the nature of my role as teacher and as woman, but now those issues are focused in dialogue with others who teach. I joined with five classroom teachers several years ago to investigate the possibilities of collaborative and reciprocal versions of teacher-as-researcher. As we continue our collaborative investigations, we also continue to challenge not only our taken-for-granted conceptions of research, teaching, and curriculum, but also those political and social constructs, including gender, which still influence our notions of collaboration, of subjectivity, of schooling. We continue to grapple with the forms of research that are authorized in both schools and universities as those that can predict and control. Our versions of ourselves as teacher-researchers of our own underlying assumptions and expectations challenge those authorized versions, and, at the same time, exemplify the difficulties that frame collaborative ventures between university and classroom teachers. Working together to challenge issues of hierarchy and imposition in collaborative inquiry, we now understand too that finding voices and creating spaces for such work are not definitive, bounded events, but rather are constantly emerging and contradictory processes (Miller, 1990).

And so as I continue to examine underlying assumptions and expectations for myself within these constructs, I also work now to incorporate possibilities for such examinations within the teaching, writing, and research in which I engage with teachers in both university and inservice settings. These examinations are aspects of curriculum, as we together work to excavate the habitual, the routine, the taken-for-granted that mask oppressive contexts, relations, and contents within our our educational lives.

Donna and I talked about ways in which such perspectives could enable both students and teachers to examine "official" versions of curriculum and teaching and research, even as they are engaged in processes that both replicate and resist such versions. We settled ourselves into lobby chairs and Donna said, "You know, maybe I can turn this pressure on me for standardized testing of the writing-across-the-curriculum program into departmental discussions of curriculum—whose versions of knowledge are we asking kids to write about? And what ways are we saying that those knowledges can be known?

She wondered if her questions would be heard by those who would make final decisions on the testing. Together, we acknowledged that, even in our present positions, we still struggled to hear our own voices, voices that were changing almost daily and which could no longer remain silent or compliant. But, at the same time, we realized that we had just participated in conversation that enabled us both to voice our similar *and* our different experiences of the same processes and events of our undergraduate preparation to become teachers of English. And, although each of us has been able to reconsider those experiences from perspectives that incorporate issues of gender, among others, as critical lenses, neither of us told completed stories.

That day's reunion conversation provided moments stolen from the rigid conference schedule in which to renew our long-term friendship. That conversation also contained, within our overlapping and partial stories, gendered versions of our experiences and understandings of ourselves as women who teach. And finally, that conversation provided framings for our critique and analyses of a variety of related issues regarding gender and teaching. These included our participation in teaching as a "natural" extension of our supposed essential nature as nurturing caretakers, and the resulting still-gendered nature of divisions of labor in schools; the gender-biased exclusions in curriculum contents and in their very constructions as "objective" and "unitary" knowledges; and the continuing separations of public from private, the separations of teachers' voices and experiences from "official" school knowledges, forms and practices, that characterize teachers' preparation and ensuing professional development.

Further, it was apparent yet again that morning, as Donna and I filled the breakfast table with verbal and literal snapshots of our professional and personal lives, that teachers have little, if any, official space in which to gather together and to share their knowledges and practices and critiques of schooling. In our long breakfast reunion, sequestered in our restaurant booth, we were able to tell and re-tell those stories that enabled us not only to unravel the ways we have constructed and have been constructed as teachers, but also to discuss how we might work to change those constructions that have fixed or reified us in oppressive ways. Our stories thus contextualized the particular social, political, and historical conjunctions in our personal and professional lives that led to our initial acceptance and later questioning of teaching as a gendered act.

And so, by telling and re-telling these partial and on-going tales, we could sense the complexity of experience that any story necessarily reduces (Brodkey 1987; Lewis and Simon 1986). And in the tellings, we diminished the distance between the private and public poles of our experiences:

> As we study the forms of our own experiences, not only are we searching for evidence of the external forces that have diminished us; we are also recovering our own possibilities. We work to remember, imagine, and realize ways of knowing and being that can span the chasm presently separating our public and private worlds. (Grumet 1988, xv)

I think that Donna and I were recovering, in our morning conversation, our own possibilities as women and as teachers who are committed to creating just and humane educational situations for ourselves and our students. And we were trying to do so, I think, in those college courses and in our dorm study sessions and late-night talks, even though we then could not have named those attempts as such. Because we now have gender analyses with which to frame our discussions, our understandings of possibilities for ourselves as women and as teachers have enlarged with the perspectives that we have incorporated into the study of our own experiences. These perspectives constantly call attention to the ways in which curriculum and teaching are gender texts.

And so, as Donna and I talked that morning, autobiographically, we drew multiple accounts of our educational experiences, perspectives, assumptions, and situations, thus enabling ourselves to view the particularities and contingencies, the changing historical and social constructs, of our knowledges and practices. And as we incorporate those autobiographical and contextual studies into the ways in which we write and teach and research, we might also create similar conversations with our students and our colleagues in education.

For I believe that it is in conversation not only with others but also with our own histories and with the larger contexts in which those events and our relationships are located that we might begin to address the complexities of our roles as women and men who teach. As Donna and I parted, we agreed that our morning-long conversation had only touched the surface of the myriad and differing stories that we could continue to share and to examine. But in that brief morning together, we had created new knowledges about our ever-emerging possibilities. We already have a date for our next conference breakfast conversation.

Works Cited

Apple, Michael W. 1986. *Teachers and Texts: A Political Economy of Class and Gender Relations in Education.* New York: Routledge and Kegan Paul.

Berlak, Ann. 1989. Teaching for Outrage and Empathy in the Liberal Arts. *Educational Foundations*, Summer: 69–93.

———. 1991. Experiencing Teaching: Viewing and Reviewing Education 429. *Educational Foundations*, Spring: 27–46.

Britzman, Deborah P. 1991. *Practice Makes Practice: A Critical Study of Learning to Teach*. Albany: State University of New York Press.

Brodkey, Linda. 1987. Writing Critical Ethnographic Narratives. *Anthropology and Education Quarterly* 18: 67–76.

Ellsworth, Elizabeth. 1989. Why Doesn't This Feel Empowering? Working Through the Repressive Myths of Critical Pedagogy. *Harvard Educational Review* 59: 297–324.

Grumet, Madeleine R. 1988. *Bitter Milk: Women and Teaching.* Amherst: University of Massachusetts Press.

Hoffman, Nancy. 1981. *Women's "True" Profession: Voices from the History of Teaching*. New York: The Feminist Press.

Laird, Susan. 1988. Reforming "Women's True Profession": A Case for "Feminist Pedagogy" in Teacher Education? *Harvard Educational Review* 58: 449–463.

Lather, Patti. 1991. *Getting Smart: Feminist Research and Pedagogy With/In the Postmodern*. New York: Routledge.

Lewis, Magda, and Roger I. Simon. 1986. A Discourse Not Intended for Her: Learning and Teaching Within Patriarchy. *Harvard Educational Review* 56: 457–72.

Liston, Daniel and Kenneth Zeichner. 1990. Teacher Education and the Social Context of Schooling: Issues for Curriculum Development. *American Educational Research Journal* 27:4, 610–36.

Miller, Janet L. 1990. *Creating Spaces and Finding Voices: Teachers Collaborating for Empowerment*. Albany: State University of New York Press.

Miller, Jean Baker. 1986. *Toward a New Psychology of Women*, 2nd Edition. Boston: Beacon Press.

CONTINUING THE CONVERSATION: GENDER AND TEACHING

Think of the ways gender has influenced your professional work. You might start with your choice to become a teacher, and then consider your choice of the subject and grade level at which you teach. Might any of this have been different had you been of a different gender? How so?

Think about your current workplace. Who gets to decide the issues to be discussed? What issues seem never to get addressed? What issues are usually addressed by women and not by men? By men and not by women? What about the school would change if these gender-based differences were lessened?

Sketch out a plan for a piece of action research you might do, preferably with a colleague or two, that would enable you to achieve more gender balance in your professional setting. Try it out. Write it up and send it to a national or state professional journal.

Review any formal research you have done as part of your graduate studies. Are the questions addressed by that school sponsored research truly significant questions that arose from your personal knowledge of teaching and learning, or are they questions that were "manageable"? Try to remember exactly whose question you were answering. Were there any questions you wanted to study but were advised to put aside as too unwieldy or unorthodox?

When you reread the reports of your own graduate school research, do you see any of what Greenwood calls, "Voiceless Findings?" If you were to rewrite your report what would you add now in light of your readings in this book?

A Bibliography for Gender Balancing the English Curriculum

Bruce C. Appleby

The following bibliography is provided to help you choose and pursue the lines of inquiry that your thinking about gender and teaching suggest, particularly after having read or browsed through this book. Again, this bibliography does not contain all there is to read about genders issues in the teaching of English. A few years of leisure might provide you the opportunity to read all that is here, realizing that as you read you're going to be going what I like to call "spin-off bibliographies": this idea leads you to that source which takes you on to this other new source which leads into a whole new line of inquiry.

I have been working for years on this bibliography—at least since 1976. It has had a life of its own, growing and changing and gaining maturity. So many people and books and presentations and articles have had an influence on putting it together that it is impossible to give credit to any single—or multiple—source(s). As with other bibliographies I put together, I have tried to go outside the discipline of English/language arts into parallel ares that I realized could contribute.

When we were in the final throes of putting this book together, I commented to Nancy (at the same moment I accidently erased about three hours of computer time from a file whose title I misread): "It always amazes me how much there is going on outside our field even though *we* are the ones who should be most involved."

Please do attend to the articles in such journals as *Communication Education*, *Western Journal of Speech Communication*, *Language and Speech*, *Human Communication Research*, *Journal of Language and Social Psychology*, and *Language in Society*. As teachers of the language arts, we too easily forget that we are concerned with speaking and listening as much as we are with reading and writing. Although we may not teach these language arts as directly or as much as our colleagues in speech and communications, we are still constantly using these skills in the very act of teaching.

Let us never forget that "context is all" and that many of the differences between female and male patterns of using language—what Mulac calls "gender-linked language effect" (1989)—are so specific and draw on so small a sample that the conclusions must be seen as tentative. Context becomes even more important when we heed Holmes' (1984) statement that "One woman's hedge may be another man's perspicacious qualification." (169) The research on "power" and "powerless" language (such as that of William O'Barr) is just beginning to find its way into English/language arts and we need to attend to it.

Caywood and Overing's *Teaching Writing: Pedagogy, Gender, and Equity* and Flynn and Schweickart's *Gender and Reading: Essays on Readers, Texts and Contexts* are particularly helpful to English/language arts teachers. Culley and Portuge's *Gendered Subjects: The Dynamics of Feminist Education* is equally helpful in a more general way. Isaiah Smithson's excellent "Introduction: Investigating Gender, Power and Pedagogy" in the book he co-edited with Susan Gabriel, *Gender in the Classroom: Power and Pedagogy* is a particularly thoughtful analysis of the research and its shortcomings, as well as its strengths.

Finally—and again—let us know what we have missed and what you have found particularly helpful. We look for this bibliography to grow in proportion to the growth and interest in the topic of gender issues in the teaching of English. We welcome and solicit your contributions to this growth.

Abbott, ed. 1990. *Men and intimacy*. Freedom, CA: Crossing Press.

Abbott & Sapsford. 1987. *Women and social class*. New York, WY: Tavistock.

Abel, ed. 1982. *Writing and sexual difference*. Chicago: U. of Chicago P.

Abel & Abel, eds. 1983. *The signs reader: Women, gender and scholarship*. Chicago: U. of Chicago P.

Adams & Pittman. 1988. *Adolescent and young adult fathers: Problems and solutions*. Washington, D.C.: Children's Defense Fund.

Adelson. 1986. *Inventing adolescence: The political psychology of everyday schooling*. New Brunswick, NJ: Transaction Publishers.

Alishio & Schilling. 1984. Sex differences in intellectual and ego development in late adolescence. *Journal of youth and adolescence*. 13 (3), 213–24.

Alter, L. 1976. Do the NCTE Guidelines on nonsexist use of language serve a positive purpose? *English journal*. 64 (9), 10–13.

American Psychiatric Association. 1977. Guidelines for nonsexist language in APA journals. *American psychologist*. 32, 487–94.

Annas, P. 1985. Style as politics: A feminist approach to the teaching of writing. *College English*. 47 (4), 360–372.

Appleby, B. 1976. Big boys don't cry. Unpublished paper, given at NCTE Spring Conference.

———. 1981. Sexism and the English teacher: Where do we go from here? *English journal*. 70 (2), 49–50.

Aries, E. 1976. Interaction patterns and themes of male, female and mixed groups. *Small group behavior*. 7 (1), 7–18.

———. 1987. Gender and communication. In P. Shaver & C. Hendrick, eds. *Sex and gender*, 149–76. Beverly Hills: Sage.

Arnot, M., ed. 1987. *Gender and politics of schooling*. NY: Hutchinson.

Ashton-Jones, E., & D. Thomas. 1990. Composition, collaboration, and women's ways of knowing. *Journal of advanced composition*. 10, 275–92.

Ashmore, R. 1981. Sex stereotypes and implicit personality theory. In Hamilton, D., ed. *Cognitive processes in stereotyping and intergroup behavior*. Hillsdale, NJ: Lawrence Erlbaum.

Astin & Bayer. 1979. Pervasive sex differences in the academic reward system: Scholarship, marriage, and what else? In Lewis & Becker, eds. *Academic rewards in higher education*. New York, NY: Ballinger.

August. 1986–87. Real men don't: Anti-male bias in English. *University of Dayton review*: 18 (2).

Akward, M. 1988. Race, gender and the politics of reading. *Black American literature forum*. 22, 6–27.

Bailey, L. A., & L. A. Timm. 1976. More on women's and men's expletives. *Anthropological linguistics*. 18, 438–49.

Baird. 1976. Sex differences in group communication: A review of relevant research. *Quarterly journal of speech*. 62, 179–92.

Balswick. 1988. *The inexpressive male*. New York, NY: Lexington Books.

Balswick, J., & C. P. Avertt. 1977. Differences in expressiveness: Gender, interpersonal orientation, and perceived parental expressiveness as contributing factors. *Journal of marriage and the family*. 39, 121–27.

Bar-Haim, G., & J. Wilkes. 1989. A cognitive interpretation of the marginality and underrepresentation of women in science. *Journal of higher education*, 60: 371–87.

Barker. 1989. A gradual approach to feminism in the American literature classroom. *English Journal*, 78 (6): 39–44.

Baron, D. 1986. *Grammar and gender*. New Haven, CT: Yale UP.

Barthel. 1988. *Putting on Appearances: Gender and Advertising*. Philadelphia: Temple UP.

Basow. 1986. *Gender stereotypes: Traditions and alternatives*. Pacific Grove, CA: Brooks/Cole.

Bate. 1978. Nonsexist language use in transition. *Journal of communication*. 28 (1), 139–49.

Bate & Taylor. 1988. *Women Communicating: Studies of Women's Talk*. Norwood, NJ: Ablex.

Bauer. 1990. The other "F" word: The feminist in the classroom. *College English*. 52, 385–96.

Beattie. 1981. Interruption in conversational interaction, and its relation to the sex and status of interactants. *Linguistics*, 19: 15–35.

Beck, K. 1971. Sex differentiated speech codes. *International journal of women's studies*, 1: 566–72.

Becker & Greer. 1970. Participant observation and interviewing: A comparison. 133–142 in *Qualitative methodology*. Filstead, ed. NY: Rand McNally.

Belenky, M. F., B. M. Clinchy, N. R. Goldberger, & J. M. Tarule. 1986. *Women's ways of knowing: The development of self, voice, and mind*. NY: Basic Books.

Benderly. 1987. *The myth of two minds: What gender means and doesn't mean*. NY: Doubleday.

Beneke. 1982. *Men on rape*. NY: St. Martin's Press.

Bernard, *et al*. 1981. Sex-role behavior and gender in teacher-student evaluations. *Journal of educational psychology*, 73: 681–96.

Berryman & Eman, eds. 1980. *Communication, language, and sex: Proceedings of the first annual conference*. New York, NY: Newbury House.

Berryman, C. L., & J. R. Wilcox. 1980. Attitudes toward male and female speech: Experiments on the effects of sex-typed language. *Western journal of speech communication*, 444: 50–59.

Berryman-Fink, C. L., & J. R. Wilcox. 1983. A multivariate investigation of perceptual attributions concerning gender appropriateness in language. *Sex roles*, 9: 663–81.

Bertilson, Springer, & Fierke. 1982. Underrepresentation of female referents as pronouns—Examples and pictures in introductory college textbooks. *Psychological reports*, 51: 923–31.

Blaubuergs, J. 1980. An analysis of classic arguments against changing sexist language. In Kramarae, C., ed. *The voices and words of women and men*, 135–47. Oxford: Pergamon.

Bleich, D. 1986. Gender interests in reading and language. 234–66. In Flynn & Schweickart.

———. 1989. Genders of writing. *Journal of advanced composition*. 9, 10–25.

———. 1990. Sexism in academic styles of learning. *Journal of advanced composition*. 10 (2) 231–47.

Bleier, ed. 1984. *Science and gender: A critique of biology and its theories on women*. Oxford: Pergamon.

Bly, R. 1990. *Iron John: A book about men*. NY: Addison-Wesley.

Bodine, A. 1975. Androcentrism in prescriptive grammar: Singular "they," sex-indefinite "he," and "he or she." *Language in society*. 4 (2), 129–46.

Boersma et al. 1981. Sex differences in college student-teacher interactions: Fact or fantasy? *Sex roles*. 7, 775–84.

Boice & Kelly. 1987. Writing viewed by disenfranchised groups: A study of women and women's college faculty. *Written communication*. 4 (3), 299–309.

Bolker. 1979. Teaching Griselda to write. *College English*, 40 (8): 906–908.

Borisoff, D., & L. Merrill. 1985. *The power to communicate: Gender differences as barriers*. Prospect Heights, IL: Waveland Press.

Bradac, J. J., M. R. Hemphill, & C. H. Tardy. 1981. Language style on trial: Effects of "powerful" and "powerless" speech upon judgments of victims and villians. *Western journal of speech communication*, 45 (4): 327–41.

Bradac, J. J., & A. Mulac. 1984(a). Attributional consequences of powerful and powerless speech styles in a crisis-intervention context. *Journal of language and social psychology*, 3 (1): 1–19.

Bradac, J. J., & A. Mulac. 1984(b). A molecular view of powerful and powerless speech styles: Attributional consequences of specific language features and communicator intension. *Communication monographs*, 51 (4): 307–19.

Bradley, P. H. 1981. The folk-linguistics of women's speech: An empirical investigation. *Communication monographs*, 48: 73–90.

Briere & Lanktree. 1983. Sex-role related effects of sex bias in language. *Sex roles*, 9: 625–32.

Brod, ed. 1987. *The making of masculinities: The new men's studies*. Concord, MA: Allen and Unwin.

Brodsky. 1987. *Academic writing as social practice*. Philadelphia: Temple UP.

Brody. 1985. Gender difference in emotional development: A review of theories and research. *Journal of personality*, 53: 102–149.

Bronstein & Cowan, eds. 1987. *Fatherhood today*. NY: Wiley & Sons.

Brooks. 1982. Sex differences in student dominance behavior in female and male professors' classrooms. *Sex roles*. 8, 683–90.

Broverman, I., S. Vogel, D. Broverman, F. Clarkson, & P. Rosekrantz. 1972. Sex-role stereotypes: A current appraisal. *Journal of social issues*, 28: 59–78.

Brouwer, D., M. Gerritsen, D. & DeHaan. 1979. Speech differences between women and men: On the wrong track? *Language in society*. 8, 33–50.

Brown, P. & S. Levinson. 1978. Universal in language usage: Politeness phenomena. 56–289 in Goody, E. ed., *Questions and politeness: Strategies in social interaction*. Cambridge: Cambridge UP.

Brownell, W., & D. Smith. 1973. Communication patterns, sex, and length of verbalization in speech of four-year-old children. *Speech monographs*. 40, 310–16.

Brush. 1980. *Encouraging girls in mathematics: The problems and the solution*. Lanhan, MD: Abt Books.

Burtuff, D., & E. L. Epstein, eds. 1978. *Women's language and style*. Akron, OH: L & S Books.

Butler & Paisley. 1980. *Women and the mass media: Sourcebook for research and action*. New York, NY: Human Sciences Press.

Campbell & Wirtenburg. 1980. How books influence children: What the research shows. *Interracial books for children*. Bulletin 11.

Cambridge. 1987. Equal opportunity writing classrooms: Accommodating interactional differences between genders in the writing classroom. *The writing instructor*. 7 (1), 30–39.

Cameron, D. 1985. *Feminism and linguistic theory*. NY: St. Martin's Press.

Cannon, G. & S. Robertson. 1985. Sexism in present-day English: Is it diminishing? *Word*. 36, 23–35.

Capek. 1987. *A women's thesaurus: An index of language used to describe and locate information by and about women*. NY: Harper and Row.

Carlson, D. 1980. *Boys have feelings too: Growing up male for boys*. NY: Atheneum.

Carlson, M. 1989. Guidelines for a gender-balanced curriculum in English, Grades 7–12. *English journal*. 78 (6), 30–33.

Carpenter. 1981. Exercises to combat sexist reading and writing. *College English*. 43, 293–300.

Carter, M. 1991. What's wrong with using generic terms? *Illinois English Bulletin*. 78 (3), 23–30.

Carter & Spitzak, eds. 1989. *Doing research on women's communication: Perspectives on theory and method*. Norwood, NJ: Ablex.

Catano. 1990. The rhetoric of masculinity: Origins, institutions, and the myth of the selfmade man. *College English*, 52 (4): 421–36.

Cayton. 1990. What happens when things go wrong: Women and writing blocks. *Journal of advanced composition*. 10, 322–37.

Caywood, C., & G. Overing. eds. 1987. *Teaching writing: Pedagogy, gender and equity*. Albany, NY: SUNY P.

Chapman, A. 1988. *The difference it makes: A resource book on gender for educators*. Washington, DC: National Association of Independent Schools.

Cheepen. 1988. *The predictability of informal conversation*. NY: Columbia UP.

Cherry. 1987. *WomansWord: What Japanese words say about women*. New York, NY: Kodansha International.

Chesler. 1978. *About men*. San Diego. CA: Harvest/HBJ.

Children's Rights Workshop. 1976. *Sexism in children's books: Facts, figures and guidelines*. Washington, D.C.: Writers and Readers Co-op.

Chodorow, N. 1978. *The reproduction of mothering: Psychoanalysis and the sociology of gender*. Berkeley: U. of California Press.

———. 1984. Gender, personality and the sexual sociology of adult life. In Jaffar & Rothenberg (see below) 358–67.

Christian, B. 1985. *Black feminist criticism: Perspectives on black women writers*. NY: Permagon.

Clapp, O. L. Coy, N. Harty, R. Lysne, eds. 1976. *Responses to sexism*. Urbana, IL: NCTE.

Coates, J. 1988. *Women, men and language: A sociological account of sex differences in language*. NY: Longman.

Coates, J. & D. Cameron, eds. 1988. *Women in their speech communities*. NY: Longman.

Cole & Stokes. 1985. *Sex and the American teenager*. NY: Harper & Row.

Collier, M. J. 1986. Culture and gender: Effects on assertive behavior and communication competence. In M. McLaughlin, ed. *Communication Yearbook*, 9. Beverly Hills: Sage.

Cooper, M. 1989. Women's way of writing. In M. Cooper & M. Holzmaan, eds. *Writing as social action*, 141–56. Portsmouth, NH: Boynton/Cook.

Cooper, P. 1989. Children's literature: The extent of sexism. In Lont & Friedley, eds. (see below) 233–249.

Cornillon, S., ed. 1972. *Images of women in fiction: Feminist perspectives*. Bowling Green, OH: Bowling Green UP.

Cowell, P. 1987. Valuing language: Feminist pedagogy in the writing classroom. In Caywood & Overing (see above) 147–49.

Crosby, F., & L. Nyquist. 1977. The female register: An empirical study of Lakoff's hypotheses. *Language in society*, 6 (3), 313–22.

Culley, ed. 1985. *A day at a time: The diary literature of American women from 1764 to the present*. New York, NY: Feminist Press at CUNY.

Culley & Portuges, eds. 1985. *Gendered subjects: The dynamics of feminist teaching*. London: Routledge and Kegan Paul.

Cummins, J. 1986. Empowering minority students: A framework for intervention. *Harvard educational review*. 56, 18–36.

Daly. 1989. Laughing *with*, or laughing *at* the young-adult romance. *English journal*, 78 (6), 50–60.

Daly, M. 1978. *Gynecology: The metaethics of radical feminism*. Boston: Beacon.

D'Angelo, D. 1989. Developmental tasks in literature for adolescents: Has the adolescent female protagonist changed? *Child study journal*, 19 (3), 219–37.

David & Brannon, eds. 1981. *The 49% majority: Readings on the male sex role*, 2/e. Reading, MA: Addison-Wesley.

Davies & Harre. 1990. Positioning: Conversation and the production of selves. *Journal for the theory of social behaviour*, 20 (1), 43–63.

Davis, A. 1983. *Women, race and class*. NY: Vintage Books.

Davis, B. 1989. Feminizing the English curriculum: An international perspective. *English journal*. 78 (7), 45–49.

Deaux, K., & B. Major. 1990. A social-psychological model of gender. In Rhode, D., ed. (see below) 89–99.

Dehler, K. 1989. Diaries: Where women reveal themselves. *English journal.* 78 (7), 53–54.

deKlerk, V. 1990. Slang: A Male Domain? *Sex roles.* 22 (9–10), 589–606.

Delpit, L. 1988. The silenced dialogue: Power and pedagogy in educating other people's children. *Harvard educational review.* 58, 280–98.

DeShazer, M. 1981. Sexist language in composition textbooks: Still a major issue? *College composition and communication.* 32, 57–64.

DeSole & Hoffmann, eds. 1981. *Rocking the boat: Academic women and academic processes.* MLA.

Diamond, I. & L. Quinby. 1988. American Feminism and the Language of Control. In *Feminism & Foucault: reflections on resistance.* 193–206. Diamond & Quinby Boston: Northeastern UP.

Dinnerstein, D. 1976. *The mermaid and the minotaur: Sexual arrangements and human malaise.* NY: Harper Colophon.

Dixon. 1977. *Catching them young: Sex, race and class in children's books.* Pluto Press.

Donelson & Nilsen. 1989. *Literature for today's young adults*, 3/e. Glenview, IL: Scott, Foresman.

Douvan, E. 1969. Sex differences in adolescent character processes. In Rogers, ed., 437–45. *Issues in adolescent psychology.* NY: Appleton.

Doyle. 1983. *The male experience.* Dubuque, IA: Wm. C. Brown.

Dubois, B. L., & I. Crouch. 1975. The question of tag questions in women's speech: They don't really use more of them, do they? *Language in society* 4, 289–94.

Dubois, B. & I. Crouch. eds. 1976. *The sociology of the languages of American women.* Trinity UP.

Dudovitz, ed. 1984. *Women in academe.* NY: Pergamon.

Duley & Edwards, eds. 1986. *The cross-cultural study of women: A comprehensive guide.* The Feminist Press.

Dworkin, A. 1974. *Woman-hating.* Dutton.

Dworkin & MacKinnon. 1988. *Pornography and civil rights: A new day for women's equality.* Organizing Against Pornography.

Eakins, B. & Eakins, G. 1978. *Sex differences in human communication.* Boston: Houghton-Mifflin.

Eckert. 1990. Cooperative competition in adolescent "girl talk." *Discourse processes.* 13, 91–122.

Edelsky, C. 1981. Who's got the floor? *Language in society.* 10, 383–421.

Edwards & Spence. 1987. Gender-related traits, stereotypes and schemata. *Journal of personality and social psychology.* 54, 146–54.

Elgin. 1984. *Native tongue.* New York, NY: DAW.

Ellsworth, E. 1989. Why doesn't this feel empowering? Working through the repressive myths of critical pedagogy. *Harvard educational review*, 59, 335–56.

Emerson. 1985. *Some American men*. NY: Simon and Schuster.

Enos, T. 1990. Gender and journals, conservers or innovators. *PRE/TEXT* 9, 209–214.

Eschholz, P., A. Rosa & V. Clark, eds. 1990. *Language awareness*. NY: St. Martin's Press.

Eubanks, S. 1975. Sex-based language differences: A cultural reflection. In Ordoubadian, R. & von Raffler Engel, W., eds., 109–120. *Views on language*. Murfreesboro, TN: Inter-University Publishers.

Fairclough, N. 1989. *Language and power*. London: Longman.

Farrell, T. 1979. The female and male modes of rhetoric. *College English*, 40 (8), 909–921.

Farrell, W. 1975. *The liberated man*. NY: Random House.

———. 1986. *Why men are the way they are*. NY: McGraw-Hill.

Fasteau, M. 1974. The Male Machine. NY: McGraw-Hill.

Fausto-Sterling. 1986. *Myths of gender: Biological theories about women and men*. New York, NY: Basic Books.

Fetterley, J. 1978. *The resisting reader: A feminist approach to American fiction*. Bloomington: Indiana UP, 1978.

Filene. 1986. *Him/her/self: Sex roles in modern America*, 2/e. Johns Hopkins UP.

Fillmer, H. T. & Haswell. 1977. Sex-role sterotyping in English usage. *Sex roles*, 3 (3), 257–63.

Fine, M. 1987. Silencing in public schools. *Language arts*, 64, 157–74.

———. 1988. Sexuality, schooling, and adolescent females: The missing discourse of desire. *Harvard educational review*, 58, 29–53.

Fishman, P. 1978. Interaction: the work women do. *Social problems*, 25, 397–406.

———. What do couples talk about when they're alone? 11–22 in Burtuff & Epstein, eds. (See above.)

Fisher, S., & A. Dundas. 1988. *Gender and discourse: The power of talk*. Norwood, NJ: Ablex.

Fisk. 1985. Responses to "neutral" pronoun presentations and the development of sex-biased responding. *Developmental psychology*, 21 (3), 481–85.

Fitzpatrick. 1983. Effective interpersonal communication for women of the corporation: Think like a man, talk like a woman. In *Women in Organizations: Barriers and Breakthroughs*. Prospect Heights, IL: Waveland Press.

Flemming, L. 1988. New visions new methods: The mainstreaming experience in retrospect. In Aiken *et al.*, eds., *Changing our minds: Feminist transformations of knowledge*. Cambridge: Harvard UP.

Flore & Elsasser. 1982. "Strangers No More": A liberatory literacy curriculum. *College English*. 44, 115–28.

Flynn, E. 1988. Composing as a woman. *College composition and communication*. 39 (4), 423–35.

———. 1990. Composing "Composing as a woman": A perspective on research. *College composition and communication*, 41 (2), 83–89.

Flynn, E. & E. Schweickart, eds. 1986. *Gender and reading: Essays on readers texts, and contexts*. Baltimore, MD: John Hopkins UP.

Fontaine, S., J. Peavoy, & S. Hunter. 1990. Unprivileged voices in the academy of the privileged. *Freshman English news*. 19, 2–9.

Foster, J. 1985. *Sex variant women in literature*. Tallahassee, FL: Nalad Press.

Frances, S. J. 1979. Sex differences in nonverbal behavior. *Sex roles*, 5, 519–35.

Frank, F. & A. Ashen. 1984. *Language and the sexes*. Albany, NY: SUNY Press.

Frank, F. & P. Treichler. 1989. *Language, gender, and professional writing: Theoretical approaches and guidelines for nonsexist usage*. NY: MLA.

Franklin. 1984. *The changing definition of masculinity*. New York, NY: Plenum.

Freed, A. 1987. Hearing is believing: The effect of sexist language on language skills. In Caywood & Overing (see above) 65–79.

Frey, O. 1990. Beyond literary Darwinism: Women's voices and critical discourse. *College English*. 52 (5), 507–526.

Friedan, B. 1971. *The feminine mystique*. NY: Dell.

Gabriel, S. & I. Smithson, eds. 1989. *Gender in the classroom: Power and Pedagogy*. Urbana, IL.: U of Illinois P.

Gannett, C. 1991. Genders and the journal. Albany, NY: SUNY Press.

Gappa & Pearce, eds. 1982. *Sex and gender in the social sciences: Reassessing the introductory course*. Washington DC: Women's Educational Equity Act Program.

Gardner, H. 1983. *Frames of mind: The theory of multiple intelligences*. NY: Basic Books.

Garfinkel. 1985. *In a man's world: Father, son, brother, friend and other roles men play*. New York, NY: New American Library.

Gearhart. 1979. The womanization of rhetoric. *Women's studies International Quarterly* 2 (2), 195–201.

Gere, A. 1987. *Writing groups: History, theory and implications*. Carbondale, IL: Southern Illinois UP.

Gerlach, J., & V. Monseau, eds. 1991. *Missing chapters*. Urbana, IL: NCTE.

Gershuny, A. 1974. Sexist semantics in the dictionary. *A review of general semantics*, 31 (2), 159–69.

Gerzon. 1982. *A choice of heroes: The changing faces of American manhood*. Boston: Houghton Mifflin.

Giddings, P. 1984. *When and where I enter: The impact of black women on race and sex in America*. NY: William Morrow.

Gilbert, S. & S. Gubar. 1985. Sexual linguistics: Gender, language, sexuality. *New literary history*. 16 (3), 515–43.

———. 1987. *The war of the words*. V. 1 of *No man's land: The place of the woman writer in the twentieth century*. New Haven, CT: Yale UP.

———. 1989. *Sexchanges*. V. 2 of *No Man's Land: The Place of the woman writer in the twentieth century*. New Haven, CT: Yale UP.

Gillette, D., & R. Moore. 1990. *King, warrior, magician, lover: Rediscovering the archetypes of the mature masculine*. San Francisco: Harper.

Gilley, H., & C. Summers. 1970. Sex differences in the use of hostile verbs. *Journal of psychology*. 76, 33–37.

Gilligan, C. 1982. *In a different voice: Psychological theory and women's development*. Cambridge, MA. Harvard UP.

Gilligan, C., N. Lyons, & T. Hanmer, eds. 1989. *Making connections: The relational world of adolescent girls at Emma Willard School*. Troy, NY: Emma Willard School.

Gilligan, C., J. Ward, J. Taylor, & B. Bardige. 1988. *Mapping the moral domain: The contributions of women's thinking to psychological theory and education*. Cambridge: Harvard UP.

Gilmore. 1990. *Manhood in the making: Cultural concepts of masculinity*. New Haven, CT: Yale UP.

Gleser, G. C., L. A. Gottschalk, & W. John. 1959. The relationship of sex and intelligence to choice of words: A normative study of verbal behavior. *Journal of clinical psychology*. 15, 182–91.

Goldberg, P. 1968. Are women prejudiced against women? *Transaction*, 5, 28–30.

Goodwin, M. (in press) *He-said-she-said: Talk as social organization among black children*. Bloomington: Indiana UP.

Goodwin. 1990. Tactical uses of stories: Participation framework within girls' and boys' disputes. *Discourses processes*. 13, 33–71.

Gornick. 1983. *Women and science: Portraits from a world of transition*. NY: Simon & Schuster.

Graddol & Swann. 1989. *Gender voices*. London: Basil Blackwell.

Greif, E. 1980. Sex differences in parent-child conversations. *Women's studies international quarterly*, 3 (2 & 3), 253–58.

Grumet, M. 1981. Pedagogy for patriarchy: The feminization of teaching. *Interchange*, 12, 165–84.

Guidelines for nonsexist use of language in NCTE publications. 1990. Urbana, IL: NCTE.

Guttentag & Bray. 1976. *Undoing sex stereotypes: Research and resources for educators*. NY: McGraw-Hill.

Haas. 1979. Male and female spoken language differences: Stereotypes and evidence. *Psychological bulletin*, 86 (3), 616–26.

Hall & Dawson. 1989. *Broodmales*. Dallas, TX: Spring Press.

Hall & Halbertstadt. 1981. Sex roles and non-verbal communication skills. *Sex roles*. 7 (3), 273–87.

Harding. 1986. *The science question in feminism*. Ithaca, NY: Cornell UP.

Harding & O'Barr, eds. 1987. *Sex and scientific inquiry*. U of Chicago P.

Harrigan, J., & K. Lucic. 1988. Attitudes about gender bias in language: A reevaluation. *Sex roles*, 19, 129–40.

Harrison & Passero. 1975. Sexism in the language of elementary school textbooks. *Science and children*, 12 (4), 22–25.

Hartman, M. 1976. A descriptive study of the language of men and women born in Maine around 1900 as it reflects the Lakoff hypotheses in *Language and women's place*. In Dubois, B., and I. Crouch, eds. (see above) 81–90.

Harvey, G. 1986. Finding reality among the myths: Why what you thought about sex equity in education isn't so. *Phi delta kappan*. 67 (7), 509–512.

Haslett, B. 1983. Children's strategies for maintaining cohesion in their written and oral stories. *Communication education*. 32, 91–105.

Heilbrun, C. 1974. *Toward a recognition of androgyny*. Harper & Row.

———. 1988. *Writing a woman's life*. Norton.

Helgeson. 1976. The prisoners of texts: Male chauvinism in college handbooks and rhetorics. *College English*, 38, 296–406.

Henley, N. 1973. Power, sex and noverbal communication. *Berkeley journal of sociology*, 18, 1–26.

Henley. 1985. Psychology and gender. *Signs: Journal of women in culture and society*, 11 (1), 101–119.

Henley & Freeman. 1989. The sexual politics of interpersonal behavior. In *Women: A feminist perspective*, Freeman and Henley, eds. Mountain View, CA: Mayfield Pub.

Hernton, C. 1987. *The sexual mountain and black women writers: Adventures in sex, literature, and real life*. NY: Anchor Press.

Hewlett, S. 1986. *A lesser life: The myth of women's liberation in America*. NY: Morrow.

Hiatt, M. 1977. *The way women write*. NY: Teachers College Press.

———. 1978. The feminine style: Theory and fact. *College Composition and communication*, 29, 222–26.

Hill. 1986. *Mother tongue, father time: A decade of linguistic revolt*. Bloomington: Indiana UP.

Hinds. 1980. Japanese expository prose. *Papers in linguistics: International journal of human communication*, 13, 117–58.

Hirschman, L. 1973. Female-male difference in conversational interaction. Paper given at Linguistic Society of America, San Diego, CA.

Holbrook, S. 1991. Women's work: The feminizing of composition. *Rhetoric review*, 9 (2), 201–29.

Holland. 1987. A radical approach to educating young black males. *Education week*, 6 (26).

———. 1989. Fighting the epidemic of failures: A radical strategy for educating inner-city boys. *Teacher magazine*, Sep./Oct.

Holmes, J. 1984. Women's language. A functional approach. *General linguistics*. 24, 149–78.

———. 1986. Functions of "you know" in women's and men's speech. *Language in society*, 15, 1–22.

Howe, F. 1971. Identity and expression: A writing course for women. *College English*, 32, 863–71.

———. 1984. *Myths of coeducation: Selected essays, 1964–1983*. Bloomington, IN: Indiana UP.

Hubbard. 1988. Science, facts and feminism. *Hypatia*, 3, 5–17.

———. 1990. *The politics of women's biology*. East Rutherford, NJ: Rutgers UP.

Hughes. 1988. But that's not what I *really* mean: Competing in a cooperative mode. *Sex roles*, 19 (11–12), 669–87.

Hull, et al., eds. 1982. *All the women are white, all the blacks are men, but some of us are brave: Black women's studies*. NY: Feminist Press.

Hunt, K. W. 1960. *Grammatical structures written at three grade levels*. Champaign, IL: NCTE.

Hunter, et al. 1988. Competing epistemologies and female basic writers. *Journal of basic writing*, 7 (1), 73–81.

Hunter, S. 1991. A woman's place *is* in the composition classroom: Pedagogy, gender, and difference. *Rhetoric review*, 9 (2), 230–45.

Hyde. 1984. Children's understanding of sexist language. *Developmental psychology*. 21 (3), 697–706.

———. 1984. How large are gender differences in aggression? *Developmental psychology*. 20 (4), 722–736.

Hyde & Lynn. 1988. Gender differences in verbal ability: A meta-analysis. *Psychological bulletin*, 104, 53–69.

Ickes. 1988. Narrative social cognition: Intersubjectivity in same-sex dyads. *Journal of non-verbal behavior*, 12 (Spring) 58–83.

Iglitzin. 1973. *A child's eye view of sex roles and sex role stereotyping in the schools*. Washington, DC: National Education Association.

Jacobus, ed. 1979. *Women writing and writing about women*. NY: Harper & Row.

Jacobus, Keller, & Shuttleworth, eds. 1989. *Body/Politics: Women and the discourse of science*. New York, NY: Routledge.

Jaggar & Bordo, eds. 1989. *Gender/body/knowledge: Feminist reconstructions of being and knowing*. East Rutherford, NJ: Rutgers UP.

Jaggar & Rothenberg, eds. 1984. *Feminist frameworks*. McGraw-Hill.

Jaraid & Randall. 1982. *Women speaking: An annotated bibliography of verbal and non-verbal communication*, 1970–1980. New York, NY: Garland.

Jardine & Smith, eds. 1987. *Men in feminism*. New York, NY: Methuen.

Jenkins & Kramer. 1978. Small groups processes: Learning from women. *Women's studies international quarterly*. 5, 767–72.

Jeske, J. & K. Overman. 1984. Gender and the official language. *International journal of women's studies*. 7, 322–35.

Johnson, C. 1987. An introduction to powerful and powerless talk in the classroom. *Communication education*. 36 (2), 167–72.

Johnson & Fine. 1985. Sex differences in uses and perceptions of obscenity. *Women's studies in communications*. 8, 12–23.

Jordanova. 1989. *Sexual visions: Images of gender in science and medicine between the eighteenth and twentieth centuries*. U of Wisconsin P.

Josselson. 1987. *Finding herself: Pathways to identity development in women*. San Francisco, CA: Jossey-Bass.

Juncker, C. 1988. Writing (with) Cixous. *College English*. 50, 424–36.

Kagan & Lamb, eds. 1987. *The emergence of morality in young children*. Chicago: U of Chicago P.

Kaschak. 1981. Another look at sex bias in students' evaluations of professors: Do winners get the recognition that they have been given? *Psychology of women quarterly*, 5, 767–72.

Kass-Simon & Farnes, eds. 1989. New York, NY: *Women in science*.

Kavanaugh. 1970. *There are men too gentle to live among wolves*. San Francisco, CA: Sunrise.

Keen, S. 1991 *Fire in the belly: On being a man*. NY: Bantam.

Kehr. 1986. Gender research and education. *American psychologist*. 41 (10), 1161–168.

Keller. 1985. *Reflections on gender and science*. New Haven, CT: Yale UP.

———. 1987. Feminism and science. In Harding and O'Barr (see above), 233–46.

Keller & Moglen. 1987. Competition and feminism: Conflicts for academic women. *Signs: Journal of women in culture and society*, 12 (3), 493–11.

Kelly. 1988. Gender differences in teacher-pupil interactions: A meta-analytic review. *Research in education*, 39, 1–23.

Keroes. 1986. But what do they say? Gender and the content of student writing. ED 269 802.

Key. 1975. *Male/female language*. Metuchen, NJ: Scarecrow Press.

Kimmel, ed. 1987. *Changing men: New directions in research on men and masculinity*. Newbury Park, CA: Sage.

Kissel. 1988. But when at last she really came, I shot her: *Peter Pan* and the drama of gender. *Children's literature in education*, 19, (1), 32–41.

Klee. 1987. Different language usage patterns by males and females in a rural community in the Rio Grande Valley. In *Language and language use: Studies in Spanish*. Morgan, ed. Lanham, MD: U. Press of America.

Klein, S., ed. 1985. *Handbook for achieving sex equity through education*. Baltimore: John Hopkins UP.

Koblinsky, Cruse, & Sugawara. 1978. Sex role stereotypes and children's memory for story content. *Child development*, 49, 452–58.

Koenigsknecht, R., & P. Friedman. 1976. Syntax development in boys and girls. *Child development*. 47, 1109–115.

Kolba & Widmayer. 1989. Running the minefield of gender-fair language. *NWSA journal*. 1 (4), 689–96.

Kolodny, A. 1975. *The lay of the land*. Chapel Hill: U of NC P.

Komarovsky, M. 1976. *Dilemmas of masculinity*. Norton.

Kramarae, C., ed. 1980. *The voices and words of women and men*. Pergamon Press.

———. 1981. *Women and men speaking* Rowley MA: Newbury House.

———. ed. 1988. *Technology and women's voices*. London: Routledge and Kegan Paul, Ltd.

Kramarae, C., Schulz, & O'Barr, eds. 1984. *Language and power*. Newbury Park, CA: Sage.

Kramarae, C., & P. A. Treichler. (with assistance of Ann Russo). 1985. *A feminist dictionary*. Concord, MA: Allen and Unwin.

———. 1990. Power relationships in the classroom. In Gabriel & Smithson (see above) 41–59.

Kramer, C. 1975. Women's speech: Separate but unequal. In Thorne & Henley (see below).

———. 1977. Perceptions of female and male speech. *Language and speech*, 20, 151–61.

———. 1978. Women's and men's ratings of their own and ideal speech. *Communication quarterly*, 26 (2), 2–11.

Kramer, C., B. Thorne, & N. Henley. 1978. Perspectives on language and communication. *Signs: Journal of women in culture and society*, 3 (3), 638–51.

Kramer. 1990. No exit: A play of literacy and gender. *Journal of advanced composition*, 10, 305–19.

Lake, P. 1988. Sexual stereotyping and the English curriculum. *English journal*, 77 (6), 30–34.

Lakoff, G. 1987. *Women, fire, and dangerous things: What categories reveal about the mind*. Chicago: U of Chicago P.

Lakoff, G., & M. Johnson. 1980. *Metaphors we live by*. Chicago: U of Chicago P.

Lakoff, R. 1975. *Language and woman's place*. NY: Harper and Row.

———. 1989. Talking like a lady. In S. Miller, ed. *The written world: Reading and writing in social contexts* 533–42. NY: Harper & Row.

Lamb, C. 1989. Less distance, more space: A feminist theory of power and writer/audience relationships. In C. Kneuper, ed. *Rhetoric and ideology: Compositions and criticisms of power* 99–104. Arlington, VA: Rhetoric Society of America.

———. 1991. Beyond argument in feminist composition. *College composition and communication*, 42 (1), 11–24.

Lamb, ed. 1981. *The role of the father in child development*. New York, NY: John Wiley.

Language and Gender Working Party. 1985. *Alice in genderland*. London: NATE.

Lapadat, J., & M. Seesahai. 1978. Male vs. females codes in informal contexts. *Sociolinguistic newsletter*, 8, 7–8.

Lassner, P. 1990. Feminist response to Rogerian argument. *Rhetoric review*, 8, 220–32.

Lauter, P., ed. 1983. *Reconstructing American literature: Course, syllabi issues*. NY: The Feminist Press.

Lawlor. 1989. *Earth honoring: The new male sexuality*. Rochester, VT: Inner Traditions/Park St. Press.

Lay. 1989. Gender's effect on collaborative writing. Unpublished paper given at CCCC, March.

Lengermann & Wallace. 1985. *Gender in America: Social control and social change*. NY: Prentice-Hall.

Lenz, E., & B. Myerhoff. 1985. *The feminization of America*. Los Angeles: Jeremy P. Tarcher, Inc.

Levinson. 1978. *The seasons of a man's life*. NY: Knopf.

Lewis & Sussman, eds, 1986. *Men's changing roles in the family*. Binghamton. WY: Haworth.

Lewis, M., & R. Simon. 1986. A discourse not intended for her: Learning and teaching within patriarchy. *Harvard educational review*. 56, 457–72.

Lockheed. 1985. Women, girls and computers: A first look at the evidence. *Sex roles*. 13 (3, 4), 115–22.

Lont, C., & S. Friedley, S., eds. 1989. *Beyond boundaries: Sex and gender diversity in communication*. Fairfax, VA: George Mason UP.

Lowe & Hubbard. 1983. *Women's nature: Rationalizations of inequality*. Elmsford, NY: Pergamon.

Lu. 1987. From silence to words: Writing as struggle. *College English*, 49, 437–48.

Lundsford, A., & L. Ede. 1990. Rhetoric in a new key: Women and collaboration. *Rhetoric review*, 8 (2), 234–41.

Lynch. 1987. Mauve washers: Sex differences in freshmen writing. *English journal*, 76 (1), 90–94.

Maccoby & Jacklin. 1974. *The psychology of sex differences*. Standford UP.

Mackay. 1980. Psychology, prescriptive grammar, and the pronoun problem. *American psychologist*, 35, 444–49.

———. 1983. Prescriptive grammar and the pronoun problem. In Thorne, Kramarae & Henley, eds., *Language, gender and society*. Newbury House.

Maher, F. 1985. Pedagogies for the gender-balanced classroom. *Journal of thought*, 20 (3), 48–64.

Maggio, R. 1987. *The nonsexist word finder: A dictionary of gender-free usage*, Boston, MA: Beacon Press.

Makino. 1979. Sexual differences in written discourses. *Papers in Japanese linguistics*, 6, 195–217.

Malamuth & Donnerstein, eds. 1984. *Pornography and sexual aggression*. San Diego, CA: Academic Press.

Maltz & Borker. 1982. A cultural approach to male-female miscommunication. In Gumperz, ed., *Language and social identity*. 195–216. New York, NY: Cambridge U. Press.

Martin, J. 1982. Excluding women from the educational realm. *Harvard educational review*, 52, 133–48.

———. 1985. *Reclaiming a conversation: The ideal of an educated woman*. New Haven, CT: Yale UP.

Martin, W. 1972. The sex factor in grading composition. *Research in the teaching of English*, 6, 36–47.

Martyna. 1978. What does "he" mean?: Use of the generic masculine. *Journal of communication*. 28 (1), 131–38.

———. 1983. Beyond the "he/man" approach: The case for nonsexist language. In Thorne, Kramarae & Henley, eds. (see below).

May. 1980. *Sex and fantasy: Patterns of male and female development*. New York, NY: Norton.

McClelland, K. 1991. Clearinghouse on Gender and Education: Center for the Study of Gender and Education. Kent, OH: Kent State U.

McCracken, N. 1990–91. Penelope talks back to her anthology. *Ohio Journal of English language arts*, 31 (2), 14–17.

McCracken, N., L. Green, & C. Greenwood. (in press). Resisting gender in composition research: A strange silence. In Hunter & Fontayne, *Unheard voices: Writing ourselves into the story*. Carbondale, IL: Southern Illinois UP.

McConnell-Ginet, S. 1978. Intonation in a man's world. *Signs: Journal of women in cultures and society*. 3 (3), 541–54.

McConnell-Ginet, S., R. Borker, & N. Furman, eds. 1980. *Women and language in literature and society*. New York: Praeger.

McMillan, J., A. Clifton, D. McGrath, & W. Gale. 1977. Women's language: Uncertainty or interpersonal sensitivity. *Sex roles*, 3, 545–59.

Meditch. 1975. The development of sex-specific patterns in young children. *Anthropological linguistics*, 18 (9), 421–433.

Meese. 1990. Women and writing: A re/turn. *College English*. 52, 376–76.

Meisenhelder. 1985. Redefining "powerful" writing: Toward a feminist theory of composition. *Journal of thought*, 29 (3), 184–95.

Miller. 1983. *Men and friendship*. Boston: Houghton Mifflin.

Miller. 1986. *The poetics of gender*. NY: Columbia UP.

Miller, C., & K. Swift. 1976. *Words and women: New language in new times*. New York, NY: Anchor/Doubleday.

———. 1980. *The handbook of nonsexist writing: For writers, editors and speakers*. NY: Harper and Row.

Miller, G., & M. McReynolds. 1973. Male chauvinism and source competence: A research note. *Speech monographs*, 40, 154–55.

Millman & Burchell, eds. 1989. *Gender issues in secondary education: Agenda for change*. Taylor & Francis.

Mills. 1987. The male sentence. *Language and communication*, 12, 189–98.

Mines, J. 1989. Young adult literature female heroes do exist. *ALAN review*, 17 (1), 12–24.

Mischel, H. N. 1974. Sex bias in the evaluation of profession achievements. *Journal of educational psychology*, 66, 157–66.

Moi, T. 1985. *Sexual/textual politics: Feminist literary theory*. Methuen.

Moore, L. 1989. One on one: Pairing male and female writers. *English journal*, 74 (3), 54–59.

Moore & Gillette. 1990. *King, warrior, magician, lover: Rediscovering the mature masculine*. NY: Harper/Collins.

Moraga, C. & G. Anzaldua, eds. 1983. *This bridge called my back*. NY: Kitchen Table: Women of Color P.

Morahan. 1981. *A woman's place: Rhetoric and readings for composing yourself and your prose*. Syracuse: SUNY Press.

Morgan, R. 1988. *The demon lover: On the sexuality of terrorism*. Norton.

Morgan, R., ed. 1984. *Sisterhood is global*. NY: Anchor Books.

Moulton, J. 1981. The myth of the neutral man. In Vetterling-Braggin, ed., *Sexist language: A modern philosophical analysis*. 100–115. Totowa, NJ: Rowman & Littlefield.

Moulton, *et al*. 1978. Sex bias in language use: Neutral pronouns that aren't. *American psychologist*, 33, 1032–1036.

Mulac, A. 1989. The gender-linked language effect. Paper given at Speech Communication Association, San Francisco, CA.

Mulac, A., S. Blau, & L. Bauquier. 1983. Gender-linked language differences and their effects in male and female students' impromptu essays. Paper given at Speech Communication Association, Washington, D.C.

Mulac, A., J. J. Bradac, & S. K. Mann. 1985. Male-female language differences and attributional consequences in children's television. *Human communication research*, 11, 481–506.

Mulac, A., C. Incontro, & M. James. 1985. Comparison of the gender-linked language effect and sex-role stereotypes. *Journal of personality and social psychology*, 49, 1098–1109.

Mulac, A. & T. L. Lundell. 1980. Differences in perceptions created by syntactic-semantic productions of male and female speakers. *Communication monographs*, 47, 111–118.

Mulac, A., & T. L. Lundell. 1982. An empirical test of the gender-linked effect in a public speaking setting. *Language and speech*, 25, 243–56.

Mulac, A., & T. L. Lundell. 1986. Linguistic contributors to the gender-linked language effect. *Journal of language and social psychology*, 5, 81–102.

Mulac, A., T. L. Lundell, & J. J. Bradac. 1986. Male/female language differences and attributional consequences in a public speaking situation: Toward an explanation of the gender-linked language effect. *Communication monographs*. 53, 115–29.

Mulac, A., J. M. Wiemann, S. J. Widenmann, & T. W. Gibson. 1983. Male/female differences and their effects in like-sex and mixed-sex dyads: A test of interpersonal accommodation and the gender-linked language effect. Paper given at Second International Conference, Social Psychology and Language, Bristol, England.

Murray, S. 1985. Towards a model of members' methods for recognizing interruptions. *Language in society*, 14, 31–40.

Nelson. 1990. Gender communication through small groups. *English Journal*, 79 (2), 58–61.

Newcombe, N., & D. Arnkoff. 1979. Effects of speech style and sex of speaker on person perception. *Journal of personality and social psychology*, 37, 1293–1303.

Nicholson. 1984. *Men and women: How different are they?*. Oxford: Oxford UP.

Nadler, Nadler, & Todd-Mancillas, eds. 1987. *Advances in gender and communication research*. Lanham, MD: University Press of America.

Nilsen, A. P. 1979. *Changing words in a changing world*. Tempe, AZ: Arizona State U.

———. 1984. Winning the great he/she battle. *College English*, 46, 151–57.

———. 1987. Guidelines against sexist language: A case history. In *Women and language in transition* 37–64. Albany: SUNY.

———. 1990. Sexism in English: A 1990's update. In Eschholz, Rosa, & Clark (see above), 277–87.

Nilsen, A. P., H. Bosmajian, L. Gershuny, and J. P. Stanley, eds. 1977. *Sexism and language*. Urbana, IL.: NCTE.

Nye. 1991. Computers and gender: Noticing what perpetuates inequality. *English Journal*, 80 (3), 94–95.

O'Barr, W. M. 1983. *Linguistic evidence: Language, power and strategy in the courtroom*. NY: Academic Press.

O'Barr, W. M., & B. K. Atkins. 1980. "Women's language" or "powerless language." In McConnel-Ginet, Borker & Furman, eds. (see above).

Olgivie. 1986. *Women in science*. Boston: M.I.T. Press.

Olsen, T. 1965. *Silences*. NY: Delta/Seymour Lawrence.

Osborn, S. 1987. Revisioning the argument: An exploratory study of some rhetorical strategies of women student writers. *Praxis*. 1, 113–33.

———. 1991. Revision/re-vision: A feminist writing course. *Rhetoric review*, 9 (2), 258–73.

Osherson. 1986. *Finding our fathers: The unfinished business of manhood*. New York, NY.: Free Press/MacMillan.

Ostriker, A. 1986. *Stealing the language: The emergence of women's poetry in America*. Boston: Beacon Press.

Page, C. 1989. Bad-news barometer for black men. *Chicago Tribune*, 26 Feb.

Paglia, C. 1990. *Sexual personae: Art and decadence from Nefertiti to Emily Dickinson*. New Haven, CT: Yale UP.

Parham & McDavis. 1987. Black men, an endangered species: Who's really pulling the trigger? *Journal of counseling and development*. 66, 24–27.

Parke. 1981. *Fathering*. London: Fontana Open Books.

Pearson. 1985. *Gender and communication*. Dubuque, IA: Brown Publishing.

Pearson, C., & K. Pope. 1981. *The female hero in American and British literature*. NY: Bowker.

Penelope, J. 1990. *Speaking freely: Unlearning the lies of the father's tongues*. Elmsford, NY: Pergamon.

Persing. 1983. *The nonsexist communicator: Solving the problems of gender and awkwardness in modern English*. NY: Prentice-Hall.

Pfeiffer. 1985. Girl talk-boy talk. *Science, '85*. Washington, DC: American Assn. for the Advancement of Science.

Phillips, S., S. Steele, & C. Tanz, eds. 1987. *Language, gender and sex in comparative perspective*. Cambridge: Cambridge UP.

Pigott. 1979. Sexist roadblocks in inventing, focusing, and writing. *College English*. 40 (8), 922–27.

Pittman & Adams. 1988. *What about the boys: Teenage pregnancy prevention strategies*. Children's Defense Fund.

Pleck. 1981. *The myth of masculinity*. Boston: MIT Press.

Pleck & Pleck, eds. 1980. *The American man*. NY: Prentice-Hall.

Pleck & Sawyer, eds. 1974. *Men and masculinity*. NY: Prentice-Hall.

Plamin. 1989. Environment and genes. *American psychologist*, 44 (2), 105–119.

Poole, M. 1979. Social class, sex, and linguistic coding. *Language and speech*, 22, 49–67.

Pottker & Fisher, eds. 1977. *Sex bias in the schools: The research evidence.* Associated University Presses.

Preisler. 1986. *Linguistic sex roles in conversation: Social variation in the expression of tentativeness in English.* Berlin: Mouton de Gruyter.

Price, G. B. & R. L. Graves. 1980. Sexs differences in syntax and usage in oral and written language. *Research in the teaching of English*, 14 (2), 147–53.

Purcell, P. & L. Stewart, L. 1989. Dick and Jane in 1989. *Sex roles*, 22 (3–4), 177–84.

Purves, ed. 1988. *Writing across languages and cultures: Issues in contrastive rhetoric.* Newbury Park, CA: Sage.

Quina, K., J. A. Wingard, & H. G. Bates. 1987. Attitudes toward a hypothetical male or female presidential candidate—A research note. *Political psychology*, 9 (4), 591–98.

Raphael. 1988. *The men from the boys: Rites of passage in male America.* U. of Nebraska Press.

Ray, K. 1985. The ethics of feminism in the literature classroom: A delicate balance. *English journal*, 74 (3), 54–59.

Rich, A. 1979. *On lies, secrets, and silence: Selected prose: 1966–1978.* New York, NY: Norton.

Richardson & Damron. 1981. Gender, descriptive language and scientific reporting. *Perceptual and motor skills*, 53, 483–89.

Risch. 1987. Women's derogatory terms for men: That's right, "dirty" words. *Language in society*, 16 (3), 353–58.

Robinson & Barret. 1986. *The developing father.* New York, NY: Guilford.

Roemer, J. 1989. Celebrating the black female self: Zora Neal Hurston's American classic. *English journal*, 78 (7), 70–72.

Roop. 1989. The English teacher as midwife: Gender sensitivity in teaching methods. *English journal*, 78 (6), 90–91.

Rosaldo, M., & L. Lamphere, eds. 1974. *Women, culture, and society.* Stanford: Stanford UP.

Rose. 1986. Culture shock: Men's and women's myths of literacy in academe. ED 277 043.

Rosenblatt, L. 1938/1968. *Literature as exploration.* NY: Noble and Noble.

———. 1978. *The reader, the text, the power: The transactional theory of the literary work.* Carbondale: Southern Illinois UP.

Rosenthal, J. 1990. Gender benders. In Eschholz, Rosa, & Clark (see above), 303–305.

Rosser. 1988. Girls, boys and the SAT: Can we even the score? *NEA Today*, 6 (6), 48–53.

Rossiter. 1982. *Women scientists in America.* Baltimore: John Hopkins UP.

Rubie, T. L. 1983. Sex stereotypes: Issues of change in the 1970's. *Sex roles*, 9, 397–402.

Rubin. 1983. *Intimate strangers: men and women together*. NY: Harper & Row.

Ruddick, S. 1989. *Maternal thinking*. Boston: Beacon.

Rush & Allen. 1989. *Communications at the crossroads: The gender gap connection*. Norwood, NJ: Ablex.

Russ. 1983. *How to suppress women's writing*. Austin, TX: U. of Texas P.

Russett. 1989. *Sexual science: The Victorian construction*. Cambridge: Harvard UP.

Sacks, H., E. Schegloff, & G. Jefferson. 1974. A simplest of systematics for the organization of turn-taking in conversation. *Language* 50, 696–735.

Sadker & Sadker. 1980. *Beyond pictures and pronouns: Sexism in teacher education textbooks*. Washington DC. U.S. Department of Education, Women's Educational Equity Program.

———. 1982. *Sex equity handbook for schools*. NY: Longman.

———. 1986. Sexism in the classroom: From grade school to graduate school. *Phi delta kappan*, 67 (7), 32.

Sanders. 1984. The computer: Male, female or androgynous. *The computer teacher*, 11 (8), 31–34.

Sandler. 1988. The classroom climate: Chilly for women? In Deneef *et al*, eds., *The academic's handbook*. Durham, NC: Duke UP.

Sause, E. F. 1976. Computer content analysis of sex differences in the language of children. *Journal of psycholinguistic research*, 5, 311–24.

Schiffrin, D. 1987. *Discourse markers*. Cambridge: Cambridge UP.

Schneir, M., ed. 1972. *Feminism: The essential historical writings*. NY: Random House.

Schuster, M., & S. Van Dyne, eds. 1985. *Women's place in the academy: Transforming the liberal arts curriculum*. Totowa, NJ: Rowman & Allanheld.

Schiebinger. 1989. *The mind has no sex?* Cambridge: Cambridge UP.

Schneider & Hacker. 1973. Sex role imagery and the use of generic "man" in introductory texts: A case in the sociology of sociology. *American sociologist*, 8, 14.

Scott-Jones, D., & M. Clark. 1986. The school experience of black girls: The interaction of gender, race, and socioeconomic status. *Phi delta kappan*, 67 (7), 499–503.

Schwager. 1987. Educating women in America. *Signs: Journal of women in culture and society*, 12 (2), 333–72.

Sears, P., & D. Feldman. 1974. Teachers interactions with boys and with girls. In Stacey, Bereaud, & Daniel, eds. (see below), 147–158.

Serbin & O'Leary. 1975. How nursery schools teach girls to shut up. *Psychology today*, 9, 57–58, 102–103.

Selfe, C., & P. Meyer. 1991. Testing claims for on-line conferences. *Written communication*, 8 (2), 163–92.

Shapiro. 1984. *Manhood: A new definition* New York, NY: Putnam.

Sheldon. 1990. Pickle fights: Gendered talk in preschool disputes. *Discourse processes*, 13, 5–13.

Shinar, C. 1978. Person perception as a function of occupation and sex. *Sex roles*, 4, 679–93.

Showalter, E. Critical cross-dressing: 1987. Male feminists and the woman of the year. In A. Jardine & P. Smith, eds. *Men in Feminism*, 116–132. NY: Methuen.

———. 1985. *The new feminist criticism*. NY: Pantheon.

Showalter, E., ed. 1989. *Speaking of gender*. New York, NY: Routledge.

Siegler, D., & R. Siegler. 1976. Stereotypes of males' and females' speech. *Psychological reports*, 39, 167–70.

Sirc. 1989. Gender and "writing formations" in first-year narratives. *Freshman English news*, 18 (1), 4–11.

Sklar. 1983. Sexist grammar revisited. *College English*, 34 (4) 348–56.

Skolnick, et al. 1982. *How to encourage girls in math and science*. Englewood Cliffs, NJ: Prentice-Hall.

Smith. 1985. *Language, the sexes and society*. Cambridge, MA: Blackwell.

Smithson, I. 1990. Introduction: Investigating gender, power, and pedagogy. In Gabriel & Smithson, eds. (see above), 1–27.

Sorrels B. 1983. *The nonsexist communicator: Solving the problems of gender and awkwardness in modern English*. Englewood Cliffs, NJ: Prentice-Hall.

Spender, D. 1982a. *Invisible women: The schooling scandal*. London: Wheaton

———. 1982b. *Men's studies modified: The impact of feminism on the academic disciplines*. NY: Pergamon.

———. 1982c. *Women of ideas and what men have done to them: From Aphra Behn to Adrienne Rich*. Boston: Routledge & Kegan Paul.

———. 1986. *Mothers of the novel: 100 good women writers before Jane Austen*. London: Pandora Press.

———. 1985 (sec. ed.) *Man made language*. Boston: Routledge & Kegan Paul.

———. 1989. *The writing or the sex? or why you don't have to read women's writing to know it's no good*. NY: Pergamon Press.

Spender, D., & Sarah, eds. 1980. *Learning to lose: Sexism and education*. London: Women's Press.

Stacey, J., S. Bereaud, & J. Daniels, eds. 1974. *And Jill came tumbling after: Sexism in American education*. NY: Dell.

Staley, C. M. 1982. Sex-related differences in the style of children's language. *Journal of psycholinguistic research*, 11, 141–58.

Stanford, B., & K. Amin. 1978. *Black literature for high school students*. Champaign, IL: NCTE.

Stanger, C. 1987. Sexual politics of the one-to-one tutorial approach and collaborative learning. In Caywood & Overing, eds., (see above), 31–44.

Stanley J. 1978. Sexist grammar. *College English*, 39, 800–811.

Stannard, U. 1977. *Mrs. man*. San Francisco, CA: Germain Books.

Stanworth. 1983. *Gender and schooling: A study of sexual divisions in the classroom*. London: Century Hutchinson Ltd.

Staples, R. 1986. *Black masculinity: The black male's role in American society*. San Francisco: The Black Scholar Press.

Steedman, Urwin, & Walkerdine, eds. 1985. *Language, gender and childhood*. Boston: Routledge & Kegan Paul.

Stensland, A. 1984. Images of women in recent adolescent literature. *English journal*, 73 (7), 66–72.

Stern. 1985. *The interpersonal world of the infant*. New York, NY: Basic Books.

Sternburg. 1980. *The writer on her work*. Holt Rinehart.

Sternglantz & Lyberger-Ficek. 1977. Sex differences in student-teacher interaction in the college classroom. *Sex roles*, 3, 345–52.

Stewart & Ting-Toomey, eds. 1987. *Communication, gender, and sex roles in diverse interaction contexts*. Norwood, NJ: Ablex.

Stinton, ed. 1979. *Racism and sexism in children's books*. New York, NY: Writers and Readers Publishing Co-op.

Stitt, B., et al. 1988. *Building gender fairness in schools*. Carbondale, IL: Southern Illinois UP.

Stoller. 1975. *Sex and gender*. (Vol. 11). Northvale, NJ. Jason Aronson.

Stoltenberg. 1989. *Refusing to be a man: Essays on sex and justice*. Portland, OR: Breitenbush Books, Inc. (p.b.: Meridian).

Stump. 1985. *What's the difference? How men and women compare*. NY: Morrow.

Sunday. 1981. *Female power and male dominance: On the origin of sexual inequality*. Cambridge: Cambridge UP.

Swann, J. 1988. Talk control: An illustration for the classroom of problems in analyzing male dominance of conversation. In Coates and Cameron (see above), 122–140.

Swann, J. & E. Graddol. 1988. Gender inequalities in classroom talk. *English in education*, 22 (1), 48–65.

Switzer, J. 1990. The impact of generic word choices: An empirical investigation of age-and-sex-related differences. *Sex roles*, 22 (1 & 2), 69–81.

Szirom. 1988. *Teaching gender? Sex education and sexual stereotypes*. Concord, MA: Allen & Unwin.

Tannen, D. ed. 1982. *Spoken and written language: Exploring orality and literacy*. Norwood, NJ: Ablex.

———. 1984. *Conversational style: Analyzing talk among friends*. Norwood, NJ: Ablex.

———. 1986. *That's not what I meant! How conversational style makes or breaks your relations with others*. NY: Morrow.

———. 1990a. Gender differences in conversational coherence: Physical alignment and topical cohesion. In Dorval, ed., *Conversational coherence and its development*, 167–206.

———. 1990b. Gender differences in topical coherence: Creating involvement in best friends' talk. *Discourse processes*, 13, 73–90.

———. 1990c. *You just don't understand: Women and men in conversation*. NY: Morrow.

Tate, ed. 1985. *Black women writers at work*. New York, NY: Continuum Publishing.

Tavris & Wade. 1984. *The longest war: Sex differences in perspective*, 2nd ed. Orlando, FL: Harcourt Brace Jovanovich.

Tedesco, J. 1991. Women's ways of knowing/women's ways of composing. *Rhetoric review*. 9 (2), 246–56.

Tejirian. 1990. *Sexuality and the devil*. Boston: Routledge & Kegan Paul.

Tetreault, J. 1987. Rethinking women, gender, and the social studies. *Social education*. 51 (3), 170–78.

Theroux. 1985. Being a man. In *Sunrise with seamonsters*. Boston: Houghton Mifflin.

Thompson. 1991. *To be a man*. Tarcher.

Thorne, B. 1986. Girls and boys together ... but mostly apart: Gender arrangements in elementary schools. In Hartup & Rubine, eds. *Relationships and development*, Hills dale, 167–84. Erlbaum.

Thorne, B., & N. Henley, eds. 1975. *Language and sex: Difference and dominance*. Rowley, MA: Newbury House.

Thorne, B., C. Kramarae, & N. Henley. eds. 1983. *Language, gender and society*. Rowley, MA: Newbury House.

Todd & Fisher, eds. 1988. *Gender and discourse: The power of talk*. Norwood, NJ: Ablex.

Todd-Mancillas, W. 1981. Masculine generics-sexist language: A review of literature and implications for speech communications professionals. *Communication quarterly*, Spring, 107–114.

Treichler & Kramarae. 1983. Women's talk in the ivory tower. *Communication quarterly*, 31, 118–132.

Trudgill, P. 1983. Language and sex. In *Sociolinguistics: An introduction to language and society*, 78–99. London: Harmondsworth: Penguin.

Vandell, K. 1990. *Restructuring education: Getting girls into America's goals*. Rockville, MD: A.A.U.W.

Vetterling-Braggin, ed. *Sexist language: A modern philosophical analysis*. Savage, MD: Littlefield, Adams, and Co.

Vogel. 1990. Gender differences: Both/and, not either/or. In Moran & Penfield, eds. *Conversations: Contemporary critical theory and the teaching of English*. Urbana, IL: NCTE.

Walker, A. 1983. *In search of our mother's gardens*. NY: Harcourt Brace Jovanovich.

Walker, C. & D. Elias. 1987. Writing conference talk: Factors associated with high and low rated conferences. *Research in the teaching of English*, 21, 266–85.

Walker. 1984. Sex differences in the development of moral reasoning: A critical review. *Child Development*. 55, 677, 91.

Wandor, ed. 1983. *On gender and writing*. London: Pandora Press.

Ware & Stuck. 1985. Sex-role messages vis-a-vis microcomputer use: A look at the pictures. *Sex roles*, 13 (3,4), 205–214.

Warhol, R. 1989. *Gendered interventions*. New Brunswick, NJ: Rutgers UP.

Warshay, D. W. 1972. Sex differences in language style. In C. Safilios-Rothschild, ed. *Toward a sociology of women*, 3–9. Lexington, MA: Xerox College Publishing.

Waxman. 1989. Politics of the survey course: Feminist challenges. *English in the two-year college*, 16 (1), 17–22.

Weiler, K. 1988. *Women teaching for changes: Gender, class and power*. South Hadley, MA: Bergin & Garvey.

West, C., & D. H. Zimmerman. 1975. Sex roles, interruption and silences in conversation. In Thorne & Henley (see above), 105–129.

West, C., & D. H. Zimmerman. 1983. Small insults: A study of interruptions in cross-sex conversations between unacquainted person. In Thorne, Kramarae & Henley, eds. (see above) 102–117.

Westmoreland, R., D. P. Starr, K. Shelton, & Y. Pasadeos. 1977. News writing styles of male and female students. *Journalism quarterly*, 54, 599–601.

White. 1989. The power of politeness in the classroom: Cultural codes that create and constrain knowledge construction. *Journal of curriculum and supervision*, 4 (4), 298–321.

Whyld, ed. 1983. *Sexism in the secondary school curriculum*. NY: Harper and Row.

Wiley, M., & A. Eskilson. 1985. Speech style, gender stereotypes and corporate success: What if women talk more like men? *Sex roles*, 12, 993–1007.

Williams, J., & S. Bennet. 1975. The definitions of sex stereotypes via the adjective check list. *Sex roles*, 1, 326–37.

Willinsky. 1987. Learning the language of difference: The dictionary in the high school. *English education*, 19 (3), 146–58.

Wilson. 1978. Teachers' inclusion of males and females in generic nouns. *Research in the teaching of English*, 12 (2), 155–61.

Wodak, P. 1981. Women relate, men report: Sex differences in language behavior in a therapeutic group. *Journal of pragmatics*, 5, 261–65.

Wodak, R., ed. 1988. *Language, power and ideology: Studies in political discourse*. White Plains, WY: John Benjamin's Publishers.

Women on Words and Images. 1974. *Dick and Jane as victims: Sex stereotyping in children's readers*. Washington, D.C.: Resource Center on Sex Roles in Education.

Wolfram. 1991. *Dialects and American English*. New York, NY: Prentice Hall/C.A.L.

Wood, M. M. 1966. The influence of sex and knowledge of communication effectiveness on spontaneous speech. *Word*, 22, 112–37.

Woods, N. 1989. Talking shop: Sex and status as determinants of floor apportionment in a work setting. In Coates and Cameron (see above), 141–57.

Worby. 1979. In search of a common language: Women and educational texts. *College English*, 41, 101–105.

Wright, J. W. II, & L. A. Hosman. 1983. Language style and sex bias in the courtroom: The effects of male and female use of hedges and intensifiers on impression information. *The southern speech communication journal*, 48 (2) 137–52.

Youniss & Smollar. 1985. *Adolescent relations with mothers, fathers and friends*. Chicago: U. of Chicago P.

Zahn, C. J. 1989. Sex-linked language revisited: A critical review of research on gender and language. Paper given at Speech Communication Association, San Fransisco, CA.

Zahn, C. J., & R. Hopper. 1987. The bases for differing evaluations of male and female speech: Evidence form ratings of transcribed conversation. Paper given at Speech Communication Association, Boston, MA.

Zellman. 1984. *Connections between sex and aggression*. Hillsdale, NJ: Erlbaum Assocs.

Zimmerman, D. H., & C. West. 1975. Sex roles interruptions and silences in conversations. In Thorne & Henley, eds. (see above), 105–129.

Contributors

Nancy Mellin McCracken is Assistant Professor of Curriculum and Instruction and English and Coordinator of the English Education program at Kent State University. She has published a number of essays on the teaching of literature, language, and composition and conducts workshops with teachers on writing across the curriculum, whole language assessment, collaborative learning, and teaching response to literature.

Bruce C. Appleby is Professor of English and Professor of Curriculum and Instruction at Southern Illinois University at Carbondale. He has taught at all grade levels from pre-school through graduate school and now does in-service and pre-service teacher education for all levels. He has published widely and does workshops and speeches nationally and internationally in such diverse areas as multi-media, computers and composition, gender issues, teaching literature, whole language in the secondary school, and reading and writing across the curriculum.

David Blakesley is Assistant Professor of English at Southern Illinois University at Carbondale. He has published on rhetoric and literacy and is completing a book on Kenneth Burke's rhetoric.

Cynthia Ann Bowman is an English teacher at Father Lopez High School in Daytona Beach, Florida. She received the 1991 James Britton Award for Inquiry in English Language Arts for her study of "The Effectiveness of the Learning Log on High School Literature Achievement."

Nancy R. Comley is Associate Professor of English and Co-Director of Composition at Queens College of the City University of New York. She has published articles on the pedagogy of literature and composition and on modernist literature and has collaborated with Robert Scholes, Gregory Ulmer, and others on *The Practice of Writing* (1989), *Elements of Literature* (1990), *Fields of Writing* (1989), and *Text Book* (1988).

Claudia M. Greenwood is Associate Professor of English and Coordinator of Regional Campusses English faculty for Kent State University. She has directed the Women's Studies program at the Ashtabula campus. She conducts writing workshops for teachers.

Lisa J. McClure is Assistant Professor of English and Director of General Education in English at Southern Illinois University at Carbondale. She has taught writing courses ranging from basic writing to graduate seminars in theory. She works in computers and composition, gender issues, and—with her experience at the secondary level—the training of secondary school English teachers. She has published chapters in several books and articles in several journals.

Janet L. Miller is Associate Professor in the Department of Curriculum and Teaching at Hofstra University. Her research interests include curriculum studies, gender issues, and teachers' knowledges. She serves as Managing Editor of *JCT: An Interdisciplinary Journal of Curriculum Studies* and also serves on the Executive Committee of the Conference on English Education.

Duane H. Roen is Associate Professor of English at the University of Arizona, where he serves as director of the graduate program in Rhetoric, Composition, and the Teaching of English, and as Coordinator of Graduate Studies for English. In addition to dozens of articles, he has co-authored (with Stuart Brown and Robert Mittan) *Becoming Expert: Writing and Learning in the Disciplines* and co-edited (with Gesa Kirsch) *A Sense of Audience in Written Communication*. His research interests include collaborative scholarship and writing, writing across the curriculum, audience awareness in writing, and gender in writing.

Jean Sanborn is Associate Professor of English at Colby College in Waterville, ME. Her research interests are in gender and writing, and the history of the essay. She has published on teaching writing, writing with ESL students, and gender.

Lois Stover taught high school English in rural Vermont and junior high English and Drama in Virginia Beach. Currently, she is Assistant Professor of Education at Towson State University where she supervises English student teachers and teaches courses in Curriculum and Instruction. Her husband is an author of young adult novels who works at home and cares for their four-year-old daughter.